DBT PRINCIPLES IN ACTION

DBT Principles in Action

Acceptance, Change, and Dialectics

Charles R. Swenson

foreword by Marsha M. Linehan

THE GUILFORD PRESS

New York   London

Library of Congress Cataloging-in-Publication Data

Names: Swenson, Charles R., author.
Title: DBT principles in action : acceptance, change, and dialectics /
   Charles R. Swenson.
Description: New York : The Guilford Press, [2016] | Includes bibliographical
   references and index.
Identifiers: LCCN 2015049503 | ISBN 9781462526727 (hardback : acid-free paper)
   ISBN 9781462536108 (paperback : acid-free paper)
Subjects: LCSH: Dialectical behavior therapy. | BISAC: MEDICAL / Psychiatry /
   General. | SOCIAL SCIENCE / Social Work. | PSYCHOLOGY / Psychotherapy /
   Counseling.
Classification: LCC RC489.B4 S94 2016 | DDC 616.89/142—dc23
LC record available at http://lccn.loc.gov/2015049503

About the Author

Charles R. Swenson, MD, is Associate Clinical Professor of Psychiatry at the University of Massachusetts Medical School and maintains a private practice in psychiatry and psychotherapy with adults, families, and adolescents in Northampton, Massachusetts. He has over 25 years of experience in the practice, supervision, training, and implementation of dialectical behavior therapy (DBT) in a wide range of mental health systems in Canada, the United States, and Europe. Dr. Swenson was the first professional authorized by Marsha M. Linehan to deliver intensive DBT training, is cofounder of the International Society for the Improvement and Teaching of DBT (ISITDBT), and has published numerous articles and book chapters on DBT. He is a recipient of the Cindy J. Sanderson Outstanding Educator Award from ISITDBT and is a Distinguished Life Fellow of the American Psychiatric Association. His website is *www.charlesswenson.org*.

Foreword

Charlie Swenson called me in 1987 for the first time. I was conducting the first randomized controlled trial of dialectical behavior therapy (DBT) and continuing to fine-tune the treatment, which at that point did not exist outside of my lab at the University of Washington. Charlie explained that he was a psychiatrist in New York, an Associate Professor of Psychiatry at Cornell University Medical School, and that he was the director of a long-term inpatient treatment unit for individuals with severe personality disorders. His mentor and medical director was Otto Kernberg, a psychoanalyst widely known for his theories on personality disorders. Charlie's treatment program was based on Kernberg's treatment model, now known as transference-focused psychotherapy (TFP).

Having learned about my work from a colleague, Charlie asked if he and his wife, Meredith, a clinical psychologist, could visit me in Seattle and learn about DBT. At that stage, as the developer of an as-yet-unpublished treatment approach for suicidal individuals, I was shocked that a psychiatrist who was head of a highly respected treatment program at a famous New York hospital would stop everything to visit a nobody psychologist simply because someone else had told him that she had the most effective treatment for the clients he was treating. Very unusual, I must say. More importantly, he had enormous humility and provided passionate care for his patients. I invited Charlie and Meredith to my lab, and they soon visited for about a week. Given his psychoanalytic treatment background, I was even more impressed by Charlie's willingness to open his eyes to a very different model, based on behaviorism, Zen, and dialectics. After their visit, Charlie went on to develop an inpatient treatment program based entirely on DBT. This was no small task, as I had developed a treatment that was entirely outpatient. Charlie's was the first DBT inpatient program, and served as the inpatient DBT model for many years to come.

While I was on sabbatical at Charlie's hospital and program, as I wrote my DBT treatment manual, I visited his unit each day and worked with him and his staff and patients. Charlie had become a believer in DBT, a monumental change for a psychoanalyst. Along with his team, Charlie was one of 20 therapists in the very first 10-day DBT intensive training in 1993. He eventually began his own intensive trainings, which he has done ever since. When I did my first training program with him, I found that he not only knows the treatment but is also a very effective, creative, compassionate, and charismatic teacher of DBT. By now, he is a teacher's teacher, a model for other experts in how to make DBT clear and accessible to experts and practitioners at all levels. When my students and I decided to found the International Society for the Improvement and Teaching of DBT (ISITDBT), Charlie was right there with us and was the program director for the first 2 years of its annual conference, in 1996 and 1997. In 2003, Charlie received the first Cindy J. Sanderson Outstanding Teacher Award bestowed by ISITDBT. For the past 20 years, he has played a huge role in the implementation of DBT across a range of treatment settings throughout North America and Europe.

Having done all of this for thousands of students in workshops, seminars, consultations, and supervisions, Charlie has now put it together for readers of this book, *DBT Principles in Action: Acceptance, Change, and Dialectics*. There is no book out there quite like this: clear, deep, compelling, and at times funny. It is true to the model of DBT and at the same time personal, seeming as if you are in a supervision with him. I'm sure it will strengthen your practice of DBT, wherever you may be.

MARSHA M. LINEHAN, PHD, ABPP
Professor and Director
Behavioral Research and Therapy Clinics
University of Washington

Preface

I was in the sixth grade in my elementary school in Albany, Oregon. I was an incredibly slow runner. In physical education class, when we all lined up to run as fast as we could across the gymnasium floor, I finished an embarrassing last. It might have been less humiliating had I not harbored one, and only one, goal in life at that time: to be a professional basketball player. As a gym rat, I sought out open gyms on nights and weekends to play basketball as much as possible. I had some advantages: I was tall, intelligent, ambitious, and with all of the practicing, could shoot accurately. But it would all come to naught if I remained so slow.

Following specific advice from the track coach at the University of Oregon, over the next 2 years, I trained morning and night to increase my speed, quickness, and power. By the time I was in high school, I had very strong legs, but was not much faster. As my high school years unfolded, and while other players had growth spurts, my snail-like pace became an increasing disadvantage. By age 16, my dream had collapsed. When I turned to golf as an alternative sport, and to academics where I had some advantages, my central experience at the time was that my life-long dream was crushed.

Fast-forward to 1978, 18 years after finishing last in my gym class. By then, I had graduated medical school, become a doctor, and was in a residency training in psychiatry at Yale University. While there, I did my psychoanalytic training and was involved in experiencing my own psychoanalysis, as was required by the program. I went over the painful details of the collapse of my dream with my psychoanalyst. As I told him the story, I indicated my slow pace was genetically determined by my parents, who had burdened me with biological disadvantages. He asked an odd question: "What makes you think you are so slow?" I responded, "Because I *was* slow! I'm still slow. My times for a 100, a 440 [quarter mile], or a mile are too embarrassing to mention." After a pause, he inquired again, "But what makes you *think* you are so slow?" I was surprised and irritated. "I told you; it's because I *am* slow! I am a slow runner. I run slowly, and I have the times to prove it." By then I regretted bringing the topic to his attention, having already had the impression that he had no interest in athletics. After another pause, he repeated for the third time, "But what makes you think you are so slow?" At this point, I wasn't sure how to respond. My surprise was now shock, my irritation was outright anger; in addition, I experienced some concern for him. What was going on? Did he not hear me? Was he trying to annoy me? Was he having a stroke? I resolved to stop talking about it; it was too aggravating! I moved on.

But outside of my psychoanalytic sessions four times a week, I did not "move on" from the topic. During my usual bouts of jogging for exercise, which included running around a track at Yale University's athletic fields (the "Yale Bowl," as it was called), I noticed a track athlete who frequently worked out there who was clearly serious about running. I built up my courage, approached him, and asked, "I've seen you here a lot. You are clearly a runner, and I'm not. I have always wanted to increase my speed, and in the past I worked hard at it but without results. Would you be willing to watch me run and give me tips?" He seemed pleased to be asked. He asked me to run 40 yards as fast as I could. Over the next several weeks, several times per week, he tutored me in running. He made suggestions, monitored my times, and gave me encouragement. What was so helpful, in addition to his willing, even devoted attitude, was the specificity of his suggestions.

- "You are a tall guy, so you have to shorten your steps."
- "You need to feel as if your steps are really short."
- "Pound your legs into the ground as if they were pistons in an engine."
- "Look straight ahead, down the track, not from side to side."
- "You need to lean forward in the direction you are running, almost as if you are going to fall on your face, which will tell your legs to speed up."
- "You have to focus on the ground in front of you, and nowhere else, and just tell yourself, 'faster, faster, faster.'"

I implemented his coaching tips and worked out with more intensity. He reinforced my efforts with his suggestions, and within a few weeks I was running faster than ever before. I ran a mile in 5 minutes, 35 seconds—more than 2 minutes faster than any previous mile I had run. I was almost 30 years old by then, and it was too late for a career move to the NBA, but it was amazing and wonderful to have found that I could so dramatically increase my running speed.

Meanwhile, I did not talk about my efforts and exploits with my psychoanalyst. I remained angry with him for his repetitive question and his failure to convey empathy. I didn't want to give him the impression that his remarks had motivated me. In fact, his obnoxious persistence had planted seeds of doubt in my mind about the inevitability of my running deficit. His comments motivated me to wonder, push myself, ask for coaching support, and ultimately improve my speed. Time and again, I reflected upon his repetitive question. Obviously, he wasn't stupid. I really don't think he was insensitive, and it became clear that he had not had a stroke. I don't even think he was trying to provoke me. I concluded that he was in fact genuinely wondering what made me *think* I was so slow. He must have perceived, as he listened to my "inner voice," that I myself was in fact perplexed about my own lack of progress in running. He must have heard, while listening with his "third ear," a crack in my convincing "genetic" explanation. I don't think he cared whether I ran faster; his concern was the story of my inner life, and the way I represented and understood myself. He intervened the way he did because he could hear, or sense, a discrepancy in my storyline.

For me, as time passed and I reflected on how I had been able to change such a stubborn behavioral pattern, the take-home lesson was the following: *In order to change, I needed an analyst and a coach.* I needed one person who attended to my story in sufficient detail, listened more carefully than anyone else, and had the courage to challenge my compelling explanation. I needed another person who was an expert in the mechanics of running, someone who could watch me run, pay attention to the details of running, offer suggestions, monitor my progress, and provide reinforcement. Maybe the same person could have performed both roles—I don't know. What stuck with me, though, and what has remained with me up to this moment, was the message that we are indeed capable of changing very stubborn behavioral patterns, and that it may require both an "analyst" and a "coach" to do so.

By 1987, I was in my fifth year as the unit chief of a long-term psychoanalytically oriented inpatient program at New York Hospital–Cornell Medical Center, Westchester Division, in White Plains, New

York. We based our work on the ego-psychological, object relations model of Otto Kernberg, who also was our medical director and my mentor and supervisor. During that year, we were treating a young woman who made relentless efforts to harm herself and kill herself. For months on end, she remained on constant one-to-one supervision, 24 hours a day, and still she frequently lost control and was placed in restraints. I was perplexed and troubled at our ineffectiveness in finding a solution.

One day, as she sat in the security room under close observation, I reviewed her history and treatment again. Downstairs, a conference on personality disorders was taking place. I wandered down to the meetings. I saw a senior colleague there named Allen Frances, who was also on the Cornell psychiatric faculty and an expert on personality disorders. I asked him if he would be willing to come upstairs and join me in an informal consultation regarding the treatment of this patient. He readily agreed, and within minutes the two of us were seated on the floor of the security room opposite the patient in question. Dr. Frances interviewed her in some detail. After perhaps 45 minutes, he surprised me by saying to her, "I have a suggestion for you. In Seattle, Washington, is a psychologist named Marsha Linehan. She has developed a treatment program for patients with problems like yours, all on an outpatient basis. It's a new approach and I think it would be a good fit for you. Why don't you get your act together, get out of here, and make your way out to Seattle to meet her?"

At first I was irritated that Dr. Frances delivered this recommendation directly to the patient without talking with me first. Didn't he realize that this could worsen the situation for my staff and me, working with a patient who now had been told that she would be better off somewhere else? As it turned out, he was not too concerned with my staff; he was more concerned about the patient finding what she needed. It was the first time I had heard of Marsha Linehan.

Curious about Linehan's work and program, I learned that she was a cognitive-behavioral therapist and an expert on suicide and self-harm behaviors. I was not familiar with cognitive-behavioral therapies. Furthermore, I had absorbed the psychoanalytic bias at the time, in which behavioral treatments were considered superficial in their impact, bringing "mere" behavioral change rather than the far more desirable "structural intrapsychic change." I located Linehan's (1987) first report of her treatment program for patients with borderline personality disorder in the *Bulletin of the Menninger Clinic*, a psychoanalytically oriented journal. It was fascinating to read about applying a behavioral approach on an outpatient basis to the kinds of individuals we were treating with psychoanalytic psychotherapy on an inpatient unit.

As quickly as we could arrange it, I traveled to Seattle with my wife, Meredith Gould, herself a clinical psychologist and an expert in Kernberg's model of treatment. We spent more than a week at Linehan's lab at the University of Washington, which at the time was the only location in the world where dialectical behavior therapy (DBT) was under way. It would still be 4 years before the publication of Linehan's (Linehan, Armstrong, Suares, Allmon, & Heard, 1991) first randomized controlled trial, and 6 years before the publication of her treatment manual and skills training manual on DBT (Linehan, 1993a, 1993b). We had the opportunity to have lengthy discussions with Dr. Linehan about the treatment and to witness her treating her patients on videotape and behind a one-way mirror.

I was fascinated. Linehan's model was clearly behavioral, which included specific behaviorally defined treatment targets, skills training, and role playing, all of which were at odds with a psychoanalytic approach. Moreover, she conducted her treatment in a deliberately validating and compassionate atmosphere, quite at variance with the objectivity, boundaries, and technical neutrality of a psychoanalytic approach. Yet I could see that Linehan's approach had a lot in common with Kernberg's style. They were both rigorous in their adherence to their theoretical and practical treatment models; they both established intense relationships with patients within clear frameworks of agreements; they organized session agendas according to hierarchies of thematic priorities or target priorities; and they were talkative, direct, and even confrontational with patients. In 1989, I tried to specify the similarities and differences between the two approaches in an article published in the *Journal of Personality Disorders*. I valued the elegance of Kernberg's model for understanding and intervening with "primitive states of mind." I valued Linehan's attention to behavioral detail and the model for coaching individuals to replace maladaptive behaviors with skills. Once again, I saw the value of having an analyst and a coach. I resolved to introduce DBT skills and coaching within my psychoanalytic inpatient program.

My senior staff would have none of it. From their perspective, the incorporation of elements of behavioral treatment, especially within psychotherapy, would contaminate and undermine the theoretically consistent psychoanalytic model. Having preceded me in their work with Kernberg, they adamantly maintained a kind of theoretical purity. I was momentarily stymied, but my supervisor and administrator, Richard Munich, found an alternative. Noting that the chief of another inpatient unit under his administration was leaving her post, he proposed that I develop a DBT-based inpatient program. I jumped at the offer, and I directed both units for the next 18 months, going back and forth several times each day, shifting from one model to the other as I went. It was an amazing opportunity to explore these two approaches, to learn DBT, and to find more ways to treat these patients. I recruited six colleagues to join my senior staff on the DBT unit, and we undertook the journey together. As it turned out, our first task was to learn to practice cognitive-behavioral therapies. Slowly but surely, I came to understand that DBT contained within it the role of the analyst (the psychotherapist who focused on motivation) and the coach (the skills trainer). I was happy to have found my niche.

By 2013, I was practicing DBT with patients and had implemented it in several different settings where I worked. I provided 10-day intensive training to more than 400 treatment teams and consulted on the implementation of DBT in more than 500 programs, ranging from inpatient to outpatient, adult to adolescent, day treatment to residential, case management to emergency room, and substance abuse to eating disorders. Having to apply DBT in so many different circumstances required rigor and flexibility: rigorous adherence to the evidence-based model, and flexibility in adapting it to different populations and contexts (Koerner, Dimeff, & Swenson, 2007). Where adaptations were needed, I learned to keep them within the treatment principles and I spelled them out in more detail for myself. By heightening my focus on DBT's principles in psychotherapy and teaching, I found myself to be more fluid and creative than before, while still adhering to the model. The dialectic of adopting DBT with rigor while adapting it within the principles became my trademark. I decided to write this book in hopes that my evolution and my discoveries would help others.

I have been cautious in writing this book, trying to make it very clear that a principle-based focus in therapy is not an alternative to a protocol-based approach. They go hand in hand, and a correct use of principles will deepen and broaden the reach of the therapist whose work adheres to the DBT manual. It will help the therapist to navigate and transform challenging moments, to stay on track, and to maintain movement when stalemates arise.

Acknowledgments

I have so many amazing people to thank for what I have learned, for what I have taught, and for the opportunity I have had to write this book.

Cindy Sanderson was my closest friend outside of my marriage until she died at age 49 of breast cancer. She was my DBT buddy, having helped me to develop the first inpatient DBT program. We were co-teachers of DBT workshops for a decade. We were rabid basketball fans together. Never has there been such a blend of intellect, passion, and wit in the teaching of DBT. Never have I had more fun teaching. I will never forget the day, as she faced the end, when she said, "Charlie, for the past 11 years I have asked about my cancer, 'Why me?' Today, as I sat on my porch looking out at the beauty of the world, I thought, for the first time, 'Why not me?'" Cindy, thank you, you are an amazing being wherever you are, and we both know that you would have written this book with me.

Marsha Linehan has been a friend, colleague, mentor, and model to me for almost three decades, and her generosity has enriched my life more than I can explain here. Her work has created the context for my work. Details from sessions of supervision with her stick with me 25 years later. The story of her life, and her relentless pursuit of getting other people out of hell, has inspired me. Her capacity to move between fierce constructive criticism at one moment, and compassion, empathy, and laughter in the next moment, is extraordinary. Obviously this book could not have been written without her, and any accuracy in my understanding of DBT is due to her.

Shireen Rizvi is a dear friend, a wonderful and precise teacher, a DBT scientist, a fellow sports fan, and a karaoke performer who catalyzed my DBT songwriting career. Along with her students at Rutgers University, Shireen read several early chapter drafts and provided invaluable feedback.

My gratitude goes out to many therapists, trainers, and other heroes. Three have influenced me profoundly. With her open mind and courageous heart, Kelly Koerner has enhanced my own courage. Alec Miller has consistently modeled extraordinary teaching and great fun, in spite of his passion for the New York Yankees. Perry Hoffman has dedicated her time and abundant talents to individuals with borderline personality disorder and their families, and has been a fount of balance and wisdom to me. My most important teachers have been my patients.

Having never written and published a book, I did not know what to expect of an editor. I think I have had an unusual and blessed experience in working with Kitty Moore at The Guilford Press. Kitty was excited about this book well before it existed. She read every chapter in each revision, was gentle but incisive with suggestions, was patient when life intervened to slow down my progress, and, most of all, was explicitly and believably encouraging at moments when I was convinced that my writing was terrible and the project was doomed. I was lucky to have the chance to work with her.

Edward Emery, a learned psychoanalyst, has been a relentless supporter and constructive critic of my work, and as my therapist has helped me locate my voice.

I have loved being a teacher, and have taught and learned alongside a talented, committed, compassionate cast of characters in my DBT journey; all of them have contributed to this book in one way or another. It is a tribute to Marsha Linehan that so many amazing people have remained loyal and passionate about DBT. I am choosing not to name all of them here, but they include every person with whom I have taught DBT over the past 30 years, some 30 or 40 individuals from across the United States and Europe. Thank you all.

Meredith Gould, PhD, my wife and the love of my life, is not a DBT therapist. Nevertheless, more than any other psychotherapist, she has been my model. She brings a level of generosity, devotion, directness, irreverence, genuineness, and compassion toward which I can only strive. She has delivered many from hell during her practice. She's my closest friend, my dearest love, and my sounding board. Our two sons and I have been lucky to receive her care and affection at home. She has supported the writing of this book and made it possible. My gratitude to her goes beyond any words.

My two sons, Max and Ruben, mean everything to me. Thank you, guys.

Contents

Contents

CHAPTER 1

Getting Started in Therapy

Pretreatment and the Life-Worth-Living Conversation

Even while adhering closely to dialectical behavior therapy's (DBT's) treatment manuals (Linehan, 1993a, 2015b), the therapist still encounters thousands of choices per session. For instance, although the manual specifies that the therapist begin a session by reviewing the diary card with the patient, it cannot tell the therapist whether to be cool, firm, and insistent or warm, validating, and encouraging in the process. It cannot tell the therapist whether to do an assessment of the therapy-interfering behavior of noncompliance, or whether to have the patient fill out the card right then and there. And the manual cannot tell the therapist when, if ever, to allow diary card noncompliance, in deference to other priorities.

In the treatment of a severe, chronic, and complex condition, it is a blessing to have such a comprehensive manual, loaded with goals, stages, and targets; functions and modes; agreements and assumptions; prescribed protocols; dozens of skills; and upward of 80 different strategies. And it is the job of the DBT therapist to learn and practice all of these elements to a level of adherence. Given the substantial and growing evidence base for DBT (Feigenbaum et al., 2011; Gutteling, Montagne, Nijs, & van den Bosch, 2012; Harned, Jackson, Comtois, & Linehan, 2010; Harned, Korslund, & Linehan, 2014; Hill, Craighead, & Safer, 2011; Koons et al., 2001; Linehan et al., 1999, 2002, 2006; Linehan, Armstrong, Suares, Allmon, & Heard, 1991; Linehan, Heard, & Armstrong, 1993; Linehan, McDavid, Brown, Sayrs, & Gallop, 2008; Lynch, Morse, Mendelson, & Robins, 2003; Mehlum et al., 2014; Neacsui, Rizvi, &

Linehan, 2010; Rathus & Miller, 2002; Safer, Robinson, & Jo, 2010; Safer, Telch, & Agras, 2001; Telch, Agras, & Linehan, 2001; Turner, 2007; van den Bosch, Koeter, Stijnen, Verheul, & van den Brink, 2005; van den Bosch, Verheul, Schippers, & van den Brink, 2002; Verheul, van den Bosch, & Koeter, 2003), the responsible course is to practice the treatment as specified. But even the experienced therapist practicing DBT to adherence might notice that he still is not sure what to do *most of the time*. In other words, every one of the prescribed steps, protocols, and strategies can be carried out in hundreds of different ways, and the interstices lying between the steps are bigger than the steps themselves. A behavioral chain analysis of the same behavioral episode can be carried out in at least a million different ways.

But of course this is exactly why Linehan (*www.nimh/nih.gov/news/media/2011/bpd1/shtml*) described DBT as a *principle-based treatment* with protocols. Determining how to carry out the prescribed steps, and navigating the interstices between them, requires unblinking clarity about goals and targets; tact, timing, and agility; persistence, patience, and courage; and an overlearned grasp of DBT's strategies. In the background of these moment-to-moment clinical judgments, the therapist is guided by a deep and precise working understanding of DBT's principles. This is true from the very beginning of treatment. The first stage of treatment is called *pretreatment*, but to be quite clear, pretreatment is already treatment, even in the first minute. The therapist must be ready with the whole DBT treatment package from the outset. In this chapter, I introduce the role of paradigms and principles in DBT by considering the principle-based management of the pretreatment stage. The principles, from which the strategies and protocols flow, are derived from the three paradigms underlying DBT: acceptance, change, and dialectics. In the next four chapters I present the paradigms more formally and the principles that follow from each.

PRETREATMENT STRATEGIES AND THE LIFE-WORTH-LIVING CONVERSATION

The patient entering DBT is in a stalemate. She may have considered suicide and perhaps even attempted it, though not successfully. She has undoubtedly made efforts to improve her life, with limited, temporary, or no success. Failing to find a way out, either by ending her life or by building a better life, she is in a holding pattern. She tries to avoid emotional triggers, but it's nearly impossible to do so. She tries to block or escape from painful emotions, using behaviors to bring relief, but many of the behaviors are self-destructive and the relief is temporary. Time stands still. Efforts to get relief override efforts to build a life. One of my early mentors, Otto Kernberg (1984), routinely referred to a subset of impulsive patients with borderline personality organization as having suicide and hospitalization as a way of life. Similar statements could be made about those whose "ways of life" revolve around self-injury, substance abuse, eating disorders, violence, dissociation, and other "escape" behaviors. The suffering is intense, the hopelessness grows, and the ability to imagine a life worth living fades. In pretreatment, from the first minute of therapy, efforts are under way to strengthen the patient's motivation to live and commit to a treatment plan.

In her treatment manual (Linehan, 1993a, pp. 438–448), Linehan has described the "contracting strategies" for starting DBT. She clearly and crisply defines the steps to be taken, which typically take at least the first four sessions and constitute the pretreatment stage. After a diagnostic assessment, the therapist sequentially (1) presents the biosocial theory to the patient, (2) orients her to the distinctive features of DBT, (3) helps in orienting the patient's social–professional network to the treatment, (4) reviews treatment agreements and rules, (5) uses commitment strategies to elicit the patient's commitment to DBT, (6) conducts initial analyses of major target behaviors, and (7) begins to develop a collaborative treatment relationship. The primary goal of pretreatment is to gain the patient's agreement on a treatment plan involving a prioritized set of behavioral targets, and to elicit the strongest possible commitment to the plan. The manual specifies the steps to be taken and provides an excellent framework for getting started.

In cognitive-behavioral therapy of less severe disorders, the prescribed contracting strategies generally work well to orient the patient, arrive at a rational and specific treatment plan, and establish the credibility of the treatment and the therapist. In other words, the manual-prescribed steps *suffice* to chart the early course, to get the treatment off to a good start. However, when working with individuals with chronic, severe emotional dysregulation—individuals whose valid responses have been pervasively invalidated by the familial, social, and or professional environment—the pretreatment stage, indeed even the first minute of it, can be challenging. The therapist adheres to the step-by-step intervention sequence in the contracting protocol, but navigating these early difficulties, while holding DBT's principles in mind, allows for flexibility and improvisation. The therapist can remain adherent to the manual, attuned to the patient, and skillful in the moment.

DBT PRINCIPLES AND THE
LIFE-WORTH-LIVING CONVERSATION

I recently started therapy with a 30-year-old woman who had made a suicide attempt after months of repetitive, daily episodes of nonsuicidal self-injurious behavior. She had been diagnosed with borderline personality disorder in the hospital and was referred to DBT with me upon discharge. Over the phone, she said she would "give therapy a try." When she arrived to our first meeting, she struck me as poised, intelligent, perceptive, and cautiously willing to get started. I asked her, "What would you hope to accomplish in therapy?" It was as if I had flipped a switch; she went from receptive and conversational to angry and forceful. It seemed like I had insulted her. "That's a stupid thing to ask me! You don't know a thing about me! Why would you assume I can accomplish anything?! My life is over! I have tried everything, and it's only made me worse! I have been damaged . . . irreparably!"

Less than 1 minute into our relationship, we were already encountering difficulty. On the one hand, this difficulty was fortuitous because I was already experiencing, firsthand, some of the problematic behaviors I would be assessing and treating. On the other hand, it was difficult to know what to do, how to respond. What I could not have known yet was that my question about her hopes for her future had set off intense feelings of shame and hopelessness. In her childhood she had been treated as someone who was a failure and would never amount to anything. To avoid the shame and hopelessness, she had learned to avoid thinking about the future in optimistic terms and to block active efforts to improve her life. That is, I was encountering a blockade that had been many years in the making, the sources of which were a mystery to me. I had not yet built a relationship, and we had made no agreements about what to target or how to work together. Yet we were already in DBT.

It is in this kind of moment that a conscious preoccupation with strategies, protocols, and skills will inhibit the therapist. Ideally all of these maneuvers are overlearned, ready to go when needed. But the therapist has to move in response to the patient. Therapy is a dance, not a seminar, and to stand still while considering among strategies is to miss opportunities and to create gaps in the session, gaps in the relationship. My recommendation throughout this book is that the therapist, in such moments, is wise to consider which way to move by wondering which of three paradigms to follow: acceptance, change, or dialectics. Each of the three represents a basic direction, and if the therapist moves in one of those directions, principles and strategies will follow. The *acceptance paradigm* prescribes just being there, in that moment, listening, inquiring, validating, elaborating, conveying objectivity, emanating compassion, and providing clarity. The *change paradigm* promotes the push for behavioral change by designating goals and target behaviors, assessing obstacles, finding solutions, insisting on action, and encouraging the patient to close the gap between designated targets and current functioning. The *dialectical paradigm* focuses attention on balance, synthesis, and movement: balance between acceptance and change interventions, balance between opposing positions by finding the wisdom on each side, and synthesis of the contradictory positions. When the therapist moves toward acceptance, he engages DBT's acceptance-based strategies. When he moves toward change, he engages the problem-solving strategies derived from CBT. And when he moves dialectically, he engages in dialectical thinking and uses dialectical strategies.

When the patient's anger was triggered by my question about her hopes for the future, I moved immediately into a stance of acceptance. I refrained from "doing" anything, opting for just "being there" with her. I tried to be open, curious, without assumption or judgment. Pushing for change seemed inadvisable, given that I had so little connection or information, and improvising with dialectical thinking seemed premature. After a pause, I spoke, saying, "I'm so sorry. It's true that I don't know you yet. I need to know all about the damage before we go any further." The patient seemed to appreciate the apology, seemed to feel validated, became more regulated, and proceeded to tell me about the tragedies that had befallen her during the prior 3 years.

In another case, my initial stance of acceptance quickly set the stage for a gentle movement toward change. I began my assessment of a 44-year-old woman who had a chronic relapsing–remitting case of bulimia, a profound sense of emptiness, a relentless preoccupation with suicide, and a diagnosis of borderline personality disorder, by asking what her goals might be for treatment. She responded, "My only goal is to get through today, and I'm never sure whether I will make it. I can't think about the future any more. I can't even think about thinking about it." I started with acceptance: "You are telling me that your daily life is just about too much to bear. The future barely exists as long as the present is impossible." She felt understood. "I haven't thought about the future since I was probably about 15 years old. There's no such thing." I extended her sentence by adding " . . . yet." It was a gentle challenge, and it represented a slight shift from acceptance toward asking for change (i.e., change in her thinking). I continued in the change-oriented vein as I followed up her suggestion that she once had a vision of her future. "I wonder what the future was going to be when you were 15, or before that?" She promptly answered, "I wanted to be an actress." I told her that I was trying to envision her as an actress, hoping she could elaborate. Quickly she disavowed the possibility: "That was then. This is now. There's nothing left!" At least we had one image of the future, even if it had been buried in a distant past. Note that from a principle-based perspective, I responded at first with validation, an acceptance strategy; and having succeeded in reducing the distance between us, I shifted over to change, challenging her disavowal of the future, and even though she disavowed it again, I thought it was a step forward just to remember that she used to have a dream.

On some occasions the therapist moves quickly and boldly to a change strategy as the conversation about a life worth living gets under way. Having done the assessment, I began therapy with a woman whose problems included self-harm and alcoholism. Her style was reserved and polite, though she was brutal to herself and others when she was intoxicated. I asked what goals she might have for treatment. "I'm a victim of my own stupidity. I really can't say I deserve any better than what I've got. You seem like a nice man, but I have to tell you, there's no way out for someone like me." The content was demoralizing, but something in her tone irked me. Her description of me struck me as dismissive. It felt like a veiled insult, as if she were saying I was the kind of "nice man" who would be passive and ineffectual with her. In fact, her comment kindled a feeling in me that was hardly "nice." These are uncertain moments for a therapist, especially when just starting with a new patient, wondering whether to challenge a response or to wait and let things unfold. In this case I pushed back right away with an irreverent tone. "You actually don't know me yet. It might be a big mistake for you to assume that I am a nice man. I don't know you yet either, and it could be a big mistake for me to assume that you don't deserve a better life, to assume that there is no hope." Her facial expression tightened. Her tone suggested annoyance toward me, as she went on to defend her claim that she was hopeless and undeserving of help. Her energetic defense of her hopelessness hardly seemed consistent with hopelessness. Paradoxically, she acted like someone who thought she deserved to be believed when explaining why she was so undeserving. I backed down a little bit. I said I was willing to wait and see what the truth was as we got to know each other. I told her I was sorry if I had offended her, and I appreciated that she could stand up for herself. As is often the case when a therapist uses irreverence, I felt energized and liberated instead of feeling defeated by her helpless presentation. I had the impression that we had already encountered and navigated a choppy moment, and that we were each left with energy and possibly a sense of pride.

The conversation about what would make life worth living is a natural starting point and a perfect accompaniment to the step-by-step contracting protocol. By attending to it as it weaves its way in and out of the treatment, the therapist works to ally himself with the patient's ultimate goals and values, even while spelling out the problem behaviors that interfere. In addition, as we have seen in these examples, initiating the conversation provides a window into the patient's capacity to envision a positive future and work toward it. If we dutifully follow the steps of the pretreatment protocol, we sometimes bypass the opportunity to engage the patient around the big picture and the motivating forces. Furthermore, this conversation provides an opportunity for the therapist to respond genuinely, personally, constructively, and in a way that already models the treatment.

Not every patient entering DBT presents such challenging responses at the beginning. In some cases the therapist can follow the step-by-step prescriptions of the contracting protocol with little need for improvisation. One patient of mine, having spent the better part of 3 years in a state hospital due to suicidal behavior, readily responded to the goals question: She wanted to work toward having an apartment, having an intimate partner, and going back to school to become a paralegal professional. She wanted to assist those with mental illnesses to navigate the legal system. In other words, she had the capacity to envision some aspects of a life worth living, to work collaboratively on spelling out a plan for treatment, and to make a commitment to the plan. We completed the pretreatment stage in four sessions and moved right on to DBT's Stage 1, the goal of which is to establish better behavioral control. Rather quickly, as her early momentum was slowed by her reluctance to attend the skills group, her episodes of dissociation, and her urges to kill herself, the sense of collaboration and mutual commitment collapsed. She seemed overtaken by intense emotions. Things seemed more black and white, and we seemed more like adversaries than partners. In one session she was yelling at me and covering her ears, at which point my capacity to improvise was tested. I had to shift gears and focus my attention on the assessment and understanding of these in-session behavioral problems. Momentarily I believed that I had overestimated her level of commitment to the treatment plan. As it turned out, this patient was actually quite firmly committed to the treatment goals but had become overwhelmed by fear, triggered by our disagreement into a dissociative episode and longstanding suicidal urges. Within that session, as I attempted to make sense of her emotional and interpersonal dysregulation, she regained better emotional control and restated her commitment to treatment and her image of building a life worth living.

I have worked with a sizable number of patients who *seemed* able to negotiate the initial contracting steps but who also presented noticeable cues that not all was as it seemed. A 33-year-old woman entered treatment after a decisive suicide attempt in which she had jumped from the balcony of a hotel room. She presented in my office as well mannered, sweet, and easy to engage, disconcertingly at odds with the image of her leaping from a balcony. She had graduated from college, but in her family of very accomplished professionals, she still was the underachiever and was treated as something of an embarrassment. When I asked how she thought treatment could help her improve her life, she said she had always wanted to be a mutual funds manager and that she needed to "get myself stable first." Although I know that some young people can get excited about being a mutual funds manager, her manner of communicating this to me seemed hollow and disembodied, as if it were rehearsed. When I asked further about her life goal, intimating that there was something unconvincing about it, she started crying and said that no one ever takes her seriously. Little did I know at the time that the dialogue happening between us already provided a microscopic window into the central catastrophe of her life: her tendency to disavow some of her unique qualities while casting herself in terms provided by her family. Although the remainder of the session seemed to go fairly smoothly, she went directly to the bathroom after the session to cut herself, which I discovered when I was on the way to the waiting room to meet my next patient. Not all was lost. I had learned rather quickly that it was typical for her to mask her distress, that she could appear competent and comfortable when in fact she was upset, that self-cutting was her primary and nearly automatic affect regulation strategy, and that her sense of shame was unbearable. Months later, after successfully establishing behavioral control and reducing her suffering, I was to learn that what would make her life worth living, among other things, was to be a gardener and homemaker. Following a complete course of DBT, she realized that dream. One of the take-home lessons was that many *patients do not have access to an image of a life worth living at the beginning of treatment.*

For some, as we have seen, the challenge comes in the first minute of conversation. For others, it arises during pretreatment around the discussion of one of the agreements or expectations of treatment. For still others, things go fairly smoothly until the therapist pushes for a stronger commitment. In any case, the management of this initial stage will establish a pattern of working together that will endure throughout the rest of the treatment; it becomes, looking back later, the "early life history" of the working relationship. The therapist learns a great deal from the initial encounters about the patient's sensitivities, skills, strengths, vulnerabilities, and capacities to recover. The patient, likewise, learns a great deal about the therapist's sensitivities, skills, strengths, vulnerabilities, and capacities to improvise and stay the course. As a therapist, one almost hopes to run into significant difficulty early on, in order to set the stage for successfully encountering challenges together.

THREE TASKS IN THE
LIFE-WORTH-LIVING CONVERSATION

As must be clear by this point, I see the life-worth-living conversation, weaving itself implicitly and explicitly through the pretreatment stage, as rife with difficulties and rich with opportunities. A large number of those opportunities revolve around three important therapeutic tasks. The DBT therapist who is on the lookout for these three tasks early in treatment and is prepared to address them in a principle-based manner stands a better chance of addressing them with awareness and precision, getting therapy off to a good start. The first task is *dialectical*, in that the therapist will intervene in the patient's dialectic, or ambivalence, between wanting to build a life worth living, on the one hand, and wanting to die, on the other. The second task is *behavioral*, in that the therapist can work to strengthen the patient's capacity to vividly envision a life worth living and to translate that vision into realistic goals and treatment targets. The third task is *relational*, in that the therapist works toward the establishment of a strong and flexible patient–therapist attachment, enhanced through encountering and solving adverse experiences together during pretreatment. It may be significant that these three tasks are suggested by the three words in the name of the therapy: there is a *dialectical* task, a *behavioral* task, and a *therapy* (relationship) task. As we now consider each of these three tasks, each being integral to the life-worth-living conversation, keep in mind that each task is addressed *while* following the contracting strategies with adherence to the manual, not *instead* of doing so.

The Dialectical Task in the
Life-Worth-Living Conversation

When the therapist starts out by asking about the patient's goals for treatment, as a way of getting a picture of what would make life worth living for this individual, she is likely to activate what we might call the suicide-versus-life-worth-living dialectic. This "destinational dialectic," as I call it, pertains to where the patient's life is going, the ends in view. The more commonly discussed "interventional" dialectic in DBT pertains to the strategic means for getting there: a synthesis of the opposing forces of acceptance and change. To illustrate what I mean by the suicide-versus-life-worth-living dialectic, I invite you to picture an American football field. Obviously a football game consists of a dialectic: the tension between two teams, each wanting to win, going in opposite directions, playing against each other. In this metaphor, the goal at one end of the field represents suicide and death; the goal at the other end is the life-worth-living goal. The opposing teams are pursuing, respectively, suicide versus a life worth living. This is the DBT football field, and the entire course of treatment is played out between the two end zones.

Naturally, and commonly, the DBT therapist enters the DBT football field on the side of the life-worth-living team, opposing the suicide-and-death team led by the patient. In doing so, however, the therapist is not acting in a dialectical manner and could thereby contribute to an unnecessarily adversarial transaction with the patient. It's simply more complicated than that. The patient has, within her own being, the whole dialectic already going on before the therapist enters the field. She has ambivalence. She wants to die, to end the unbearable suffering. She wants to live, hoping that somehow someone will help her get out of hell and build a life worth living. It's even possible that in her life history there were those who really wanted her to die and those who wanted her to live a good life. In other words, when the therapist enters the "game" on the field, the two teams (two aspects of the patient) are already opposing each other, it's a high-stakes game, and the therapist needs to find the optimal position for influencing the outcome.

Of course the DBT therapist is far from neutral in regard to the outcome. DBT therapists, beginning with Linehan, take the side of life, advocate for the building of a life worth living. Yet, thinking strategically, to simply take the side of life in transactions with the patient runs the risk of forcing the patient to the other side of the ambivalence. I have consulted with several patients who were in DBT treatment with therapists from whom the patients had each gotten the impression, probably correctly, that the therapists were insisting that they "take suicide off the table." Although it is often clinically indicated to get the patient to commit to "take suicidal actions off the table," it is more troublesome to insist that the patient "take suicidal thoughts and feelings off the table." Asking the patient to suppress suicidal thoughts and feelings is likely to result in their intensification.

It requires balance, and at times courage, for the therapist to enter the field siding with both "teams," genuinely seeking to understand the "wisdom" of the direct and indirect forms of self-destructiveness and, at the same time, initiating and promoting conversations about hopes and dreams. The patient's ambivalence certainly runs deeply, has a painful history, and should be approached dialectically, highlighting the wisdom of both sides. Not long ago I consulted with a young woman who was diagnosed as meeting criteria for borderline personality disorder. She was in a DBT program with individual therapy and a skills training group but seemed to be at a lengthy standstill. She had been subject to sexual abuse by her father when she was a latency-age child, and was raped several times by a neighbor in her teenage years. She began a decade of polysubstance abuse as a teen, and became just as addicted to frequent self-injury of a moderate severity in her 20s. She clearly saw that the use of substances and cutting was her arsenal to bring temporary but reliable relief from emotional suffering, but also understood that both "addictions" were ruining her life. She was pretty sure that if she had not had these two emotion regulation "strategies" (substance use and self-harming behaviors), she would have killed herself long ago. I asked her to tell me what her goals were, what her vision was of a life worth living. There was a long pause; in fact, I had the impression that she had entered a dissociative state. I called her name and she seemed to return to the present. She asked me what I had asked her. I repeated the question. She said she had no idea how to answer it, that she didn't really think about the future.

We were momentarily stuck between two opposing poles of a dialectic: at one end was the inevitability of suicide and the goal of doing whatever was necessary to eliminate pain; at the other end was the hypothetical concept, impossible even to think about at that point, of a life worth living. As many times as I have had these conversations, I still found it stunning that she could not come up with one idea that might be related to the future. It was as if the concept of future had been amputated from her consciousness, and all that remained was an agonizing present, penetrated by a disturbing past, managed by extreme behaviors that would numb or distract her. Returning to my metaphor, she could not see downfield toward the life-worth-living end zone, not even one yard. She had managed to avoid ending up dead by engaging in behaviors—addictions, cutting, and dissociative episodes—that were not far from the suicide end zone, and that served to prevent death but not move further from it. The metaphor offers this additional insight about problematic behavioral patterns that are self-destructive but not (quite) suicidal: They may prevent death, but they keep the patient stuck near the suicidal end of the field, which keeps her from moving toward the life-worth-living end.

I tried various ways to elicit some elements of a positive image of the future from her. I asked her to consider what she might have hoped for when she was a child, trying to recover a future orientation buried in her past. But she had no memory of her past except for a few horrible episodes in which she was frightened or abused. I tried to elicit her strengths, accomplishments, and values, hoping that we could build a vision of the future that might be compelling and realistic. She did acknowledge that if she were to have a future, she would want a cat with her, and a place to live, and would want "people to be nice to each other." It was a foggy and indistinct image, but it felt like a beginning. Having used a good deal of problem-solving strategies (from DBT's change paradigm) to elicit some kind of direction, and a great deal of validation (from DBT's acceptance paradigm) to authenticate some of the horrible events of her life and to express my understanding of her desire to die, I still felt stuck.

In DBT, when paralysis remains even in the face of change or acceptance strategies, the therapist naturally shifts to principles and strategies from the dialectical paradigm. Liberated by taking a "both . . . and" position that validates both sides of the dialectic and allows for speed, movement, and flow, I opened my mind to the strategic possibilities. One of DBT's dialectical strategies is to use a metaphor that captures the dilemma and opens new avenues for conversation. I suggested to the patient that she was standing at the edge of a landmass where life had been incredibly painful, a place with conditions that had driven her toward suicide. And she was looking across the vast waters in front of her, and it was a foggy day, and she couldn't see very far. And I suggested that there was an island out there, beyond the fog, and on that island was a home for her, a cat, and a life in which people were treated decently. To get there would require that she get into a boat and row toward that island without knowing exactly where it was or what it looked like. That boat was her DBT treatment. Because she had informed me that she kept a special razor blade in her apartment, which she called her "saving grace," I suggested that if she saw her DBT treatment as the boat, and her therapist as a fellow passenger, it would be important to leave the razor blade on shore and not take it with her. She was able to engage with the metaphor. She said that if she didn't have the razor blade, she absolutely needed something else, something that could help her get through the unbearable times, especially when she was overtaken by flashbacks of sexual abuse. I agreed entirely, and we began to consider what kinds of strategies could replace the razor blade.

The therapist simply cannot bypass, suppress, or overrule the essential life-versus-death ambivalence without making the problem worse. While staunchly holding out for a life worth living, sticking with a hopeful attitude in any way that works, the therapist also has to allow space and time for the patient to communicate the thoughts, feelings, and wishes related to suicide, without endorsing them as a plan. Linehan has said that DBT therapists have to accomplish two overarching essential tasks in working with the suicidal individual with borderline personality disorder: They have to be able to "get into hell" with the patient and see what it looks and feels like, and to help the patient "find a way out of hell." It's a dialectical metaphor, acknowledging the validity of both sides: the side of wanting to die and the side of wanting to find a way out without dying. It's a synthesis of acceptance and change. The work of "finding a way out of hell" begins with the work of envisioning a life worth living that works for that patient.

It's interesting to see that this middle path concept, although not named as such, was central to the thinking of Schneidman (1996, pp. 59–61), commonly referred to as the "father of suicidology" and the founder of the American Association of Suicidology. He posited that the thinking of the suicidal individual, who finds life unbearable and unfixable, narrows down to only two options: (1) the option of living with unbearable misery (which Schneidman termed *psychache*); and (2) the option of killing oneself. Once things get to that point, suicide risk is high. In Schneidman's view, the therapist somehow must insert a third option into the equation. That option can take many forms, but it has to provide a genuine alternative to the other two, a different direction. In some cases that third option comes about through the attachment to the therapist or to someone else. Many patients who are dying to die rue the day they began to get attached to their therapist (or to someone else). In other cases, the third option is a pursuit of some kind.

I remember a persistent DBT therapist who inserted herself into the miserable existence of a young woman whose life had come down to the choice of a life of unrelenting misery or suicide. Emerging out of a protracted and contentious suicide-versus-life-worth-living conversation, in the context of a growing mutual attachment and with the support of the DBT consultation team, the two of them arrived at a stunning agreement. The patient, who had always wished that she had been more athletic and hated the thought of dying without ever experiencing greater physical strength, agreed that she would take on a certain task "before I kill myself." The task, impressive given that she had never been a runner, was to complete the Boston Marathon. She seemed to make the decision in "rational mind," like making a bargain with the therapist (devil), but then she stuck to it. She committed to train for a year, and it was agreed that if things were no better at the end of that year, she could kill herself. Given her poor physical condition at that point, and her continued misery, it required amazing effort day-by-day and step-by-step. Her therapist framed the treatment around the life-worth-living goal of running the Boston Marathon. It was perfect for DBT, or any CBT treatment. She could visualize this long-term goal, it was compelling and might be realistic, the progress on it would happen step-by-step, and it could be monitored objectively. Suicide was on her mind all year, but the focus on a positive task helped her to inhibit the associated urges, to increase her resilience, and eventually to complete the marathon. By that time other things had changed. Her life, although still hard, seemed bearable; the relationship with the therapist was stronger, and she began to consider meaningful goals in her life.

The Behavioral Task in the Life-Worth-Living Conversation

I discussed the patient who was unable to envision any positive future outcome through the dense fog, or to name any goal beyond daily survival. The fact that she could not envision a better life, and that she could not name any goals toward a better life, was itself disabling. Without a life-worth-living goal to compete with the seductive magnetism of suicide, treatment loses a huge ally. These are skills—the skill of envisioning a positive and realistic future state, and the skill of articulating realistic goals that lead to that future—that are familiar within a larger set of capabilities known as *executive functions*. In fact, the capacity to envision a desired future state (visually, if possible) is an executive function that recruits all of the other executive functions in the course of getting things done. (Other executive functions that follow include marshaling resources toward the goal, monitoring progress toward the goal, inhibiting alternative pursuits that will interfere, and maintaining a level of cognitive flexibility that facilitates problem solving in the face of various obstacles.) Once we conceptualize the failure to envision a positive and motivating image of the future, and the deficiency in setting goals toward such an image, as capability deficits, we can organize our thinking and interventions around a familiar task in DBT: capability enhancement, or skills training.

When my older son was 13 and I was helping him to plan his summer, I asked him what mattered the most to him about this particular summer. For the first time in his life, as far as I could remember, he identified a goal that would affect the planning of the whole summer, several months in advance of it. He was on a youth hockey team, and he was, as he put it, "in the middle of the pack." He wondered aloud whether spending several weeks in hockey camps in the summer would translate into getting "up toward the top of the pack." We agreed that it might, and he asked if I could sign him up for some hockey camps. This would mean cutting down on many of his favorite summer activities. He had a vision that we were able to spell out in the form of concrete goals, which in turn helped him to inhibit alternative activities that would have interfered with this vision, and he was able to stick to the plan. He began the next hockey season closer to the "front of the pack."

When our patients have little or no capacity to dream, to envision, or to set a non-mood-dependent goal, it is an invisible handicap. We can't simply ignore this deficit. We need to assess it and to use our skills training knowledge to address it. And if we tackle this deficit at the very beginning of treatment, we might help to build or strengthen essential executive functions, to provide an *in vivo* demonstration of the value of skills training, and to begin a collaborative treatment relationship focused on acquiring capacities and improving motivation.

How can we optimally understand this kind of skills deficit in individuals with borderline personality and related disorders? Seen within the context of DBT's biosocial theory, these deficits are among the consequences of the larger transaction in the patient's life between her biologically based emotional vulnerabilities and the pervasively invalidating environment with which she interacted. Our patients, having survived and having been shaped by environments in which they were disregarded, denigrated, criticized, punished, and scorned, were usually not encouraged to dream or to convert their unique ideas and qualities into unique life paths. In fact, in an invalidating environment, to communicate a big dream might result in criticism and humiliation. Over time, painful transactions such as these can establish a link between envisioning the future and experiencing scorn and disappointment. The pervasive invalidation by the environment is transformed over time to a syndrome of self-invalidation; individuals learn to automatically invalidate and criticize themselves, to suppress hopes and dreams, and to discount the expectation of real support or the prospect of success. They learn that dreaming, and getting there, is for others. And as a result, they fail to build this specific and powerful life skill set: envisioning a positive future and setting a goal in that trajectory.

When the patient enters treatment and we ask her what she wants to accomplish, or more pointedly what would make life worth living, we encounter all varieties of dysfunction, many of which pointedly expose this deficit. It is a challenge for assessment to tease out to what degree the incapacity to envision the future and establish a goal is actually due to the *absence* of the capacity or to the *weakness* of it. In most cases, we can eventually locate the presence of a weakened or distorted capacity to dream and set goals, but it has been rendered invisible or ineffective due to one or more of several factors: Dreaming or goal setting may be associated with *problematic assumptions or beliefs*, may automatically trigger *intense negative emotions* based on prior traumatic or invalidating responses, or may result from other *associated skills deficits* (consider the impact of deficits in emotion regulation in general, in distress tolerance, or in the mindfulness skills). Furthermore, a lifetime of unfortunate reinforcement patterns may have extinguished or punished the activities of dreaming and goal setting, and may have reinforced more dysfunctional ways to handle the question about life goals.

Because of all of this, the pretreatment stage, beginning with the first conversation, can provide the *in vivo* context for assessing these skills deficits, beginning to understand the nature and impact of this individual's invalidating environment, and working to remedy the exposed skills deficits. If the capacity is truly missing, there is an opportunity to build it "from scratch," that is, to intervene with skill acquisition. This intervention involves (1) orienting the patient to the presence and the consequences of the deficit, (2) using instruction and modeling to help the patient move through the steps of building a vision of the future and establishing associated goals, (3) reinforcing the early steps, and (4) ensuring that the patient practices these crucial skills. In those cases where the skill is present but other factors have interfered, the therapist can work toward a formulation of the factors that interfere and approach them with needed change procedures, such as cognitive restructuring, exposure, stimulus control techniques, and contingency procedures to strengthen the diminished capacity.

One of my former patients recalled being emotionally sensitive throughout her life, including as a young child. She was the only child of two very busy and self-absorbed parents. She endured years of dinner table conversations in which the parents completely ignored her, talking to each other as if she were invisible or not in the room. If she spoke up, she was told to stop interrupting; if she played her flute (she was a prodigy), she was told to go into the basement. When she communicated an emotional response, she was told to stop trying to get attention. The home atmosphere was tense, parental attitudes were severe. She began cutting herself for emotional relief at age 8, and she made her first suicide attempt at age 13. When therapy began, and she was asked what she hoped to accomplish through her therapy, she could barely speak. She stared at me as if I were speaking a foreign language. She looked perplexed and couldn't respond; this rather brilliant person who had the discipline to become an outstanding flautist could not come up with one word about her life goals. My impression was that she was baffled and perhaps mistrustful of an individual showing sincere interest in helping her to have a good life. Moving through the steps of pretreatment was a slow, halting, and torturous process. The pervasive invalidation she experienced from her environment had transformed into self-loathing. In moments of uncertainty or ambiguity, in the relationship with the therapist and others, she anticipated the imminent recurrence of environmental invalidation.

I oriented her to the problem from a skills deficit perspective. I explained that I could only assume that in the course of her life she had not been taught or encouraged to have a dream, to share that dream, and to set some goals in a relationship context like this current one. She agreed, elaborating on how her family had shown no interest in her schoolwork (she was a really good student), her music, her sports, or a social life. What she accomplished, she accomplished on her own, and she lived a high-achieving but achingly isolated life that led her to want to die. We began to work, with baby steps, in having her communicate to me what she would like to accomplish in treatment. At first she could not make eye contact when she was communicating any hopes. It was an *in vivo* exposure exercise that triggered fear and shame and elicited damaging self-talk about how she should not expect any help from anyone. She never became comfortable with expressing life dreams and goals, but she acquired the capacity to do it, albeit in a stilted and inhibited way. She learned quickly that DBT was all about working your way toward positive goals, all about strengthening motivation, and all about learning and strengthening skills. We were off to a good start.

What if the patient, even with all of this effort, cannot come up with a vision of a positive future or with a positive goal at which to aim? This happens. There are several possible strategies. One is simply to shift away from the effort to get a life-worth-living statement or associated goals, and to focus instead on smaller, more immediate, practical steps. In one case, a young male patient was unable to articulate any larger goals, but he could get motivated to get his once-beloved bicycle back into riding condition, right away. In another case, treatment focused on helping a female patient overcome her fears of taking her cat to the veterinarian. Experiencing success with smaller tasks, even the task of learning new skills in the group, begins to reinforce the effort exerted, and ultimately might lead to the capacity to set bigger goals. In these cases, we need to recast a "life worth living" into more immediate, minute, practical life goals—what the individual will be doing today, tonight, or tomorrow—and to defer the effort to look beyond the immediate future, a practice that might activate barriers that will not yield in the short run.

Another approach to helping the patient build her image of a life worth living on memories of better days and earlier hopes or previously suppressed dreams is to begin a conversation with her about her values, her strengths, and her talents. One patient of mine with borderline personality disorder and a major depressive disorder with psychotic features was sure that her life was over. She could not imagine "starting from scratch" and generating a meaningful life that included workable relationships. As we considered her values and strengths, she spoke with admiration about those who serve in the military and the police force, those who put their lives on the line to protect others. Because she had suffered several psychiatric hospitalizations, she assumed (correctly, I think) that these options were not available to her. But this discussion, to which we returned several times, and during which she was increasingly explicit about her desire to protect others, led her to concretely investigate the possibility of helping to train dogs to locate unexploded land mines in third-world countries. From that moment on, the life-worth-living conversation became very focused, practical, and motivating.

The Relational Task in the Life-Worth-Living Conversation

A third task that can be approached through the life-worth-living conversation during pretreatment is the development and strengthening of a collaborative relationship between therapist and patient. The initial discussions about goals allow the therapist to do several helpful things. He allies with hope, change, the patient's dreams and goals, and a life worth living. He validates the patient's suffering, validates the urge to commit suicide, and comes to understand the patient's narrative within which suicide makes sense, all without validating suicide as a solution. He can (1) spell out the dialectic—the opposition between pursuing suicide and pursuing a life worth living, (2) validate parts of each side of the dialectic, and (3) demonstrate patience and respect in collaboratively trying to arrive at a synthesis. In conceptualizing the associated problems of picturing the future and identifying goals as skills deficits, he points the way to remediation of the deficits in a practical manner, with concrete instructions and deliberate practices. He can demonstrate how validating the patient's suffering and sensitivity can be done without treating her as fragile. The goal is to help the patient experience the therapeutic atmosphere as one that encourages openness, genuineness, honesty, and courage, and that will tolerate disagreement and conflict. Even though these conversations can be challenging, can "shake things up" a bit, for the therapist they are an opportunity to engage and to combine hopes for the patient, passion for the treatment, and respect for the patient's positions.

Linehan has outlined the optimal characteristics of a DBT therapist as finding the middle path between polarized positions along three dimensions. As spelled out in the manual (Linehan, 1993a, pp. 109–111), the therapist can (1) insist on behavioral change in the context of deep acceptance, (2) stand with unwavering centeredness while engaging with compassionate flexibility, and (3) benevolently demand collaboration while being unconditionally nurturing. The life-worth-living conversation is an excellent task and framework in which the therapist can find and practice the middle path between these dimensions. He insists on moving the patient toward a life worth living while conveying genuine validation of the wish to die, staying centered on the life-worth-living goal while remaining flexible enough to move back and forth with the patient's ambivalence, and demanding that the patient work toward a higher quality of living while offering nurturance along the way. Obviously, a DBT therapist who can genuinely offer a dialectical position, finding the right synthesis of these polarities in the clinical moment, has an advantage in navigating toward a stronger relationship with the patient.

For many patients, the difficulty in responding to the goals question results in their first *in-session therapy-interfering behavior*. As such, it is the perfect opportunity for the therapist to bring the whole treatment package to bear, and to model the approach that will be used throughout the treatment when facing challenging situations in life and within the therapy relationship. It's like the first chapter in a book or the prelude to a large piece of music. And although the step-by-step process of using the contracting strategies, as outlined in the manual, provides an excellent framework or skeleton for the first sessions, these protocol-driven steps do not tell the therapist what to do when it doesn't go well. This is both a *principle-based* and a *protocol-based* treatment, and it starts that way from the beginning. Often the therapist needs the whole treatment package in the first minute. If entering DBT were entering a swimming pool, there is no shallow end.

Finally, the life-worth-living conversation is the best illustration to the patient that DBT is not primarily a "suicide-prevention" treatment, it is a treatment focused on building a life worth living. It is so much more motivating to strive toward something that results in a better life, than to aim only to reduce a variety of dysfunctional behaviors. If the patient succeeds in improving the quality of her life, the plan, the urge, and the idea to commit suicide becomes naturally less compelling and less necessary. In the football field metaphor, if the patient is advancing down the field toward the life-worth-living end zone, she is simultaneously moving away from the suicide end zone, however gradually, and she is moving out of the zone in which addictions, dissociation, eating disorders, and non-suicidal self-injury are so entrapping.

CONCLUDING COMMENTS

When treating the patient who wants to die, or who is living a life of deadly stagnation centered around direct or indirect self-destructive behaviors, one naturally encounters the dialectic between wanting to escape misery through death and wanting to have a life of meaning, a life worth living. During the pretreatment stage in DBT, while carrying out the prescribed contracting strategies, the life-worth-living conversation weaves its way in and out of the process. To the degree that the therapist can perceive and engage in this important conversation, he has several opportunities to address pervasive therapeutic tasks. He has the opportunity (1) to take a dialectical stance with respect to the suicide-versus-life-worth-living dialectic, (2) to assess and remedy a skills deficit in envisioning a positive future and establishing goals to get there, and (3) to build a stronger attachment between patient and therapist through the compassionate and effective handling of early adversity in therapy.

Now, having discussed the central mission of DBT—that is, to help the patient build a life worth living, enhanced by a principle-based approach—we turn to a detailed discussion of the three fundamental paradigms of DBT—change, acceptance, and dialectics—and the principles that arise from each.

CHAPTER 2

Introducing DBT's Three Paradigms

Several years ago, I saw my first college hockey game. Even though I didn't know much about the rules, the strategies, or the players, it was obvious to me that there was one particularly outstanding player. First, he possessed technical mastery of the fundamentals of skating, puck handling, passing, shooting, and checking (legally hitting opposing players when they are handling the puck). His technical skill set was so overlearned and automatic that he seemed not to have to think about it. Second, he seemed to possess a heightened sense of awareness, as if his perspective, from a level above the game, allowed him to see in all directions and to see things exactly as they were. He seemed calm, balanced, and prescient, as if he knew where the puck was going before any other player knew. Finally, he could move in almost any direction in response to the constantly changing circumstances around him. In other words, while maintaining his technical skill set and his "rink awareness," he could improvise skillfully and move rapidly, as needed.

These three qualities—a *technical skill set*, *heightened awareness*, and the *capacity to improvise*—are integral to the transformative work of any superlative performer, whether in sports, art, music, dance, public speaking, entrepreneurship, or almost any other human endeavor. It is no different for a highly competent DBT therapist.

THE DEVELOPMENT OF DBT AND THE
THREE-PARADIGM PERSPECTIVE

DBT began with Linehan's efforts to bring the *technical skill set* of behaviorism to bear on the problem of suicidal behaviors. Behaviorism became the basis of DBT's initial treatment paradigm, the paradigm of change. But clients diagnosed with borderline personality disorder were emotionally sensitive and reactive, had long histories of having been pervasively invalidated, and found the change-oriented treatment difficult to tolerate. In response, while maintaining her conviction that behavioral change strategies would be effective if they could be tolerated, Linehan began to add in interventions of a different nature. She listened more, explored patients' experiences further, acknowledged the reality of those experiences, and validated the "kernels of truth" in otherwise dysfunctional behavioral patterns. When these shifting interventions were done with accuracy and compassion, patients felt understood, felt safer and closer to their therapists, and usually became more regulated emotionally. Then, Linehan realized, it would be effective to shift back to the change agenda with behavioral techniques. Earlier in her teachings of DBT, Linehan described the cognitive-behavioral problem-solving strategies as the "bitter-tasting but effective pill," and the validation strategies as the "sugar coating" that helped the pill go down. To accept patients with compassion and to intervene with accuracy, therapists needed to develop their own *heightened levels of acceptance and awareness*. The cultivation of acceptance and awareness was grounded in the principles and practices of mindfulness.

Once able to skillfully balance change interventions with those involving acceptance, relying on behaviorism and mindfulness as the foundations, Linehan taught DBT therapists to shift back and forth between them, all in the service of helping patients move toward their life-worth-living goals. In practical terms, treatment went back and forth between pushing for change, becoming aware of the patient's reactions, communicating acceptance, pushing for change again, and so on.

Still, progress in treatment frequently came to a standstill as patient and therapist fell into rigid patterns with each other, sometimes with paralyzing passivity, sometimes with irresolvable conflicts, often on opposite sides of the fence. Balancing change and acceptance paradigms seemed to be insufficient. Linehan began to weave a third set of interventions into the treatment, strengthening the therapist's *capacity to improvise*. These interventions, which helped to counter rigidity, impasse, and opposition with flexibility, movement, and synthesis, were based in dialectical philosophy and practice. Dialectics, which has been compared to jazz music in DBT, functioned to promote improvisation. Stripped to its essence, effective DBT requires the therapist to synthesize a *technical cognitive-behavioral skill set, heightened acceptance and awareness,* and *capacity to improvise* with DBT's change, acceptance, and dialectical paradigms—all based on behaviorism, mindfulness, and dialectical philosophy—to alter entrenched behavioral patterns and "get the patient out of hell." Each paradigm gave rise to particular sets of strategies, the triadic strategic core of the treatment: *problem-solving strategies* from the change paradigm, *validation strategies* from the acceptance paradigm, and *dialectical strategies* from the dialectical paradigm.

THE CHALLENGES OF LEARNING TO PRACTICE DBT

The simplicity of this three-paradigm perspective stands in contrast to the complexity of learning to practice DBT. Early in the learning process, therapists can become flooded with choices. They have to return to behavioral assessment in nearly every session, focus on the highest-priority targets throughout the session, keep track of their patients' predominant "emotion of the moment," keep to the agreements and assumptions, apply approximately 85 strategies and a number of specialized "structural protocols," and teach and reinforce more than 100 skills. And, of course, all of this has to be done while remaining alert and aware of each patient's minute-by-minute responses, with timing and tact. As if this were not enough, DBT therapists are often doing all of this in the course of sessions that are difficult to manage, dealing with matters of life or death, and coping with their own dysregulated emotions. I have personally experienced these immense learning challenges and have come to recognize a certain "deer-in-the-headlights" look on the faces of therapists in training when they begin to suffer from information overload.

I am not just describing the challenges of therapists new to DBT. Mastering the challenge of remaining adherent to the treatment manual, responsive to the patient, true to oneself, and focused on the treatment targets requires considerable practice and expertise for highly experienced DBT therapists. Similarly, the landscape painter faces a daunting task when selecting the color for the next brushstroke from a palette that includes 150 shades. To scan and select from 150 colors would completely interrupt the flow of imagination and painting, and of course it's not what the painter does. Instead, the colors are grouped into a few color spectra, perhaps the reds, the yellows, and the blues. The painter might say to herself, "I need something with a reddish hue," then can rapidly consider a choice from among colors of that hue. She can keep her mind focused on what the painting calls for, stay in contact with her imagination, quickly and fluidly locate the best color choice, and proceed.

Similarly, faced with a given moment in a session, the DBT therapist cannot be thinking about 85 strategies, several protocols, and 100 skills. Those interventions are grouped into a handful of overarching categories: assessment strategies, structural strategies, change procedures, acceptance strategies, and dialectical strategies. The therapist might say to himself, "I need to push for behavioral change," and rapidly consider the options among the problem-solving procedures, accompanied by tonal choices from the change-oriented irreverent communication style. He can thereby keep his mind focused on the in-the-moment needs and choices, stay in contact with the destination and his imagination, quickly and fluidly locate the best strategic choice, and proceed. With study, practice, supervision, and review of one's own therapy tapes, the practice becomes more intuitive and automatic. For instance, we come to "know" when we can't push any harder for change, and we automatically add in or shift over to acceptance, augmenting or completely letting go of change (for the time being), radically accepting the moment as it is and validating the "kernel of truth" in the patient's opposition. Or in another case, say we have already shifted from change to acceptance strategies, but the impasse in the session remains, the sense of movement has ground to a halt, and we "know" to "go dialectical," drawing on principles and strategies that lay out the polarized positions, look for a middle path along which to generate movement.

This kind of flow between paradigms—the algorithmic-like movement from paradigm to principles to strategies and back to assessment again—was simply not in my mind in the early years of learning to do DBT. I was still learning the treatment strategy by strategy, skill by skill, and in coping with the fast moving world of a real live session, I know that I came across as stiff and deliberate, with my mind focused on protocols and strategies rather than on principles or the patient. I'm sure that many of my patients experienced themselves as being directed, prodded, or dragged through the prescriptions of the DBT treatment manual. I came to realize later that there had been three of us in the room: the patient, me, and the *manual*. Once I realized that I could group the myriad interventions into a few categories—assessment, change, acceptance, and dialectics—I could navigate through sessions with more intuition, speed, movement, and flow even as I remained focused on the current behavioral target, keeping track of the patient and remaining in touch with myself. I experienced greater freedom and greater confidence. In the lexicon of DBT's core mindfulness skills, I had become better able to participate effectively, one-mindfully, and nonjudgmentally. I was able to intervene with more confidence, knowing that I could shift as needed if the current intervention was ineffective. After some years of practice, I came to appreciate the huge advantages of principle-based treatment. Let's take a detailed look at how this newly grasped perspective worked in the context of a session with a young woman whom I call Tracy.

CASE EXAMPLE
OF PRINCIPLE-BASED TREATMENT

Having completed an intake assessment with "Tracy," arrived at a diagnosis of borderline personality disorder, agreed on a set of treatment targets, oriented her to the treatment, and gotten an initial commitment to the targets and the plan, we began working together in sessions in the standard way. Tracy had been in several therapies, had failed to benefit from medication trials, had become hopeless about getting help, and had come to me as her "last resort." Her prioritized target list included a number of problems: suicide attempts by overdose and self-strangulation, self-cutting behaviors of high frequency and low lethality, occasional episodes of driving at dangerously high speeds to "tempt death," inconsistent attendance in prior therapies, painfully intense emotional responses with rapid mood shifts on a daily basis, daily use of marijuana to "take the edge off" her anxieties and moods, terrible feelings of emptiness unless she was in an intense relationship, a pattern of frequent high-intensity relationships resulting in heartbreak and resentment, erratic spending patterns, and no enduring platonic friendships. She met all nine criteria for borderline personality disorder. She described herself as undirected, "sleepwalking through life," taking a new path every day, and she felt that she was "fundamentally flawed" and "out of control." When I provided the usual orientation to the problems treated in DBT, reframing the nine diagnostic criteria as representing five categories of dysregulation (emotional, interpersonal, behavioral, cognitive, and self) that are addressed in four modules of skills training, she felt temporarily hopeful—better organized, less stigmatized, and able to see a path to recovery. This more positive sense quickly slipped away as our work began.

During the first month, she arrived at sessions late, frazzled, and apologetic. She conveyed the impression of someone who was totally lost and just happened to show up in front of me. She always seemed to be in the middle of an intense emotional episode of one kind or another, and rarely did she remember what we had talked about the prior week. She began the session almost in midsentence, as if I had known what was going on in the latest troubling relationship incident. At the beginning of one such session, she walked in quickly, late as usual, dropped her purse on the floor (everything fell out of it), plopped herself down on the chair in front of me, and looked down, making no eye contact, and began speaking. She was obviously exasperated, seemed overwhelmed, and in her tone she seemed to convey, "Don't you dare say anything to me—I can't take it and I will snap at you if you do!" Within seconds the session was charged with emotionality, urgency, and impulsivity.

I began by just listening, alert to the words, the story, the tone, her body posture, and her facial expressions. I oriented myself to her in that present moment, trying to understand the realities of what had happened, seeking to make contact through listening and responding, *intervening within the paradigm of acceptance*, relying on the underlying principles of mindfulness. Within seconds I was using the first three levels of validation (completely alert and awake, reflecting her comments back to her, and articulating the unarticulated) and was using a reciprocal communication style (alert, awake, responsive to the manifest content, warm, and genuine). In myself I became aware of a small dose of the urgency and chaos reciprocal to those same qualities that she brought into the room, and I noticed an urge in myself to rescue her, to find some way to reduce her distress. Sticking with the mindfulness paradigm, emphasizing the acceptance of reality as it is in the moment, I remained in the posture of simply listening, essentially using the DBT core mindfulness skills of *observing* along with being *one-mindful*. The session was only about 45 seconds old, the problem of emotional dysregulation was present in the room, and I noted to myself that her lateness was a therapy-interfering target behavior. As mentioned, my stance was based on acceptance and awareness, using several validation strategies and mindfulness skills.

Over the next minute, she spewed out her anger at her ex-boyfriend for wanting to see her again. Having seen this pattern in her before, I could feel her emotional momentum building in a way that could become difficult to interrupt. I began to entertain a question about how to proceed. What would be consistent with DBT? I realized that there was a dialectic; I could stay within the acceptance paradigm or I could begin to push for behavioral change guided by the change paradigm. On the acceptance side I could continue to validate her. Perhaps it would result in her feeling understood as she communicated her feelings about the incident, and in regulating her emotions more effectively. But standard DBT practice would recommend that I ask to see her diary card at this point in the session, as part of assessing the prior week and determining the highest-priority behaviors to target during the session—in other words, the change direction. Once the thought occurred to me that it was time to ask for the diary card, I could feel my urge to avoid doing so. It felt to me as if asking for her diary card at that moment would be like asking a bleeding car accident victim in an emergency room for her insurance information. On the other hand, if I were to avoid asking, out of fear of her response, I might be treating her as if she were fragile, reinforcing a dysfunctional pattern of mood-dependent behavior. With a matter-of-fact tone and "acting opposite" my own urge to avoid asking for the diary card, I interrupted her, indicating that we could come back to the situation about the ex-boyfriend, and asked to see her diary card. *With respect to the paradigms, I shifted from acceptance to change and began using problem-solving strategies.*

As expected, she felt interrupted and acted as if I had thrown cold water on her. She would not look at me and took no action to locate a diary card. She looked hurt and angry but did not speak; in fact, it seemed as if she withdrew and refused to speak. I told her I was sorry to have interrupted her, and that maybe I could have done it more tactfully, but reminded her that in DBT we needed to set an agenda for the session if we were going to change her life. She remained silent and I had the impression that I had inflamed her further. Though she would not respond to inquiries, I felt as if I were being punished. Several minutes passed. I asked again if she could express her reaction to what I had done. I felt we were at a crossroads of some kind. I noticed that I was uncertain of what was going on with her and uncertain about what to do next. *Having introduced change into the session, I returned for the moment to a stance of acceptance.* I tried to remain alert to subtle changes in nonverbal communications, and tried to remain balanced. I noticed an urge to confront her, and an opposing urge to apologize to her and rescue her.

It then occurred to me that perhaps what had happened between us was not new to her, but was something that interfered with her relationships in general. I said, "Tracy, I think I was a bit clumsy the way I interrupted you, but I just wonder if this happens to you sometimes, and I wonder if we can learn something from this, both of us, that will help us hang in there with each other?" Having recognized that we were stuck, wanting to maintain movement, trying to recognize the validity both in what I had done and in her response, I tried to make "lemonade out of lemons." In DBT that is a dialectical strategy. To review: *I had begun the session within the acceptance paradigm, had shifted to the change paradigm by pressing her about the diary card, had come back to acceptance as I listened to her angry response, was feeling stuck, and had shifted into a dialectical paradigm with a lemonade-out-of-lemons strategy, highlighting our opposition and looking for synthesis.* This shift broke the logjam. Tracy yelled at me, "You are a klutz at best!" and wondered how I could be a good therapist if I interrupted people. At that point she told me she had stopped filling out her diary card this week because it was too difficult and it seemed "stupid." We proceeded to discuss the diary card, its place in the treatment, and some of the reasons she didn't want to do it. In other words, we were *back on a change-oriented agenda using orientation and recommitment*. By my count, in these first few minutes I had used about 13 treatment strategies, but my conscious awareness had been more simply focused on starting with acceptance, shifting to change, back to acceptance, onto dialectics, and back to change again. Shifting among three overarching gears, rather than considering all strategies and skills, is a more effective way of "driving" the DBT session.

CONCLUDING COMMENTS

I have now introduced the three paradigms, placed them in the context of comprehensive DBT, and considered how we move back and forth between them as we navigate sessions with clients. In the next three chapters, I examine in greater detail the principles of each paradigm and how they are woven into the treatment. But to bring the current chapter to a practical conclusion, I summarize the main factors I hold in my awareness as I move through a DBT session—numerous enough to provide me with options, few enough to help me stay organized and focused.

1. Stay focused on the primary target, which provides the overall agenda, and shift among secondary (or instrumental) targets, as needed in order to accomplish the primary target.
2. Remain alert for the presence of currently active emotions in the patient, especially those emotions that are poorly regulated; emotional dysregulation is the core construct for understanding and treating our patients in DBT.
3. Keep interventions consistent with treatment guidelines found in:
   a. Biosocial theory
   b. Therapist agreements
   c. Assumptions about patients
   d. Assumptions about therapy
   e. The current stage of treatment
4. Use the structural strategies for structuring the sessions (beginning a session, targeting, reviewing a diary card, etc.)
5. Use the suicide crisis protocol if suicidal behavior is increased or imminent.

6. Return to assessment again and again.
7. Consider which of the three paradigms—change, acceptance, and/or dialectics—is right for the moment. Use the strategies consistent with that choice.

If I have made it sound relatively simple to define one's direction as a DBT therapist by selecting among three paradigms, moment by moment, I have done the reader a disservice. Doing psychotherapy is so challenging, with so many options at every moment and so much uncertainty about the outcome of each. However, it can be useful to hold in mind the construct of the three paradigms, each with its array of strategies, especially when encountering difficulty. Each of the three provides a direction, and therapists can also rely on straightforward assessment, intuitive capacities, and wide-awake awareness and responsiveness to "feel their way" forward in the session. The therapist moves toward pushing, but senses when to push harder and when to pull back. He arrives at an accepting posture, but determines whether to actively convey understanding or whether to be still. Caught between rigid poles, he shifts into heightened movement and improvisation, but somehow intuits whether his "movements" should be big or small, fast or slow.

Finally, in determining how and when to shift among the three paradigmatic directions, the therapist is wise to remember two caveats. First, the acceptance paradigm should nearly always remain present and influential even if in the background when pushing for behavioral change. A pervasively validating environment is valuable in countering the client's pervasive self-invalidation, facilitating attachment and the leverage it provides, and supporting change-oriented work. Second, the three paradigms are not "equal" to each other in order of priority. DBT is a goal-oriented treatment, CBT is the goal-oriented paradigm and is therefore central, and the other two paradigms are, in a sense, ways to augment CBT when indicated. Having introduced the three paradigms and how therapists can draw from them during sessions, we take a closer look at the principles attendant to each in the next three chapters.

CHAPTER 3

The Acceptance Paradigm

ACCEPTANCE AND MINDFULNESS IN THE PRACTICE OF DBT

To recapitulate the DBT treatment development story, Linehan started with the change paradigm, applying problem-solving strategies from CBT to the treatment of suicidal behaviors. She added acceptance-based strategies to address the patient's suffering and to facilitate the use of CBT. To this mixture she added strategies from a dialectical perspective to address the problems of rigidity, polarization, and conflict that are typical of these therapies. But we begin our formal discussion of the three paradigms with acceptance for several reasons. First, it is the oldest of the three, the beginnings of it being traceable back to the life of the Buddha more than 2,500 years ago. It is a deep root of the "Tree of DBT" (see Chapter 6). Second, in most cases the use of acceptance-oriented interventions is a prerequisite for the effective use of cognitive-behavioral and dialectical strategies. "Getting into hell with the patient, " as discussed in Chapter 1, is essential in helping the patient find a way out of hell, and it requires careful listening and validation, essentially acceptance and heightened awareness. Third, ideally we enter into each therapy session, skills training group, telephone coaching call, and consultation team meeting with an open mind and a compassionate, accepting heart. I don't have empirical data to prove it, but my conviction, born out of clinical experience, is that I am more effective at helping my patients change when I start from an accepting—awake, alert, nonjudgmental, and fully present—stance. When I am truly and fully present at the beginning of a session, my patients notice. I can tell that they can tell. And it injects the session with a sense of relevance and immediacy. Finally, we begin here

with the explication of the acceptance paradigm because in the teaching of DBT's skills modules, the acceptance-based mindfulness skills are
central to the teaching of every module, and are thus named the *core
mindfulness skills.* Practicing mindfulness skills is integral to the learning
and practice of the others.

The acceptance paradigm in DBT is based, above all, on the principles and practices of mindfulness. Mindfulness is an innate capacity of the
human mind, the capacity to see the unfolding of reality clearly, directly,
in the here and now, moment by moment, without "delusion." Although
introduced through mindfulness meditation by the Buddha about 2,500
years ago, the basic concepts and practices can be found in every spiritual
tradition around the world, and in secular traditions as well. Mindfulness
happens unintentionally when we "wake up" in the present moment. For
instance, we suddenly become mindful, fully awake and alert to present reality, when we experience a threat to our lives or our well-being.
This same state can be cultivated intentionally by meditative practices
to bring present-moment awareness into all aspects of our lives, thereby
enhancing our well-being. In fact, the practice of mindfulness meditation
throughout the centuries has given rise to certain insights that form the
core of the principles of DBT's acceptance paradigm. Whereas the total-
ity of practices and insights from meditation provide nourishment for the
DBT therapist, five overarching principles are particularly relevant:

1. *Present-moment awareness.*
2. *Nonattachment.*
3. *Interbeing.*
4. *Impermanence.*
5. *"The world is perfect as it is."*

In concert, these principles promote awareness, acceptance, and compassion. They lay the groundwork for validation strategies and DBT's reciprocal communication style, and constitute one of the primary means with
which therapists regulate themselves during therapy.

PRESENT-MOMENT AWARENESS

Perhaps the concept and practice at the core of the acceptance paradigm—
the prerequisite for the other acceptance principles—is this one: The present moment is the only moment. When our attention is fixed on the past,
it is fixed on a memory, a story, a fiction of sorts. When our attention
is drawn to the future, it is drawn to a fantasy. In a mindfulness retreat

with Thich Nhat Hanh, he was asked how one could ever plan for the future if one's attention never left the present moment. Thich Nhat Hanh answered that the best planning for the future happens when one brings the future into the present moment, not when one abandons the present moment to enter into the future. The present moment is the host; the future is the invited guest. He went on to say that the same goes for considering the past. One can invite the memories of the past into the present moment without losing one's grounding in present-moment reality. Reality is here, it is now, and it is taking place whether we are aware of it or not. We just need to wake up and notice, and when we do, that present-moment awareness transports and transforms us, invisibly, instantly, back into reality. Thich Nhat Hanh (1975) called this state the "miracle of mindfulness."

When we inhabit the present moment, with awareness of the sensations, perceptions, thoughts, and events that reside therein, we are rooted in reality while we do whatever else we do. Whether we are hosting the past or the future, or we are engaging our DBT patients in problem solving, we try to stay grounded in the present moment. The individual who is "hijacked" by memories of a traumatic past, or who is racked with worry about the as-yet-unreal future, is not experiencing the present moment, is thereby grounded in the unrealities of the past or future, and is invisibly handicapped. Complicated grieving, posttraumatic stress, panic, intense anxiety, and worry are associated with the kind of past or future hyperawareness that eclipses the present moment. When patients are overtaken by traumatic reenactments, in some cases to the extent of dissociating from the present, "grounding" techniques are specifically aimed at helping them reclaim present-moment awareness. When patients are swept away with anxiety set off by envisioning catastrophic future outcomes, skillful therapists help reconnect them to reality by asking them to observe and describe associated sensations taking place in the here and now. When depressed patients involuntarily withdraw into cocoons of depressive ideation about the past, the future, and the world, DBT therapists help them to schedule and carry out activities that rivet their attention and awareness to the present moment. The influence of present-moment awareness—and the loss of present-moment awareness—is ubiquitous, constant, and consequential.

As one learns in DBT's Core Mindfulness Skills module, the practice of observing and describing the realities of the present moment and participating fully in it provides pathways to finding wisdom within oneself. The practice of observing and describing sensations, emotions, urges, distress, behavioral responses, and relationship events as they occur in that moment is a prerequisite for effectively participating in the three other skills modules, in which the patient is attempting to change emotional responses, tolerate distress, and change relationship patterns.

And for therapists (essentially, every one of us), who are time and time again derailed by the emotional reactions, problematic cognitions, and misperceptions of patients as they are drawn into reactions to the past, fears of the future, and sparsely based interpretations of present reality, the practice of reclaiming the present moment becomes central to clear seeing, to acceptance of reality, and to therapist self-regulation. At times, when therapists are not "residing in the present moment" and then become aware of that fact, they can reenter the present by bringing attention to their body, noticing the contact of their body upon the chair or their feet on the floor, and experiencing that their center of gravity shifts downward into the abdomen. That is, present-moment awareness is at the core of the skills at the center of each therapist's self-care, and completely necessary to the very important process in DBT of *radically accepting reality*.

NONATTACHMENT

From a Buddhist perspective, derived from more than 2,000 years of mindfulness meditation, attachment is the root cause of human suffering, and letting go of attachment is a core practice in reducing that suffering. *Attachment*, in this therapeutic context, does not refer to the attachment between beings. Attachment between patient and therapist is a crucial ingredient in DBT treatment. It refers instead to an attachment to beliefs, perceptions, possessions, preferences, and states of mind. If a person has arthritis of the hip, as I do, he experiences pain. If, in addition to that physical pain, he is attached to the belief that he should not have arthritis or that it is not fair that he has arthritis, then he is adding suffering to his pain. If a person is attached to remaining youthful, then the inevitable painful realities that accompany aging are aggravated further by the belief that it should not be so. For the person who is attached to health as if it were the only acceptable or fair state, that attachment will add suffering to the natural discomfort of illness. Those for whom the painful loss of a relationship, a person, a pet, or a job is simply unacceptable and never "should" have happened, will suffer from that nonacceptance in addition to the inevitable grieving. Having acquired the insight that life is inevitably filled with pain, and that resisting or protesting those painful realities causes additional suffering (known respectively as the First and Second Noble Truths of Buddhism), the Buddha then taught that the alleviation of suffering comes from acknowledging and accepting reality as it truly is, while letting go of attachment to beliefs, perceptions, possessions, and states of mind (Third Noble Truth of Buddhism). From these insights arises the familiar (though unattributed) saying, "Pain is inevitable; suffering is optional."

Applications of these discoveries abound in DBT. I once was asked to consult on an individual who was diagnosed with both borderline and antisocial personality disorders to provide recommendations and to consider whether he was an appropriate candidate for DBT. He was in jail (for stealing several large electronic items from a "big-box" store) and was intolerant of how he was being treated. He promptly became emotionally dysregulated and lashed out at several other inmates and a prison guard. When I saw him, he was in an isolation cell and I was not allowed to be in the same room as he. I interviewed him through a 1-by-10-inch horizontal slot in a solid door, about 3 feet off the ground. All we could see were each other's eyes. Early in the interview I asked him if he had any hopeful or meaningful image of the future, something toward which he could work. His eyes were expressive, softer than I expected, and they moistened as he pleaded with me: "All I want is to get out of this cell. It just makes me worse. I can't stand it! I can't even think about anything. Do you think you could get me back to a regular cell?" I softened as I listened to him. I felt his suffering and I noticed the urge to advocate for him. Did he really have to be in isolation? I imagined how awful it would be to be in isolation.

Alongside my empathic response to his situation, which was stronger than I expected, I also knew that he had contributed to his current status in significant part due to his deeds and his choices. Somehow he had "earned" his place in solitary. I was aware of an urge to rescue him as well as an urge to mistrust him. I was silent as I let myself take in this already-complex reaction. I just sat there, noticing him, observing my responses. I was letting my mind settle, and toward that end I brought my attention entirely to my breathing—one breath in and one breath out— then waited for a "wise mind" response to arrive. It occurred to me that in addition to the reality of being in isolation, and the realities that led to that predicament, and the reality of his discomfort, there was, *in addition*, a great deal of urgency. He wanted out of there. That was foremost on his mind. He was intolerant of his in-the-moment reality.

I said to him, "I certainly get that it is horrible for you to be in solitary. I'm sure it would be for me."

"Yeah, so get me out of here," he said in a somewhat demanding way, as if I had the authority to do so and as if he had the authority to command me. By that time in the interview I felt no pressure to rescue him or to accuse him. It was as it was.

"I don't really have the authority to get you out of here, and I don't really know the story about why you are in solitary. But I wonder if you could just settle in to where you are right now, just let yourself be where you are, and talk to me. If you spend every waking second convinced that you have to get out of there right now, you might suffer even more. If you could accept that you are where you are, for now, truly accept it, maybe you would feel less agitated. Who knows, maybe you would even end up getting out sooner if you were to stop thinking you had to get out." (This last comment, flowing easily from a mindful, accepting stance, is also an example of "entering the paradox," one of the dialectical strategies in DBT.)

I'm pretty sure I saw a cloud of anger cross his eyes, and he looked down at the floor and said, "I suppose you think I should just suck it up?"

"No," I said, "Actually that's not what I mean. I mean that if you just stop thinking you have to get out right away, stop counting the minutes and seconds, maybe you will tolerate it better. And then time will pass, and you'll be out." I thought I saw a flicker of interest come into his eyes.

This patient was attached to an outcome over which he had very little control: immediate transfer out of isolation. His attachment to getting out immediately was causing him additional suffering and increased dysregulation in his emotions and actions, further perpetuating his stay in isolation. If he could accept the reality and instead find a way to just *be in that moment*, maybe he would get out faster.

When I first began speaking with him, I experienced an immediate attachment to rescuing him, getting him out. If I had stayed attached in that way, I too would have suffered more and would have been of little use to him. To help him I had to notice, and let go of, the urge to rescue him. Although this example arose from a unique situation, visiting a patient in prison, the process of getting attached to "shoulds" or wishes happens in every session. Every session presents us with the opportunity to get hooked (attached), to suffer, to notice that we are hooked—that is, to wake up—and to let go of the attachment so that we can find our balance again.

Let's review the steps in this example for the sake of generalizing this process to other types of traps and attachments in therapy. First, I became attached. I "felt his pain," I empathized with his urgent desire to get out of isolation. His attachment became my attachment before I even thought about it. Second, and this is the key to the whole process, *I recognized that I was attached*. This need to rescue is not unusual in doing therapy with individuals who exhibit high levels of emotional dysregulation. The feeling grabs hold of us that we have to *do* something. We get attached to doing something when, in fact, nothing needs to be done. If we recognize our sense of urgency, only then are we positioned to reestablish our freedom and balance, and only then do we stand a chance of helping the patient. Third, actually letting go of the attachment, even when we see that we are attached, is not necessarily so easy. In this case I was helped by the practice of stepping back, going within myself, and observing one entire in-breath and out-breath, with full attention to the breath. We often need a vehicle like this when we are midstream in trying to get unhooked from an attachment. By analogy, if we drive a car with a manual transmission, and we want to shift from one gear to another, we need to push the clutch pedal all the way to the floor in order to shift. Engaging the clutch pedal allows us to disengage from our present gear, allowing us to then shift to the new gear. In therapy we routinely get trapped in one "gear" or another, and we need a "clutch pedal." We may be attached to preventing our patients from engaging in suicide attempts or self-harming episodes, substance use, or dissociative episodes. Or we may be attached to ensuring that our patients show visible progress. Or we may be attached to not becoming a target of their anger. The more we get attached to those things over which we don't have control, the more we get emotionally dysregulated, the more we suffer, and the less effective we become. It's an interesting paradox of DBT: If we get too attached to the outcomes, day by day, in this outcome-oriented treatment, we might become more dysregulated and less effective at accomplishing the outcomes.

To return to the example of the patient who was in isolation: (1) I had quickly become attached, as he was, to getting him out of isolation; (2) I then recognized that I was attached; (3) I managed to shift gears, to "let go" of my attachment with the assistance of one conscious breath; now (4) I could see the patient's dilemma, the suffering he was bringing on himself via his attachment, more clearly, more separately, and then I was in a position to help him cope with reality. Then the paradox occurred to me—that he might get out sooner if he stopped trying to get out—and I could communicate it to him. His puzzlement and ambivalence about my suggestion threw him off balance and opened the door to a fresh start. A quick and dirty protocol for this process might be captured as follows:

1. *Get attached* (immediate, involuntarily, automatic).
2. "*Wake up*" to the recognition of being attached.
3. "*Let go*" of the attachment, possibly with the assistance of a mindfulness vehicle.
4. *See the patient's reality as it is.*
5. *Intervene* strategically to help the patient with his or her attachment and suffering.

Sometimes the step of letting go, #3, is much more difficult than I have conveyed. Therapists might recognize that they are in a "trap," but cannot see their way out. For instance, I was once conducting a DBT family session in which an older adolescent girl with emotional dysregulation and a developmental disability was sitting between her two parents. The parents alternated in "trying to talk some sense into her" about her recent begging on the streets. She grew more and more silent and surly, and I tried everything I could think of to create movement and change in an increasingly deadly dialogue. I was getting nowhere. I was attached to changing this evolving family dynamic, which seemed to be beyond my control, and my sense of helplessness and hopelessness grew as I continued. I couldn't find a way out. I knew enough to know that I was stuck but not enough to know how to move things forward. Whereas in the prior example, I was able to let go of my attachment with one full conscious breath, that proved insufficient in this context. I needed a more substantial vehicle to clear my mind. Having never done so before, I announced a 5-minute break, stating that we were getting nowhere and would need a fresh start. I suggested that each of us take 5 minutes to do whatever it would take to clear our thinking, and then reconvene.

My office was in a mill building next to a large stream. I quickly went down to the stream, and emptying my mind of my feelings of entrapment in the family session, I just watched twigs and leaves float downstream, making their way past logs and big rocks. I entered that moment and let myself notice the details. At least for those few minutes I was able to get out of the stifling loop in which I found myself. I returned to the session, still not knowing what I would do next, but allowing for the suspended transitional state and hoping that my "wise mind" would generate a different intervention. When I sat down, I said to the adolescent that I wanted her to take over the leadership of the session. She looked puzzled and anxious. I assured her that she couldn't do any worse than I was doing. I asked her to trade seats with me, and I took the seat between her parents. She sat in my chair, placed a clipboard and a piece of paper on her lap, and announced, rather definitively, "Things are not going very well in this session; we have to change direction." She was surprisingly assertive, a radical shift from her usual passive posture. We all waited. She continued: "I think we need to talk about how parents talk to a daughter that embarrasses them." We moved into a productive discussion about how much the parents were embarrassed by their daughter's behaviors on the streets of their small town.

Honestly, upon review of my decision to make the patient into the "therapist" and move myself into her place, it is a mystery how that idea came to me. Maybe it was a "wise mind" therapeutic decision that evolved from "emptying out" my anxious mind and just observing the flowing of a stream. Maybe the value of the intervention resulted simply from "breaking set" when things had been so stuck. Perhaps positioning myself as an "observer" between the two parents was key, structurally changing the balance of power in the session so that the patient could "borrow" the power of the therapist's position. I'm not sure. But in my experience the decided shift from "doing" to simply "being" gives rise to all sorts of surprising and unpredictable openings.

INTERBEING

Ordinarily, we consider boundaries to be common and necessary ("Good fences make good neighbors"); we assume that each of us has a "self" that is unique and distinct from others' selves; and that beings, although connected to each other, are mainly separate and unique. But from another perspective—one that emerged from mindfulness meditation practices for millennia that requires a relaxation of conventional perception and thought—reality has no boundaries: *Interbeing* is the rule, and the concept of self is a delusion. We take certain "boundaries" for granted in our lives: the boundaries between life and death; between oneself and others; between the past, present, and future. The closer and more carefully we examine these assumed boundaries, however, the more blurred they become. When we deeply consider the boundary around the beginning of life, it is nearly impossible, and at times controversial, to define that moment. When we examine the boundary between life and death, we are impressed with the uncertainty about where life ends and where death begins.

　　When my father was dying, I sat alone with him, holding his hand, as his breathing became slower and slower, and I knew he was in the process of dying. I felt absolutely present and with him in a profoundly interconnected way. I recognized that he was in me, and that I was in him. His breaths began to be spaced 10, 20, 30 seconds apart. Then they seemed to totally stop . . . or did they? In my experience, he was still alive. When his breath did not return for several minutes, but he looked roughly the same, I still thought of him as being alive, yet somewhere in the process he had died. He was no longer alive, yet in another sense he was as alive within me as he had ever been. Never before had the boundary between life and death struck me as so fragile, so undefined. He was now dead, and yet he was still alive. He was somewhere, I thought: in the room, in the wall, in the atmosphere, maybe still in his body, and definitely in me. It was, to say the least, a mystery.

And when we look just as carefully at the boundary between our-selves and other people, asking exactly where we leave off and they begin, and what part of them is us, and what part of us is them, again we lose the edge, the definition of the boundary. When I teach, I generally feel as if I am having my own thoughts, presenting my ideas with my speech and gestures. It is my "self" speaking, my unique self, and the members of the audience listening, "over there." But when I have an idea, speak my idea, use a gesture, it sometimes dawns on me that all of the ideas, words, and gestures came from others. My grandfather, who was a dairy farmer for most of his adult life, traveled around to other farmers, giving lectures and leading workshops. His father had come from southwestern Sweden; in fact, I teach workshops in southwestern Sweden, perhaps to relatives of mine without my knowing it. My father was a soloist in our church choir when I was a boy, holding the attention of audiences. My oldest brother was a national champion as an orator in high school. My ideas come from the ideas of others. While teaching a workshop or seminar, I am influenced every second by my students in the ideas, words, intona-tions, and gestures that I choose. When you add it all up, literally nothing is uniquely "mine." The concept of *mine* dissolves into the recognition of *interbeing*, of profound interdependency. For Buddhist teacher Thich Nhat Hanh, this leads to an understanding of the term *emptiness* in Bud-dhism: As he explains, "In fact, the flower is made entirely of non-flower elements; it has no independent, individual existence. It 'inter-is' with everything else in the universe" (1995, p. 11). Extending that concept to the self, "Charlie Swenson is made up entirely of non–Charlie Swenson ingredients." *Interbeing* and *emptiness* go hand in hand.

Borrowing further from a metaphor of Thich Nhat Hanh, we can think of each one of us as a wave in the ocean, rolling toward the shore, from birth in the ocean to death on the shore. Each wave has its own shape, size, speed, and other features; has its unique story and form. On the other hand, every distinct wave is made up entirely of water mol-ecules, the same as all other waves. In fact, a given wave is made up of water molecules that were part of a different wave moments before. The waves are historically unique and distinct, *and* they are profoundly inter-connected and interdependent. We are waves, and we are water. Both are true, and we can shift our focus back and forth between the unique waves and the indivisible water. In fact, both "realities" are valid: the conven-tional, historical reality honoring uniqueness and separateness, and the deep truth of the interdependence of all elements all the time, as captured in the term *interbeing*.

It is but a short leap from these ideas to the idea of *non-self*. Without boundaries, without separateness, independence, or uniqueness, each of us is but a temporary, evolving, interdependent rearrangement of matter and energy. Experiencing life from this perspective, we can observe our thoughts without thinking of ourselves as the "thinkers"; feel our emotions without being the one who "has" them; and when we act, we can realize that these actions are in one respect not really our own. It can be unsettling and confusing to realize the extent to which this perspective is true; in another respect, it can be quite freeing and can contribute to deep insight about human nature. It is the wisdom of non-self, of interbeing, of no boundaries, and of *emptiness*.

When I first took note of these ideas in the teachings of meditation masters, they struck me as challenging, a bit weird, arguable, and thought provoking. But what does this set of insights have to do with the practice of DBT? Everything. Whether we choose to notice it or not, the "beginning" and "ending" of therapy are difficult to define; the boundaries between patients and therapists, between patients and their social contexts, between therapists and their DBT teams, and between patient–therapist dyads and society in general are difficult to specify; and the answer to the question "Who did what to whom?" is more complicated than it seems. When the mental health staff of an inpatient unit complains that a certain patient is "manipulating us," we can revisit the same circumstance with concepts of non-self, interbeing, and no boundaries. We realize rather quickly that the staff is supposedly in charge of establishing the conditions of the program, and that the staff, consciously or unconsciously, reinforces some patient behaviors and not others. It would be just as valid (but just as unhelpful) to argue that the staff is "manipulating" the patient to engage in certain actions by reinforcing those actions. Ultimately, the determination of who is manipulating whom becomes less meaningful and useful than adopting a transactional perspective in which both parties are considered responsible and collaboration between them is the preferred direction. In DBT, we are not so interested in who is manipulating whom, but determining how the behaviors of both parties are being reinforced.

In individual therapy, when my patient and I are at odds, not seeing eye to eye, and the session is charged with tension, struggle, or detachment, I can "drop down" from the conventional, self-oriented level of reality where I usually operate, into the place of no boundaries, no-self, interbeing, and emptiness. When I do that, everything shifts; I relax my conventional definition of what is occurring and see the interaction with the patient through a different prism. Where I saw a boundary between two independent, separate beings at odds with each other, similar to separate waves colliding in the ocean, I now see us as two interdependent forms, made of the same ingredients, both changing, both transient, each one defined in part by its relation to the other. There is no boundary, no uniqueness, nothing separating us, we are simply there. We both have our strengths, and they become collective strengths. We both have our flaws, and they become collective flaws. I stop "doing" and instead I am "being." I find it very hard to describe this different state, but it places our relationship, in that moment, on entirely different ground. It is a radical, immediate reconceptualization. I see us not as two people, each with his or her identity, at odds with each other; but instead as two parts of one entity, joined in some kind of unfolding narrative. By no means am I saying that this is "*the* truth." It is "*a* truth," a truth that is less conventional, more systemic, and that gives rise to a different approach. Through the prism of non-self, no boundaries, emptiness, and interbeing, we are all profoundly "in it" together.

One time my two young sons were fighting with each other over the control of the television remote device while I was doing something in the kitchen, very near to them. I was so aggravated by what seemed to me to be the senselessness and the unnecessary battle. My tolerance was growing short. I had the urge to repeat what I had typically done: to stand between them and the television, to raise my voice, possibly to turn off the TV, and give them a lecture about cooperating, caring for each other, or respecting that I might not want to hear their fighting. That is, I had the usual urge to "do something" about the situation, which usually had an unhappy outcome. They were "doing something" to each other, "doing something" to me, and then I would "do something" to them. But on this particular occasion, I dipped into the frame of "being." I simply observed them; observed my own thoughts, feelings, and urges; and let go of my attachment to changing the situation. Then I walked over to where they were sitting, sat between them, and continued to just observe the dance of conflict that was going on. And as I sat there, just noticing but not "doing" anything, the two of them completely stopped fighting. They asked me what I was doing, and I said I was just being there, just noticing what was happening rather than telling them what to do. The impact was immediate: They both seemed puzzled and a little uncomfortable but calmer; they continued to watch television, and the conflict ended. It lost its momentum.

Temporarily letting go of the construct of boundaries and of self during psychotherapy, and dipping into the realm of interbeing in which patient and therapist are deeply interdependent with each other, can expose the therapist, through intuition and contemplation, to another level of data about the patient. In fact, conventional and rational thought might interfere with access. A young man was describing to me the terrible experiences he was having at a new job. He was given only minimal orientation to a rather complex set of tasks for which he would be responsible, and had the impression that he should not ask many questions. Day after day, he felt overwhelmed. Faced with task after task, without the slightest understanding of how to accomplish them and without an avenue to get support, he felt that he was "going under." He thought he was becoming depressed, feeling more and more as if he were stupid and incapable. Mostly, he felt very alone. At a certain point, as he recounted another difficult week on the job, I closed my eyes for a short while, allowing myself to "fill up" with his experience, as if it were my own. The boundary between us became permeable, and I had a deep sense of loneliness and loss. I imagined being him, being stranded without help. I recalled a study I had conducted during medical school, in which I observed toddlers in the hospital without their parents, for days at a time. My thoughts went back to my own history of hospitalizations as a child, being left alone to cope. And suddenly I remembered my patient's history of having lost his mother to cancer at the age of 13. I then spoke: "I find myself thinking about loneliness and isolation, how terrible it can be to have to solve everything alone. And it reminds me that when your mother died, when you were 13, your relatives left you stranded with your little brother, and you had to figure everything out yourself. I wonder if this job situation has any flavor of that?" His eyes filled with tears and he went on to tell me more about the horrors of being stranded when his mother died. I think he felt understood, and when we returned to talking about the job situation, he seemed more resilient. To allow oneself to access the level of experience where boundaries go down and intuition goes up can add to the repertoire of the therapist with difficult-to-treat patients.

There is significant power added to our repertoires as therapists if we can move between two perspectives on the same predicament. From the perspective of the change paradigm, we act upon patients through assessment and change-oriented interventions, and patients act upon us by collaborating or opposing, making a commitment or not, carrying out assignments or not, and so on. This is the "doing" perspective at the core of the change paradigm, and it relies on the conventional understanding of self, other, and boundaries.

From the perspective of the acceptance paradigm, centered around "being" rather than "doing," we see ourselves and our patients as interdependent beings, each one part of the other, boundaries uncertain or dissolved, united in the task of therapy, sharing space, time, energy, matter, ideas, intentions, and so on. In the "doing" perspective, there is a destination or a series of destinations; there is the power of purpose. In the "being" perspective, there is no destination; there is the power of being, or interbeing, in the present moment. Out of the change paradigm perspective flow the problem-solving strategies, the irreverent style of communication, and the insistence on working with patients to solve their life problems. Out of the acceptance paradigm perspective flow validation strategies, a reciprocal style of communication, and the willingness to intervene in patients' environments on their behalf.

Perhaps even more deeply, if you can "get the feel" for it, there is a different experience from the inside out, in the body and in the mind, between these two perspectives, each with its own power (and then there is the power of moving back and forth between the two, which is captured in the discussion of the dialectical paradigm). To experience yourself within your body when "doing" is different than the experience of your body when "being." It might be the difference between leaning forward while pushing for behavioral change, versus relaxing the weight and substance of your body into the moment, into the chair, refraining from pushing. I am trying to convey that there is an experience, beyond the naming and employment of different sets of strategies, which differentiates the practicing of these two different paradigms. The internally felt experiences of "doing" versus "being" can ground you in the appropriate paradigm and set the stage for deep work on change or acceptance. The power and creativity of doing DBT effectively is to weave these two perspectives together in the service of helping your patients to build a life worth living.

IMPERMANENCE

One of the greatest challenges in treating individuals with chronic, severe emotional dysregulation arises when emotional arousal is at its most intense. The patient finds such emotions nearly intolerable and may react to them as if she is phobic of her own emotions. She has learned that a rapid escape into behaviors such as self-injury, violence, or substance abuse is an effective antidote, and she becomes trapped in a life punctuated with problematic behaviors. At the same time, by escaping quickly, again and again, in the face of emotional arousal, she acquires the belief that negative emotions are terrible, are static, and are permanent. Her rapid escapes prevent opportunities to learn otherwise.

On our inpatient unit was an 18-year-old biracial woman who was adopted by an older-than-usual Caucasian couple when she was 3 years old. Her own temperament, from the beginning, was difficult. She was moody, highly sensitive, and emotionally reactive. While her parents were devoted, kind, and generous with her, their rather laid-back, calm, low-affect intellectual styles were highly contrasting with her lively and emotional style. It is an example of the fact that even a kind and devoted environment can be invalidating for a child due to a mismatch in temperaments. By the time she was a teenager she had begun to cut herself on a regular basis as a way to deal with intense painful emotions. Without cutting, she felt that she had no way out. In addition, she came to believe that these emotions would last forever if she didn't interrupt them.

Her DBT skills group had just begun a new module, the Emotion Regulation Training module. In the first session, the teachers presented a number of basic features of emotions. One of them was that emotional responses are in fact rather brief in duration if one does not continue to retrigger them with emotional thoughts and actions. As a practice assignment, patients in the group were invited to study "the life and death of an emotion" next time an intense emotion arose.

During the community meeting on the following day, she asked me if she could be on the agenda. When I called on her, she told everyone that "a miracle happened last night." She explained that during a conversation with her mother on the telephone she had felt hurt and intense anger. She hung up on her mother and was riddled with urges to harm herself. Then she remembered the assignment from her skills group. She decided to just observe her emotions for a while. She sat for a few minutes, walked around the unit, then sat again, all the while noticing her emotions. Not only did she find that her hurt and angry feelings waxed and waned, and changed in quality over the next 20 minutes, she also found that they faded away after that amount of time, at which point she hung out with some of her peers. Her description in the meeting was exciting, as if she was reporting a newly discovered human phenomenon—which is exactly what it was for her.

Yes, emotions are impermanent, if only we let ourselves realize it. So are thoughts, actions, and the situations in which we find ourselves. The recognition that impermanence is the nature of reality can be transformative. This can be particularly helpful for therapists who feel as if they are facing, in session after session, the same unchanging patient. Frustration grows and hopelessness sets in, in part because of the growing conviction that nothing is changing, when in fact that cannot possibly be true. As therapists, we are wise to learn from our young patient's revolutionary discovery.

As with the other insights discussed in this chapter, the recognition of the impermanence of reality also informs us as therapists deeply, subtly, and constantly. It can alleviate our distress, reduce our suffering, and keep us on track in DBT if we can simply accept that things are *always* in flux. What seems unchangeable or impenetrable is actually changing.

Every moment is fresh, in fact, despite the experience of both parties that it is old, unchanging, and stagnant. In Buddhism, the term *beginner's mind* refers to the experience that the encounter with each moment is fresh and new. Like a persistent wave in the ocean, every persistent problem represents a formation or sequence, which no matter how unyielding it may seem, is made up of constantly changing ingredients, in a constantly changing context. The wave may look the same, but it consists of another, and another, and then another collection of water molecules in constantly changing orientations. Understanding this basic reality, we can say with conviction, "This too shall pass." We become more patient, more resilient, more alert to missing variables, and we learn that the "boiling point" of change could come at any moment if we keep up the heat.

Another value of recognizing impermanence as a permanent phenomenon is the recognition that if things are going well today, they probably will change for the worse tomorrow, somehow. What goes up comes down, what comes down goes up, and if we can keep this reciprocal process in mind, we will be less "thrown" by the slings and arrows of misfortune. The patient says, "But if I make things better, they will just get worse anyway, and it will be devastating." Thinking about this aspect of impermanence, the patient then avoids trying to make things better. The therapist responds: "You are right. If things get better, they will probably, in some fashion, become worse, though never the same as before. It's just a law of the universe, and if we can accept it, we can experience the gains and losses on the way to a life worth living to be speed bumps rather than brick walls."

"THE WORLD IS PERFECT AS IT IS."

This is another one of those insights that can sound rather simplistic, alien, and impossible. How could the world be perfect, when in fact there is so much suffering, wrongdoing, conflict, and misunderstanding? How can we say that everything had to be as it is, that everything should be the way it is, that everything is perfect just as it is? How can a suicide attempt, a vicious assault, or a treatment failure be "perfect"? The statement can be confusing, invalid on the face of it, until we understand that the word *perfect* is not being used in a conventional way. "The world is *perfect* as it is" does not mean that things are OK, that the world is fair and just, the environment is compassionate and forgiving. It does not mean that we approve of the world as it is, or agree with it. It simply means that the world is exactly as it is, exactly as it should be, given everything that came before. It simply means that everything is caused by what came before. Someone attempts suicide because, historically, leading into the present moment, all causes and conditions are in place to support the act of suicide. How could this moment be anything other than what it is, given the collective impact of all previous moments? This perspective is no different from the way a behaviorist thinks when assessing the controlling variables of a given behavior—that is, when assessing the causes and conditions that bestow a certain function on a behavior and maintain it.

Karma is a principle arising from Buddhism that rests upon much of the same thinking. It means that everything now was caused by prior deeds. Taking it one step into the future then means that we build our future deed by deed, by today's choices, thoughts, words, and actions. Every seed planted today has consequences tomorrow. Looking backward at how the current state came into being has to be balanced by looking at this very next moment, and all moments beyond it, in which current choices and deeds can bring about a different outcome. Finding this balance can help the DBT therapist freshly and hopefully push forward in a treatment of chronic and frustrating problems. Old deeds have brought about current outcomes; new deeds will determine new future outcomes. Things change; we plant seeds now so that new things will grow. Time may not "heal all wounds," but it definitely results in change. For the therapist working with the difficult-to-treat patient, it can be rather comforting to understand that if she can persist at the practice of DBT through thick and thin, applying its multitude of guidelines and strategies, things will indeed change. In DBT, the therapist has things to do that may help her and the patient to outlast the pathology, which is transforming constantly.

This principle that the world is perfect as it is finds its way into DBT's treatment package in several "locations." One of DBT's clinical assumptions is that, regardless of what may seem to be the case, patients are doing the best they can. Another assumption is that regardless of how patients appear to be undermining their own improvement, we assume that they want to improve. Patients may seem to be willfully and defiantly ruining their lives, ignoring their therapists, forgetting the skills, and doing the same self-destructive thing over and over again. How can they be doing the best they can? How can it be true that they want to improve? That is exactly the question at that moment for DBT. If you allow yourself to embrace the insight that "the world is perfect as it is," it will seem simple to recognize the truth of the current dysfunctional behavioral patterns; the truth that everything had to be as it is, given how it has been up to this moment; the truth that patients are doing the best they can; and the truth that they would like to improve. Then, in that moment, experiencing each patient with compassion and without judgment, the therapist can work with the patient to build a better life from that time forward.

The concept of karma finds its way into a third assumption about patients in DBT: Patients have to try harder, do better, and be more motivated to change. Even though everything is as it has to be, given everything that was, the future is not determined. Every behavior now has consequences; actions *matter*. With each action, each choice, each intervention, we are laying down stones for a path that will lead to the conditions of the future, hopefully to a life worth living. Recognizing that the "world is perfect as it is" and that we are, at every moment, laying the groundwork for the future can help the therapist to continue to "do DBT" even in the face of no immediate signs of progress.

CONCLUDING COMMENTS

I have articulated the principles of the acceptance paradigm and the practices that flow from those principles, as if they exist alongside, and in parallel with, the principles of the other two paradigms. But in practice, ideally, we are influenced by the acceptance principles all the time. As therapists, we establish and maintain a context of acceptance, within which we engage each patient in behavioral change leading toward a life worth living. We attempt to root our awareness and attention of our patients in the *present moment*, returning there again and again, as needed. We notice the ways in which patients' *attachments* (to certain perceptions, beliefs, assumptions, moods, sensations, predictions, and so on) obscure their recognition of reality "as it is," and then repeatedly attempt to help them let go of the attachments. We are informed by the recognition of the relentless *impermanence* of reality, the uniqueness of each moment, and the inevitability of change. Relaxing our investment in seeing conventional boundaries between ourselves and our patients, between any one person and all others, indeed between any phenomenon and all phenomena, we instead see the deep *interrelatedness* of all, the way in which all are one, and how in that respect we and our patients operate as one. Our ordinary convictions of the separateness of self and the uniqueness of identity gives way to a recognition that each of us is made up of all others, of all else. And in spite of the natural tendency to impose judgments on ourselves and others, we yield to the understanding that, deeply, everything emerges in response to causes and conditions of past and present, everything is as it should be, everything is *"perfect as it is."*

Influenced by these principles of acceptance, we intervene with validation strategies and a reciprocal communication style that includes warmth, genuineness, responsiveness, and self-disclosure. Ideally, we create and maintain an atmosphere in which safety, trust, and attachment emerge, providing corrective emotional experiences for all our patients.

CHAPTER 4

The Change Paradigm

Within the context of acceptance, the therapist engages the patient in the central task of the treatment: to make the behavioral changes necessary to build a life worth living. The change paradigm encompasses the theories, models, principles, protocols, strategies, and skills for bringing about behavioral change. These are incorporated from cognitive-behavioral theory and practice, and are adapted to the context of treating individuals with chronic and severe emotional dysregulation. Linehan (1993a) has organized the implementation of the change paradigm into a sequential problem-solving protocol, which is used again and again in sessions. Every DBT therapist learns this protocol. After the collaborative determination of a prioritized list of treatment targets, and the strengthening of the patient's commitment to the treatment plan, the therapist focuses the session on the highest-priority target, beginning with life-threatening behaviors.

1. The sequence then begins with a *behavioral chain analysis*, the technique used to identify the controlling variables of the target behavior.
2. Having applied one, then more, behavioral chain analyses to a given target behavior, the therapist and patient scan for relevant patterns to be found among the links in the chain. Highlighting those patterns, the therapist generates hypotheses to explain the patterns, shares them with the patient, and between them they arrive at the hypotheses that make the most sense. This process is known as *insight*.

3. Armed with insight, the therapist moves on to the next step, *solution analysis*, which involves generating and then considering a range of possible solutions that will result in the desired behavioral changes. Possible solutions are shared with the patient, and the dyad selects one or more of the solutions to implement.

4. The solutions involve variations and combinations of four categories of *change procedures*, each of which comes from a particular behavioral model or theory of change.

    a. For skills deficits, the therapist draws from skills training models and principles and applies *skills training procedures* in the session.

    b. For problematic cognitions, the therapist draws from cognitive mediation models and principles and applies *cognitive modification procedures*.

    c. For problematic contingencies, wherein maladaptive behaviors are reinforced and adaptive behaviors are not, the therapist looks to operant conditioning theory and principles and applies *contingency procedures*.

    d. Finally, for those sequences of links in the chain where cues elicit automatic and disruptive emotions based on prior conditioning, the therapist looks to classical conditioning theory and principles and applies *stimulus control and exposure procedures*.

5. Throughout the attention to behavioral change, the therapist uses *didactic interventions* to educate the patient, *orienting strategies* to clarify the respective roles of patient and therapist regarding a procedure, and *commitment strategies* to strengthen the patient's commitment to the tasks involved.

This protocol is helpful in organizing the change-oriented work of every session, and it was especially helpful to me as a newcomer to DBT and CBT, as it provided a comprehensive list of topics for my learning process. But in the heat of the moment, in sessions with difficult-to-treat patients, one cannot always count on the application of a step-by-step sequential approach to problem solving. The therapist may begin by moving through the sequence, only to be detoured into the management of dysfunctional and disruptive in-session behaviors. Or she may embark upon problem solving of a particular target behavior, then suddenly, midsession, hear about another, higher-priority target behavior. Or she may have arrived at a solution to implement, but then find that the patient is unwilling to collaborate. In other words, the often difficult and rapidly shifting clinical presentation within sessions calls for flexibility and fluidity in applying the various problem-solving activities. Consequently, the therapist needs to have overlearned the strategies so that they can be implemented at a moment's notice. Just as knowing the underlying principles of the acceptance paradigm help the therapist to create a validating environment and to pivot into validation as needed, knowing the underlying principles or processes of the change paradigm allows the therapist to push for change in circumstances that are unpredictable and changing.

While it is difficult to name a few underlying change-based principles, since problem solving involves such a wide range of strategies and stems from a number of substantial theories, I have found it possible to identify seven core processes that have helped me to apply the entire repertoire of problem-solving strategies with flexibility. The first three are foundational change-oriented tasks or processes at work in nearly every DBT session: (1) targeting and monitoring; (2) getting a commitment; and (3) behavioral chain analysis and case conceptualization. The other four are tasks or processes that flow from four underlying theories of behavioral change that are integrated into DBT: (4) skills deficit theory; (5) classical conditioning theory; (6) operant conditioning theory; and (7) cognitive mediation theory. These final four, based as they are on four rich theories of change, bring with them four respective sets of principles, four different ways of thinking, four different styles of therapeutic interaction, and four different sets of techniques.

Each of the seven core change processes in DBT gives shape to the change-oriented work, providing a set of interventions as well as a pervasive preoccupation throughout the work. For instance, although we may not be applying *targeting* strategies at a given moment, the agenda of the entire session is oriented toward a designated target, and drifting from the target can interfere with the whole enterprise. Or, to take another example, we may not be engaged in the strategy of *cognitive restructuring* at a given moment, but we are aware of the lurking presence of problematic cognitions throughout the chain and are ready, at any moment, to address them in one way or another. Keeping all seven in mind enhances our flexibility in staying connected to patients, oriented to the targets, and able to access problem-solving strategies promptly when indicated. Four of the seven (targeting and monitoring, commitment, behavioral chain analysis and case conceptualization, and skills training) are addressed in detail in separate chapters in this book and are therefore covered briefly in this chapter. The other three are discussed in more detail in this chapter after we discuss what it means to "be behavioral" in DBT.

"BEING BEHAVIORAL" IN DBT

Before dealing with each pervasive change-oriented perspective, let's first consider what it means, more broadly, to "be behavioral" in DBT, parallel to "being mindful" and "being dialectical." To describe what it is to *be behavioral* is challenging, much like describing what it is like to ride a bicycle, have a dream, or fall in love. You know it when you see it, when you feel it, and when you do it, but it's hard to really describe it without sounding trite or clumsy.

I initially encountered it during my first experience (of two) as a patient in a behavioral therapy. Having come to behavioral treatment from psychoanalytic treatment, it was a culture shock, to say the least. It was 1987. I was on the faculty of Cornell Medical School, directing a long-term inpatient program for borderline personality organization based on psychoanalytic object relations theory. My training to that point was in psychoanalytic psychotherapy. I was several years into psychoanalytic treatment for myself, which began as part of my analytic training. Knowing that I would be considered for promotion to associate professor on the medical school faculty in about 1 year, I knew that I needed to publish several more articles in refereed journals. Although I had drafts, outlines, reams of notes, and lots of ideas, they were languishing in my personal files and in my head. In my psychoanalysis, I had been exploring the fantasies, conflicts, and meanings associated with publishing (and not publishing), and although I was grateful for deepening my self-understanding, I was still not getting articles into journals.

When I explained the situation to a colleague at a social occasion, he recommended that I consult with a CBT therapist in Manhattan who had helped other faculty members with "writing blocks." I was reluctant. I couldn't imagine adding another treatment to my life, and my view at the time was that a behavioral approach was a circumscribed, superficial application of rat psychology. Still, I respected that colleague's opinion, I was curious, and I was motivated to try anything to get a jump-start. Having been exposed to DBT in the prior months, my curiosity about behaviorism was piqued. I made an appointment.

From the first moment of my meeting with Steve, the culture shock was dramatic. Accustomed to the attentive but objective stance of each of the two psychoanalysts I had seen, who would listen to me as I began to free associate, Steve was down-to-earth, matter-of-fact, direct, and welcoming. It was disarming that he asked me to address him by his first name; I wondered how competent he could be. His style was more akin to that of a car mechanic than of someone who understood people in depth. He sat opposite me with a clipboard and blank paper on his lap. "What can I help you with?" he asked. I explained that I wanted to get promoted; that I needed to publish some articles; that I had a lot of ideas, drafts, and outlines; but otherwise was making no progress. "How many articles do you need to get published?" I guessed: "It seems like I would be safe if I got six articles accepted in decent journals." He wanted a more specific goal: "By next week, find out exactly what you need." He asked for the names of the journals I was considering. Having not yet thought about that, I named a few likely candidates. He asked what the deadline was, and I suggested that I should probably submit them within 6 months and have them accepted within 1 year. He asked for specifics— goals, timelines, names of journals—and I answered with rough guesses. I came in with approximately stated intentions and hard-won insights; he narrowed in on details, on exactly what I needed to accomplish. For any cognitive-behavioral therapist, what he did was quite ordinary; for me it provided an "aha" moment regarding a problem-solving therapy. Still, it worried me. He might be too specific, too practical, too optimistic, and too naïve to do battle with the hidden forces that had blocked my progress up to that point.

I volunteered that I had explored underlying obstacles in my psychoanalytic treatment, that perhaps he would find them useful in working with me. His answer was characteristically quick and to the point, not exactly dismissive but definitely not interested. "Not really. It's great that you've learned so much about yourself, but why don't we just have you write the articles? If we run into trouble, maybe some of those insights will come in handy." Another "aha" moment: Action first, insight would follow. Still, it was troubling. I already knew how to write, and I had things to write about. Why did I need a psychologist, junior to me in age and experience, to teach me how to write? Honestly, I felt a bit like an idiot. I held my tongue, tried to soothe my wounded self, and just went with the program.

He asked me for titles and outlines for the six articles. I had ideas, I said, but he wanted titles and outlines to get me started on the concrete process of writing. My first homework assignment was to come up with six titles, to create a two-page outline for the first article, and bring them to him next week. It was so practical! I was divided within myself, one part doubt and mistrust, the other part relieved and hopeful. As I left his office after our first meeting, I asked myself, "If this is what it takes, why do I need him?" During the week I kept having the urge to cancel our next appointment and just write the articles. This was not psychotherapy as I had learned it; this was more like having a coach in golf or a teacher for playing the piano. My psychoanalysis was aimed at deepening my understanding of myself; my behavior therapy was aimed at solving an identifiable problem. For several years I compared and contrasted the approaches. In fact, one of the six articles I wrote was "Kernberg and Linehan: Two Approaches to the Borderline Patient" (Swenson, 1989).

In one session I had learned firsthand about the style and stance of pushing for change in psychotherapy. Steve was straightforward, direct, and pragmatic; his style was matter-of-fact, friendly, and optimistic. There was no mystery, no sense of exploring the depths. He asked for my goal, made it more specific, and he took it as our treatment goal. We got moving so quickly, I felt we had already embarked on a journey together. As simple as the message was, it was a surprise to me: *In order to change behavior, you have to change behavior.* I already had homework. Progress was to occur *between* sessions; sessions were to prepare for the work of the week. In contrast to my other therapists, Steve seemed impatient to get moving; over time he demonstrated patience and persistence.

I arrived at Session 2 with six titles and an outline. Steve was unabashedly pleased. I felt somewhat embarrassed, as if I were a child, but also appreciative of the overt praise. He read the outline of the first article, entitled "Projective Identification in the Inpatient Treatment of Borderline Patients." Though he was not familiar with the topic, Steve quickly (and correctly) assessed that the scope of the article was huge. "What you have here is the outline for *two* articles, at least. What are you trying to do, change the course of psychiatry or publish articles?" He gave me another homework assignment: to look at 10 decent articles in psychiatric journals and assess the scope of the contribution of each. He challenged my assumption that I had to write transformative articles, an assumption that blocked my completion of articles. He worried me. As much as I recognized the practical wisdom of his point, I was afraid that in working with him I would produce trivial articles—which I told him. He suggested I look at the 10 articles and get clear about my goals, and he reminded me that it was my choice what to write. He was pushy, but still it seemed like he respected me and that I was ultimately in charge. In fact, I did look at 10 articles, found them to be modest in their contributions, and it helped me to scale back my ambitions.

Having made progress in defining what I would write, we moved on to how I would write, what the structure would be. I explained that I did my best writing when I have 5 or 6 free hours, in which I could generate ideas, create momentum, search through other literature, and write. He challenged me again, on three counts: First, it was unrealistic to expect that I could build 5 or 6 hours into my regular schedule; second, it was a burdensome and "costly" way to write; and third, it was not a good way to create day-by-day momentum. He suggested that I write every day, 7 days a week, for 6 months, using smaller blocks of time that were scheduled at the same time every day. Furthermore, he suggested that I write the first draft of each article "straight out of my head," without the distracting and time-consuming practice of consulting other literature. As he put it, "The articles are in your head—just write them!"

He encouraged me to look ahead at the coming 6 months and cancel all "unnecessary" commitments, and to be ruthless in doing so. He wanted me to get the support of my wife and my colleagues at work, so that everyone understood that my daily writing time was to be protected and uninterrupted. I regretted that I had already made a commitment to present at a symposium 3 months hence, and that I would need time to prepare. Steve urged me to cancel. It went against my reflexes. He challenged my sense of indispensability: "People cancel out of things like that all the time." I was willing, but reluctant, afraid of disappointing. He handed me the phone: "Why don't you just take care of it right now?" I made the call, explained that unanticipated commitments had come up that required me to cancel. They were disappointed, but they seemed to understand and accept my withdrawal. After surviving the guilty feelings, I felt liberated, and it added to a sense of momentum.

I set up the "Swenson plan," as we called it. I would write every day, 7 days a week, even during vacation, for 6 months, from 8:00 to 9:30 A.M. I delegated some of my work to others. I elicited my secretary's support in insulating me from interruptions short of emergencies. I asked my wife's support in continuing the writing during a vacation we had planned. I decided not to open any mail or e-mail during those 90 minutes, or to even look at incoming messages. I confessed that 90 minutes seemed too short, but Steve suggested that if I followed this plan, I would be "writing all the time" in the back of my mind, and the 90 minutes would be enough to put it into writing. He correctly anticipated that sometimes I would want to extend the 90 minutes, if I were "on a roll." For reasons that I did not understand at first, he was opposed to any extensions. In fact, he asked me to call him if I felt strongly like continuing past 9:30 and to get his input before going ahead.

About 2 weeks later it happened, and I called him. "Steve, I'm having a lot of good ideas, and I want to keep writing." Steve got back to me shortly after I called. "Charlie, it's so great that you called. Absolutely *do not* continue to write. Anything worth preserving will stay in your mind and will return tomorrow, probably better than before." I accepted his suggestion on faith, and soon the value became clear to me. The structuring of my writing periods was so clear and so confined to the 90 minutes per morning, that I no longer felt that I "needed" to write later in the day. I wasn't plagued with the ever-present feeling that I should be writing. I experienced a sense of "flow" as I wrote, and a sense of freedom later during the day. Once the Swenson plan was in place, those 6 months were among the most productive and enjoyable of my career. *Writing* was no longer paired in my mind with *burden*. I finished about one article per month, submitted six in 6 months, and within 1 year of starting, five had been accepted. This was more than enough to get me promoted.

Not only was I surprised and pleased, I had also had my first lessons in the essentials of a behavioral approach. We began by determining my goal for treatment. We broke it down into specific objectives. We settled on a method. We created the structure in which the method could take place. We met weekly, whereupon we monitored progress, agreed on direction, and took up particular difficulties. Steve was direct in his style, bold in his expectations, and optimistic in tone. He challenged some writing-interfering assumptions, pushed me to take challenging steps that I would usually avoid, and routinely reinforced me when I was "on task." Still, he managed to convey respect for me, and I felt like we were a team on a mission. In practicing DBT, I have reflected on these lessons a thousand times.

I remember the first time I brought this kind of direct approach into a DBT treatment. I was meeting with a woman who was about to be discharged from a 3-year stay in a state hospital. Her chronic behavioral patterns were severe, including periodic high-lethality suicide attempts and chaotic episodes of binge drinking. She drank alcohol every day when she was not hospitalized, and sometimes managed to sneak it into the hospital. After we discussed her goals, I asked her for a commitment to the treatment in general terms, which she made readily. Soon I asked her to agree to not kill herself for the coming year. She surprised both of us by agreeing.

Then I asked her to refrain from alcohol or any other substances, even once, in the coming year, to go "cold turkey." Since she wanted to drink every day, this was almost unimaginable. I persisted in asking her, calmly and definitively, as Steve had done with me, to make the commitment. I told her that it would lay the groundwork for us to succeed in changing her life. She was dumbfounded and upset. She pushed back, argued, and asked me to backtrack on my request. While acknowledging the magnitude of the request, and sympathizing with her fear, I asked her to think about it. We finished the meeting with no agreement, but without an outright rejection either. I learned from her doctor at the state hospital that when she returned there from our meeting, all she could talk about was the "astonishing" request that I had made. It filled her with fear and with hope, and she soon agreed to it. Her treatment was long, challenging, and ultimately successful; looking back, it strikes me that the tone was set during that first request.

TARGETING AND MONITORING

DBT is, first and foremost, a therapy driven by the pursuit of outcomes—goals that are subdivided into specific behavioral targets to be accomplished sequentially. At the beginning of treatment, therapist and patient collaboratively reframe the presenting problem behaviors as specific behavioral targets, understood as obstacles to the achievement of the patient's goals. The targets then determine the agenda of the treatment as a whole and the agenda of each session. Progress on the targets is monitored every day by the patient with diary cards (self-monitoring forms to be completed each day), and every week by the therapist with the review of those diary cards. Therapist and patient monitor the discrepancy between targeted outcomes and current functioning, always attempting to close the gap. In this respect, targeting is not just an activity that takes place at the beginning of treatment or at the beginning of each session; it is a constant preoccupation. At any moment, if a DBT therapist engaged in a session were to be interrupted and asked the question, "What is the current target in your session?" he should have an answer. If he loses sight of his target, he is more likely to drift, influenced by other "drivers" such as the alleviation of momentary emotional distress. In sum, the practices of defining the targets, attending to them throughout treatment, and monitoring progress with regard to them are a central organizing concern in the practice of DBT. We return to this topic in two upcoming chapters: Chapter 7, on targeting, and Chapter 8, on dialectical dilemmas and secondary targets.

COMMITMENT

In the narrow sense, commitment in DBT is a process for which we utilize a set of seven defined strategies. We get a commitment to the highest-priority targets (e.g., decrease self-injurious behaviors), to the modes of treatment (e.g., attending group skills training), and to certain procedures (e.g., using exposure procedures). But as discussed with respect to targeting and monitoring, the process of getting and maintaining commitment to treatment is a preoccupation throughout therapy. The strength of the patient's commitment naturally rises and falls, yet it is always a critical variable for success, and if we fail to track its rising and falling, we are at risk of assuming that commitment is present when it has faded away. When treatment slows down or grinds to an apparent halt, which is not infrequent in treating difficult-to-treat individuals, it is not always due to diminishing commitment. But it happens sufficiently often so that we, as

DBT therapists, must have it in mind, inquire about it, and treat it with commitment strategies throughout the process of treatment. We consider the role of commitment in DBT in Chapter 10.

ASSESSMENT (BEHAVIORAL CHAIN ANALYSIS) AND CASE CONCEPTUALIZATION

In Chapters 9, on case conceptualization, and 11, on behavioral chain analysis, we consider the principles of these two practices in much greater detail, but as they are also constant and broadly applied drivers of DBT practice, I briefly discuss them here. Once we are treating a specified behavioral target, we assess the controlling variables of that target through behavioral chain analysis, and through that assessment we arrive at a case conceptualization that drives our treatment planning and implementation. Session by session, as we implement the treatment plan, we generate and encounter new data that then lead to revisions, implicitly and explicitly, in our case conceptualization. The entirely interdependent processes of behavioral chain analysis and case conceptualization become as central and constant to the work as are the interdependent processes of targeting and monitoring and the consideration of the patient's commitment. DBT therapists not only use chain analysis as a strategy for assessment and treatment; we think of our patients in terms of behavioral chains, and we envision treatment as a way of reshaping the patients' behavioral chains from dysfunctional to functional. Assessment and case conceptualization in DBT are both organized on the template provided by a behavioral chain, and problem solving during sessions is explicitly aimed at making revisions in the behavioral chain.

To proceed in therapy without an evolving case conceptualization, especially when treating an individual with chronic and severe emotion dysregulation, would be like driving to a destination in unfamiliar territory without a map. It leads to therapeutic drift and fumbling, akin to the drift mentioned above if doing therapy without specified targets and monitoring. Although instincts and intuitions are crucial to the practice of DBT, these treatments are too difficult and unpredictable to proceed without a map, or without revising that map in response to emerging data.

CLASSICAL CONDITIONING AND EXPOSURE PROCEDURES

Embedded within the larger "story" that is found in a detailed behavioral chain are a number of smaller stories in parallel with one another. Four of these smaller "stories" are manifestations of the four behavioral models. And each of these four models gives rise to a set of behavioral change procedures that are used by the therapist to problem-solve, and therefore are also considered "theories of change." The alert and well-informed therapist will recognize the presence of these stories in the chain while doing behavioral chain analysis, and as a result will scan for the presence of certain controlling variables of the targeted behavior, and will intervene to modify those stories. We begin with the story that is a manifestation of classical conditioning, also known as *respondent conditioning*.

It is a helpful oversimplification to say that there are three essential terms, or elements, of the classical conditioning story. We can organize our thinking around these three terms for purposes of assessment and intervention. The three terms are, respectively and sequentially, the *cue*, the *emotion*, and the *escape*. The *cue* elicits the emotion; the *emotion* is uncomfortable, possibly unbearable; and the individual *escapes* from the emotion into some other behavior. The escape is often the presenting problem, such as cutting or substance use. Let's consider the three terms in more detail.

The Cue

The *cue* is a particular stimulus in the present moment. Of clinical interest is that the cue has a special emotional salience for the patient, and it has the power to automatically elicit a powerful and often painful emotional response. Why does this cue in present functioning, which might be relatively benign objectively, have the power to set off such a strong emotional response? The cue of current functioning is paired in the patient's memory with an incident, or incidents, from the past that were not so benign. So, the cue of the present moment is paired with the cue of the earlier incident, now stored in memory, and therefore the response of the present moment is joined by the powerful response from the past incident. The problem, if we see it that way, is the pairing between the cue of the present, known as the *conditioned stimulus*, and the cue of the past moment, now stored in memory, known as the *unconditioned stimulus*.

The rationale for exposure procedures is that the therapist presents the cue of the present moment to the patient, again and again, in circumstances in which the outcome is relatively benign. After a number of trials, the cue of the present moment is further and further separated from the cue of the past, and the response becomes more realistic and benign. For example, the individual with PTSD, who has stored the traumatic incident(s) in memory, encounters a present-day cue that is associated in some way with the cue from the traumatic incident. The present-day cue automatically sets off a powerful emotional response that is more appropriate to the earlier traumatic incident. In using an exposure procedure, the therapist arranges for the patient to voluntarily encounter a present-day cue that sets off the traumatic response in memory, again and again, until the present-day cue loses its power to elicit the traumatic response. Essentially, exposure procedures create conditionings for *unpairing* the present-day cue from the potent cue from the past.

The Emotion

The *emotion* is the response triggered by the cue. In the case of individuals with high emotional sensitivity and reactivity, and with severe emotion dysregulation, this step in the behavioral chain can be a sudden and painful one, involving panic, terror, shame, anger, or other primary emotion, leading to dysfunctional efforts to cope with it. The fact that the powerful emotional response was triggered by what appears to be a relatively benign cue can be confusing to the patient and to those around her, sometimes confusing to the therapist, and can result in judgmental and pejorative responses to the emotionally triggered individual. The patient's repeated experience of the cue and the painful emotion may so effectively and rapidly pave the way to the escape that the emotion seems almost invisible. In other words, once this sequence is established and proves effective for avoiding emotional pain, the cue seems to elicit an escape behavior without an emotion in between. Then the therapist may need to imagine the nature of the emotion from which the patient escaped, and assess for it.

The Escape

The *escape* is the behavior in which the individual engages as a way to modify or eliminate the painful emotion. Escape can come in the form of action (e.g., self-cutting), cognition (e.g., dissociative episodes), and/ or emotion (e.g., moving from a primary emotion, such as fear or shame, to a secondary emotion, such as anger). Because the nature of the cue may be objectively benign, perhaps not even noticeable; and the intense emotional response can be so evanescent, often hidden further by suppression; the whole sequence may become noticeable only because of the escape. If it happens in a therapy session, for instance, the therapist may notice that the patient has suddenly become more withdrawn, has undergone a shift in mood, has become very angry, or threatens self-harm. The therapist who is always on the lookout for the "classical conditioning story" may then wonder whether she is encountering an escape, and may try to reconstruct the events that led up to it. She does a behavioral chain analysis of the events of the session, searching for the cue and the emotional response. Schematically, the classical conditioning story, woven into the chain, looks like this:

→ *Cue* of the present moment (which automatically and instantaneously elicits a cue in memory from past traumatic incident)

→ *Emotion* (heavily influenced by emotional response to past incident, as stored in memory)

→ *Escape* response (often a dysfunctional behavior that is one of the targets of treatment)

The alert DBT therapist is informed by this theory and is always scanning for its manifestation, searching for the cues, watching for and inquiring about unbearable emotional responses, trying to reduce or block the escapes. Our entire understanding of what we are doing in DBT can be built around the classical conditioning model, in which case the process of change can be conceptualized as centering around the procedure of exposure. One might say we are always trying (1) to block escape behaviors, which requires good cooperation, commitment, orientation, and distress tolerance skills; (2) to enhance exposure to the unbearable emotions, which requires mindfulness and emotion regulation skills that help to recognize emotions and then act opposite the urge to escape; and (3) to identify and "treat" the cues, which often include the use of interpersonal effectiveness skills and stimulus control procedures. As we will see, the other theories of change also lead to ideas about how to organize our thinking about the treatment as a whole, and the art and science of the change paradigm involves knowing all of them and integrating them into one's approach.

Now, having spelled out the three-term "anatomy" of the classical conditioning story, we can identify practical principles for the handling of each of the three terms.

Principles of Classical Conditioning in DBT

FIRST, REGARDING THE CUE

The therapist . . .

1. Determines the actual cue that triggered the patient's emotional response, the more specifically the better.

2. Ascertains that the cue used in the ensuing exposure procedure is as good a match as possible to the actual cue that usually triggers the intense response.

3. Holds the cue in place with sufficient duration and intensity so that emotional exposure can occur and new learning can take place.

4. Makes sure that the cue is not "removed" in response to the patient's escalated emotional response (a practice that reinforces the escape behavior as well as the self-construct of "fragility" in the patient).

SECOND, REGARDING THE EMOTION

The therapist . . .

1. Assesses exactly what emotion (or emotions) was set off by the cue, because it is crucial for success in exposure procedures that the problematic emotion be fully activated.

2. Distinguishes between the *primary emotion* that was set off by the cue, and the *secondary emotion* that can be set off by the reaction to the primary emotion, and thereby serve as an escape from the primary emotion.

3. Ensures sufficient duration of emotional activation so that new learning can take place (usually known as the process of *habituation*).

4. Ensures that the exposure procedure, to the degree possible, leads to a safe outcome that is discrepant from the patient's catastrophic expectation (the term for this is a *nonreinforced exposure*).

THIRD, REGARDING THE ESCAPE

The therapist . . .

1. Identifies the ways in which the patient escapes from the emotional response (e.g., escape into action, thought, or secondary emotions).

2. Works to minimize the patient's reliance on *safety signals* as a way to reduce the emotional response.

3. Elicits the patient's cooperation in *blocking* the escape; having made sure that . . .

4. The whole procedure, including the blocking of escape and the elimination of safety signals, is based in a respectful collaboration, with an agreement that the patient maintains a sense of control over the continuation of the procedure.

As mentioned, we may first be aware of the activation of the "classical conditioning story" during a session when we notice a subtle or not so subtle behavioral change. We notice the escape first, which might lead us to reconstruct the previous elements of the story. One of my patients once wept through about half of a Kleenex box. As the tissues mounted on her lap, they began to fall onto the floor. It did not occur to me that the used tissues were acting as a cue for this patient, eliciting a response of guilt and shame that was not mentioned. I did notice that she seemed generally uncomfortable with the management of the tissues, so I asked if she would like to discard them into my wastebasket. Her reaction was extreme, as she insisted that because it was my office, and my wastebasket, she would not want to "soil the wastebasket" with her tissues and tears. Realizing that her unwillingness to discard the tissues into the wastebasket was dysfunctional, much like submissive behaviors that were part of her list of treatment targets, I inquired about her response. I highlighted that it might be related to some of her submissive patterns in her relationships and that it might present an opportunity to change the pattern right then. Assuming that the cue was some aspect of her experience of dropping accumulating tissues onto the floor, and that the emotion was some version of shame or guilt, I encouraged her to "act opposite" her timid response, to discard all the tissues into my wastebasket with as much conviction as possible. She followed my suggestion, but did so timidly, as if she were just submitting to me. I asked her to do it again, this time with a batch of new unsoiled tissues from the box. She said she didn't think it was right to throw away my perfectly good tissues. I asked her to do it anyway, and to try to generate a feeling of freedom and force in doing so. She showed a little more energy and assertiveness, but was still rather restrained. On the third trial, she acted with more force, and was surprised to experience a sense of freedom. She laughed spontaneously. The main point here is that DBT therapists, in following the principles of classical conditioning (and deconditioning, or exposure), are on the alert for escape behaviors, for the emotion prompting the escape, for the cue prompting the emotion, and putting them together. When it comes up spontaneously in sessions, as in this example, the therapist finds himself "looking backward" into the chain, starting with the escape and then locating the cue and the emotion, reconstructing the three-term sequence as a way to understand and treat the "escape function" of the targeted behavior.

The work of exposure is enhanced by a certain kind of stance in therapists. We must exercise self-awareness, balance, and the capacity to self-regulate in response to cues that are difficult to hear and emotions that might be difficult to bear. Sometimes we may share the patient's urge to escape. We must be unflinching in hearing about the cues, and alert to our own urge to escape along with the patient, and pay attention to the subtle ways the patient does so. This is particularly the case when the patient is recounting life situations that were traumatic and we are helping the patient to provide the detailed story and express the associated painful emotions. It becomes the role of the consultation team to help us undergo our own exposure to the evocative cues presented by a particular patient. For instance, when I began working with a highly suicidal and intensely angry young man who was quadriplegic in the aftermath of a tragic freak accident, I benefited from my team's balanced support to my vicariously traumatic response to his presentation. With the help of the team, I was able to "go through the fire" of the emotions elicited by this patient's story, and then was able to be balanced and present for him. Using all six DBT core mindfulness skills to cultivate our own wise minds, we can then genuinely "receive" each patient while modeling openness, steadiness, and forward movement.

Needing to establish a trusting relationship and a sense that this is a safe context in which to expose to painful cues and intense emotions, the therapist acts in an objective but compassionate manner toward the patient. DBT's "GIVE" skills—those interpersonal skills that help to preserve and strengthen relationships—are excellent guidelines. The therapist is *gentle*, which allows for trust to develop; is *interested* in the patient, which promotes a sense of security; is *validating* toward the patient, which results in the patient's feeling understood; and uses an *easy manner*, which helps to encourage steadiness and persistence in spite of waves of emotion and urges to escape.

Whereas we DBT therapists need to bring balance, awareness, and compassion to bear in exposure-based work, we also need to act with clarity, purpose, and discipline regarding the task at hand. We need to "lead the way" in the procedure of exposure, knowing the technical steps to take and the obstacles to anticipate. We use precision to locate the exact cues and experience to properly engage patients in exposing them to the cue. We need to judge when it is time to help each patient advance to a more intensive version of exposure and when to hold steady. As acquired and strengthened in training and supervision, we bring a step-by-step approach to exposure procedures, whether informal or formal.

OPERANT CONDITIONING AND CONTINGENCY PROCEDURES

Operant conditioning theory, or radical behaviorism, focuses our attention on a different three-element story embedded in the larger chain. It's the story of the *context*, the *target behavior*, and the *consequences*.

Context → Target Behavior → Consequences

The Context

The *context* refers to the stimulus context, otherwise known as the *antecedent conditions*, in which the target behavior occurs. Within that context will also be the cue that we discussed in relation to classical conditioning theory, but the operant conditioning model highlights the stimulus context in all of its aspects, and one other feature in particular. As part of the "operant conditioning story," we want to discover the *discriminative stimuli*, those stimuli that signal to the patient that reinforcement may be available for engaging in a certain behavior, in this case, the target behavior. For instance, we noticed that one of the patients in our inpatient DBT program would periodically respond to her frustration by banging her head on the wall, usually during the evening shift. Upon further assessment it became clear that all such episodes took place when a particular staff member, who worked evenings, was present and was not otherwise occupied. The patient was fond of that staff member, and the episodes would lead to closer contact with her. The discriminative stimulus was the presence, availability, and responsiveness of that staff member. With that knowledge it was possible to come up with interventions that led to elimination of the head-banging behavior.

The Target Behavior

The target behavior is followed by reinforcement. The behaviors that we target for change in DBT, and for which we use contingency procedures to alter the operant conditioning story, are of two types. Most obviously, we target behaviors on the patient's list of treatment targets, developed at the beginning of treatment and modified over time. We also target behaviors of the patient that cross the therapist's personal limits; if therapists do not courageously observe their own personal limits, and target the behaviors that violate those limits, they will suffer from therapist burnout. Although most of the target behaviors of which I have spoken in this book are problematic behaviors of the patient, there are two other relevant sets of behaviors. First, we target the patient's adaptive behaviors to increase them, and in doing so, we rely on the same operant conditioning story, considering how to reinforce those behaviors. Second, we target the behaviors of the therapist that interfere with the treatment; this is done within the consultation team, and the same principles are operative.

Fortunately, the principles associated with operant conditioning are familiar. We all learn them naturalistically in our lives. We know what it is to reinforce, extinguish, and punish behaviors. We do it, and receive it, all the time. But the use of these principles in treatment with emotionally dysregulated individuals requires an enhanced awareness of them and a more disciplined understanding of how to use them.

The Consequences

The consequences of interest to the therapist in the model of operant conditioning are those that (1) are contingent upon the target behavior and (2) influence the future likelihood that the target behavior will happen again in a similar context. For the sake of illustration, let's say that, while getting coffee together, I frequently ask you for money. I never pay you back, I barely thank you, and I seem to take your generosity for granted. You get tired of this behavior, you act a little annoyed, and you ask me to stop. Your explicit request doesn't stop me. Somewhat baffled, you become curious about what is motivating me. The target behavior is my repeated request for coffee money. In the context, the discriminative stimuli might include several features: You are wealthier than me, you are a generous soul, you have money with you, and you act warmly toward me. Obviously, you have reinforced my prior requests by loaning me money in spite of your stated objections. If you decide to change my behavior, now you have all the information you need: the context, the behavior, and the reinforcer. The process of figuring out those variables central to the operant story is known as *functional analysis*. We determine the "function" of the behavior by determining what problem is solved by that behavior; in the example, the function of my asking-for-money behavior is most likely to fulfill my desire for coffee. Or it could turn out that the function is to get something, anything, from you, or to inconvenience you. Determining the function of the behavior, which requires assessment, determines what is reinforcing the behavior in that context.

At the risk of repetition for those readers with a background in operant conditioning, next I specify the kinds of consequences, or contingencies, that we use in DBT. After listing and describing them here, I consider the challenge of utilizing them in the treatment of individuals with severe emotional dysregulation.

Principles of Operant Conditioning in DBT

1. **Reinforcement** is defined as a process in which the contingent consequences of the behavior of interest, on average, increase the likelihood that the patient will engage in that behavior again in the future.

   a. In **positive reinforcement**, the reinforcing consequence is something **added** to the situation (e.g., praise, food, money).

      - Those positive reinforcers that are more immediate are likely to be more potent than those that are delayed.

      - Once a behavior is under the control of a relatively continuous or highly frequent reinforcer, the frequency of reinforcement can be reduced to an intermittent schedule. Once this adjustment has taken place, the reinforcer can be further shifted to an intermittent but also unpredictable schedule, known as *random intermittent reinforcement*. The latter is typically a powerful form of reinforcement and plays an important role when we consider how it is that certain highly dysfunctional behaviors in treatment are reinforced to the point where they are resistant to extinction.

- All other things being equal, we would prefer that the reinforcers for patients' adaptive behaviors be natural, meaning typically available in their natural environments, rather than arbitrary, meaning artificial and unlikely to be available in their natural contexts. Taking care in the selection of reinforcers increases the chance that the skillful behaviors strengthened within the treatment setting will be more easily reinforced by patients' natural environments.
   b. In **negative reinforcement**, the reinforcer is something **removed** from the situation (e.g., emotional pain, physical pain, interpersonal nagging).

2. **Shaping.** Sometimes it is unrealistic to expect that even with reinforcement, the patient can engage in a targeted behavior. In that case, the therapist might reinforce small steps on the way to engaging in the targeted behavior. This process is known as **shaping.**

3. There are two categories of approaches to the targeting of a particular behavior for reduction or weakening: **extinction** and **punishment.**

4. **Extinction** is a process in which the reinforcement for a given behavior is faded or removed, and as a result the targeted behavior declines.
   a. **Extinction burst.** When the reinforcer is no longer available or is being faded out, typically the individual initially responds with an exaggeration of the behavior that is being extinguished. This is known as an **extinction burst.** Anticipating this response when using extinction helps the therapist to avoid reinstating reinforcement for the behavior in an escalated form.

5. **Punishment** is a process by which the consequences of a targeted behavior, which are contingent on that behavior, decrease the likelihood that the patient will engage in that behavior again in the future, ultimately leading to the suppression of the behavior. Unfortunately, punishment also may lead to a sense of being judged, shamed, criticized, and/or controlled, and it is usually only effective in the presence of the person doing the punishment. It also fails to teach a new behavior to replace the old one. Punishment, if used, is most effective when . . .
   a. The therapist uses it sparingly, only when necessary.
   b. It is used with sufficient consistency, intensity, and duration to bring about the desired outcome, and no more than that.
   c. It is done from a balanced stance, ideally one that is based in compassion, not from a judgmental, angry, or punitive position.

Successfully changing behaviors of individuals with borderline personality disorder with the use of operant conditioning principles, functional analysis, and contingency procedures can be difficult. Some of the difficulties result from the patients' syndrome of severe emotional dysregulation. Others result from the lasting impact of pervasively invalidating environments. Still others arise because the therapist is human and her behaviors are subject to reinforcement, extinction, and punishment too.

Because these patients usually are highly sensitive and reactive emotionally to their sharp perceptions of others' emotions, the use of contingencies needs to be handled with care, and on a trial-and-error basis, to discover what works. It is obvious that such patients will likely have strong reactions to the aversive experiences that ensue when extinction and punishment are used. With some patients, the slightest communication of disapproval or withdrawal of warmth can set off intense emotions, including fear, shame, sadness, guilt, anger, and self-hatred. Punishment is to be used sparingly and only when the behavior *must* change (e.g., dangerous head banging) and nothing else is working. Since extinction involves taking away reinforcement, it is aversive as well. For instance, the patient in a session may engage in distractions to avoid responding to an upsetting but important topic. If the therapist remains silent, he may be inadvertently reinforcing avoidance. If instead he redirects the conversation to the upsetting topic, he may be extinguishing the avoidance behavior. In doing so, the patient could become dysregulated both because of returning to the evocative topic and because his avoidance behavior is being extinguished. As a general rule, it is wise to pair the use of extinction with soothing and validating interventions. These kinds of interventions might take the form, for instance, of saying, "I realize that this is an upsetting topic, and it makes sense that you might want to avoid it, but let's see if we can find a way to help you face it."

It can be challenging as well to use positive reinforcement of adaptive behaviors in DBT. For a number of reasons, the patient may experience standard efforts to reinforce (e.g., providing approval, warmth, praise) as uncomfortable, even frightening. For example, she may feel that if she is being praised for adaptive behavior, she now needs to be adaptive all the time. Or she may mistrust warmth or approval because in her childhood environment, such approaches were followed by exploitation or rejection. Trust is hard to win when someone has encountered such an invalidating background. The work to find those therapeutic responses that actually reinforce a patient's behaviors (i.e., that actually result in an increased likelihood of strengthening those behaviors) sometimes requires patience, ingenuity, and a trial-and-error process.

Recognizing these challenges casts light on a broader issue related to reinforcement: that is, the atmosphere of the sessions in general. Given that these patients have been invalidated and traumatized, and are usually emotionally sensitive and reactive, generally we want to establish a baseline atmosphere of warmth, concern, compassion, gentleness, and validation. We want our DBT patients to realize that they are in a safe situation in which to share their vulnerabilities. And we want them to realize that positive reinforcement for adaptive behaviors is readily available to strengthen skillful approaches. I discuss validation later; for now, it is sufficient to note that we want patients to have the experiences in which the therapist is listening, present, accurately understanding, and being as genuine as possible. Such experiences set the bar at a warm level where reinforcement for functional behaviors is not far away. If we want to extinguish or punish behaviors of any kind, it usually requires only a slight deviation from this baseline.

But this baseline can become nontherapeutic if it creates an unrealistic atmosphere of unconditional regard and warmth. The patient may feel safe, but over time the therapist may discover that whenever she pushes him for behavioral change, even when making rather normative requests and interventions, these interventions trigger intense negative responses. A baseline that conveys warmth, patience, compassion, and validation must also convey a treatment approach that pushes constantly for behavioral change. Finding this balance is sometimes not so easy. If I am too warm and approving, for example, I am treating the patient as fragile, providing temporary safety and trust that will lead to long-term paralysis in a change-oriented treatment. If I am too pushy and demanding of change, on the other hand, my approach will trigger memories of trauma and invalidation, elicit self-invalidation, and create an adversarial relationship in which pushing for change is nearly impossible.

In trying to strike the right balance of acceptance and change so that contingencies will be effective in modifying behaviors, therapists face a further challenge. Because of the distorted environments in which our patients have learned how to respond to interpersonal stimuli, we might not receive much reinforcement from them for delivering effective therapy. We might be overtly reinforced for being warm and approving (e.g., "You are the only therapist who really has listened to me"), and punished for change-oriented interventions (e.g., "How dare you ask me to try that skill? Obviously you haven't been listening to anything I have said"), and over time have trouble finding the right balance. Similarly, we may in fact find therapeutic responses that do effectively reinforce or extinguish the behaviors in the intended direction, but then cannot discern from the patient's in-session response whether the interventions are efficacious. So, based on patients' responses to interventions, therapists' behaviors are sometimes shaped into an empathic therapy approach that avoids troubling issues and behaviors, and at other times, therapists do not receive any input from patients to confirm the value of their contingency procedures. Both cases are examples of one of the most important functions of the weekly DBT consultation team meeting: Team members can reinforce each therapist for doing effective therapy, figuring out what works, helping each to stay flexible and attentive to the patient, and maintaining morale against the pressures toward burnout.

Finally, I have noticed another challenge for DBT therapists in using contingencies skillfully. As therapists, we tend to want to reinforce *any-*

thing the patient does that we think is adaptive, and to avoid reinforcing *any* behaviors that strike us as maladaptive. But in applying contingencies as a broad brush to *any* behaviors that come our way, based on whether we think they are adaptive or maladaptive in the moment, we fail to maintain our discipline in remembering that we are only targeting either those behaviors that are on the prioritized list of primary treatment targets, the secondary targets that are maintaining the specified primary targets, or those that are violating our personal limits. Countless times, when supervising staff members on my inpatient and day treatment DBT programs, and when I have reviewed sessions of my own, I find that we apply reinforcement, extinction, and punishment to any behaviors that we, personally, prefer to increase or decrease, based on our own styles and values, rather than staying focused on *those behaviors the patient needs to change in order to build a life worth living.* This kind of indiscriminate practice of contingency procedures can dilute the potency of the procedures as well as blur the awareness of what we are targeting.

A certain set of therapist qualities and a particular kind of therapeutic stance are optimal for implementing contingency procedures. First, we need to keep each patient's targets, and our own personal limits, in view throughout treatment. Simply by staying focused on specified targets and limits, we will be likely, quite naturally, to reinforce adaptive patient behaviors and to extinguish or punish maladaptive ones. Second, we must maintain a clear view of the "rules of the game": DBT agreements, treatment protocols, assumptions about patients and therapy, and rules pertaining to the context in which treatment occurs. Insofar as we are alert and firm in staying on target, maintaining limits, and delivering consequences crisply and promptly, we need the same characteristic qualities as an excellent referee in soccer or hockey. This role requires objectivity, courage, immediate responsiveness, and a sense of proportion so that the reinforcement is of appropriate potency and the "punishment suits the crime." Third, and more in keeping with the optimal qualities for an excellent personal trainer, we establish a positive, warm relationship with each patient; are attuned to the patient's way of functioning; are clear about each patient's goals, targets, capabilities, and motivational factors; and intervene with positive reinforcement promptly and inspiringly in response to behavioral progress or effort.

Finding the optimal balance in using contingencies in sessions can be challenging. We need to be clear about what we are, and are not, reinforcing, and with what degree of potency. There are so many influences on our judgment and perspective as we are in the middle of doing therapy, that it can be instructive to (1) present what we are doing in our consultation team if we are wondering, and (2) watch ourselves on videotaped sessions to get an "outside" perspective. Until I saw myself on videotape, I had no idea that my facial expressions sometimes communicated a different message than I had meant to convey.

SKILLS DEFICITS AND SKILLS TRAINING

In one of my first groups as a skills trainer, on an inpatient DBT unit, I was introducing the interpersonal skill of how to say "no" effectively. To start out, I asked each patient, in a very brief role-play exercise, to say "no" in response to my request for $3.00. I wanted each patient to have the successful experience of engaging in a role play, since we would be doing more as we went along. I was surprised when I got around to Sylvia, a 40-year-old woman who had been abused repeatedly in childhood and who had a passive interpersonal style, when she responded, "Of course, you can borrow $3.00, Dr. Swenson."

I replied, "No, Sylvia, this is just pretend. Let's try it again. Just say 'no.' Hey, Sylvia, can I borrow $3.00?"

Without skipping a beat she said, "Dr. Swenson, I wouldn't say 'no' to you if you need money."

I tried again. I couldn't get her to say "no." It was as if the word was absent from her vocabulary, could not be produced by her lips and mouth. Considering how many times she had been exploited in her adult life, it all made sense, and it seemed all the more important.

Her behavior raised the question in my mind of whether the skill was present in her repertoire, being blocked by some factor(s), or whether the skill was not within her repertoire at all. As I asked her when and where she had ever used the word "no," she came up with nothing. But a fellow patient in the group, who knew her better than I did, succeeded where I failed.

"Sylvia, what if you had a young daughter, and you had her at the playground, and she was having a good time. And a strange man came up to you and asked, 'Can I take your daughter with me down to the river?'"

Almost before her friend finished the sentence, Sylvia replied, with decisiveness and force, "No!" I certainly knew then that she had the skill in her repertoire, and could use it on behalf of a child, but not on her own behalf. It told me that she had acquired the skill, but to use it on her own behalf was blocked by other factors.

We began to work with Sylvia to use the word "no" in other contexts, with practices where she was advocating for someone else in our role plays, and then got her to begin to use it on her own behalf. It was very difficult for her, went against her "instincts," her reflexes. It felt strange. But with peer support, she began to break new ground. So she built upon the capacity to say "no," now in contexts where it had been impossible before. She had acquired the skill of saying "no," and we began to work with her to strengthen that skill. Having oriented her to the need for it, and having found her capacity to do it in one context, she practiced it again and again in the group, with considerable instruction, modeling, support, and reinforcement.

We cannot assume, however, that acquisition and strengthening of a skill in a group setting will automatically result in the person's use of that skill in life situations where it is really needed. The skill needs to be generalized into relevant contexts. As the next step, we assigned Sylvia the homework of using the skill in various situations on the inpatient unit during the day. She tried out saying no to various requests: "Sylvia, would you be willing to change rooms with me?"; "Sylvia, would you go for a walk with me?"; and so on. Her peers from the group supported her when she carried out her assignments on the unit. Next, we wanted her to practice saying "no" to others who were in positions of power and authority, since her life was filled with examples in which she had been exploited by people in authority. We assigned her the homework of saying "no" when the nurses asked her to take her medications (temporarily), and when her doctor asked if she could meet with him right then. She must have said "no" more times in 2 weeks than she had said in her entire life, and she began to acknowledge a newfound sense of self-respect alongside her fear. Obviously, the ultimate generalization of this skill would need to happen when she left the hospital.

Whereas the "stories" of respondent conditioning and operant conditioning can be broken down into three terms each, the "story" of skills deficits and their remediation is embedded ubiquitously throughout the behavioral chain, contributing to target behaviors. We find skills deficits early in the chain as well as later in the chain. We address skills deficits in regulating emotions, tolerating distress, managing oneself toward one's own goals, becoming more effective in relationships, and establishing more awareness and control through mindfulness.

As I argue in considerable detail in Chapter 14 on skills and skills training, one could reasonably posit that the entire superstructure of DBT exists to ensure the learning and application of skills where they are needed. The skills trainer may not be in a position to see that the patient who seems to learn a skill is blocked from using it by problematic cognitions (e.g., "It won't work anyway"), by intense emotions (e.g., too frightened or ashamed to try something new), or by problematic contingencies (e.g., the environment will not reinforce the patient for using the new skill, and in fact may reinforce him for using the same old problem behaviors). Hence, the individual therapist, along with any *in vivo* skills coach, works with the patient to get him to see the wisdom of the skill, to try it out, to practice it again and again, and to ferret out and solve the factors interfering with using that skill successfully. If any one of us thinks back on a time when we deliberately learned a new skill to replace an old habit, and then sustained the use of that skill over time, it will be obvious that learning and using even one new skill can be a lot of work. Yet, if accomplished, we may also recognize that one new skill can change a life.

In Chapter 14 on skills, I discuss the principles involved in skills training in more detail: skills acquisition, strengthening, and generalization. In this chapter I briefly address the need for a "readiness" to learn a skill; a skill can simply not be taught and imposed on a patient (Prochaska, DiClemente, & Norcross, 1992). The patient must have the idea, "I need this skill." Otherwise, all the best teaching in the world will go to waste. Once I was referred a 20-year old woman diagnosed with borderline personality disorder and anorexia nervosa. She was in therapy with a skilled specialist in eating disorder treatment, and she was referred to me for one-on-one skills training. The therapist, the parents, and the young woman herself could see that she needed more skills to be mindful, to regulate her emotions, and to interact more assertively in her interpersonal life. It seemed that thinness had become her main goal in life, and self-starvation her main "skill." From the beginning of our weekly meetings, she proved herself to be a good student and a quick study.

But after 4 or 5 weeks, I began to realize that she was not actually practicing the skills outside of sessions. And when I asked her what was interfering, she was rather blunt about lacking motivation. She said she thought the skills "are great," but admitted that she had little interest in using them. "I just want to get my parents off my back," and she wanted to please her therapist. She wanted everyone to leave her alone and to let her starve herself. As thin as she was (only about 5 pounds above a medically dangerous weight), she still envied those who were bone thin, close to death, *including Holocaust survivors when they were liberated from concentration camps!* She showed little readiness to learn and apply skills in the service of changing her anorexia. So I offered to work with her on skills to communicate more effectively with her parents and therapist about her true aims, but she declined. When we agreed to stop, she acknowledged that if she were ever to give up her quest for ultimate thinness, she would definitely need many of the skills we had discussed.

Needless to say, the first principle of skills training is that the patient needs to recognize that she *needs* the skill, and ascertaining this requires the therapist's attention to the "preacquisition" stage of change (Prochaska et al., 1992). Most patients with whom I have worked, unlike the example of the woman with anorexia, are aware of needing skills, are motivated to learn them, are gratified when they work, and ultimately value this part of DBT. But even with the willing patient, the effective skills trainer is aware of needing to "sell" each new skill by helping patients find their particular need for it.

The excellent skills trainer combines qualities that exemplify effective piano teachers and loving mothers. The piano teacher knows how to play what she is teaching, knows how to break down the ability to play the piano into teachable steps, knows how hard to push each student and how to provide individualized reinforcement, and shows a joy for the process of learning. The devoted and loving mother knows her child, and unambiguously knows that her child, in order to have a better life, simply has to learn to do certain things.

COGNITIVE MEDIATION AND COGNITIVE MODIFICATION

Our final theory of change, cognitive mediation, brings our attention to yet another story line embedded in the behavioral chain that surrounds a target behavior. It is the story in which we follow the impact of the process and content of thinking upon the subsequent actions and emotions in the chain.

Prompting event → Beliefs, assumptions → Actions and emotions

In essence, the idea is that our actions and emotions are mediated by our cognitive style and content. If I keep saying to myself, "Life is terrible," and I begin to believe it, I will eventually drive myself toward greater misery and hopelessness. If I keep thinking that life is dangerous outside my door, I will grow more and more anxious about leaving my room, and will probably avoid doing so. Cognitive therapy is based on this model and involves discovering the deeply held negative beliefs and related self-statements in the moment (*automatic thoughts*), bringing them to the light of day, subjecting them to testing and challenge, and trying out alternative, less dire ways of thinking.

The same model is crucial to DBT because emotionally dysregulated individuals, having learned to think in pervasively invalidating contexts, are likely to be awash in negative, harsh, blaming and self-denigrating cognitions, and to have some misunderstandings of the rules of cause and effect as they exist outside their narrow and invalidating life contexts. Consider the following cognitions, which are not unusual for those with borderline personality disorder:

"I *have* to be right; otherwise I'm a bad person."
"The more bizarrely I behave, the more interesting people will find me to be."
"If I'm alone for more than an hour, I will dissolve."
"I'm totally incompetent in everything I do."
"I'm fat, ugly, and stupid, and everyone knows it."

The beliefs can be so extreme that we might be tempted to think that treatment for such individuals should center on cognitive therapy.

In considering the relationship between cognitive mediation and the other theories of change in DBT, it is important to realize that problematic cognitions are part and parcel of every one of them. The person with posttraumatic stress disorder (PTSD) who lives in terror that around the next corner is a dangerous person, is driven by the elements of classical conditioning theory discussed earlier: the story of the cue, the (respondent) emotion, and the escape. Wrapped around that three-term story are a number of cognitions that are compatible with that predicament: "People are dangerous"; "I'm incapable of discerning whether a situation is safe"; "If I ever take a risk again, I'll probably be killed"; "The only safe place for me is death." Long-term progress for the individual with PTSD will include modification of distorted cognition. Research has shown that one can achieve effective results via cognitive therapy or exposure procedures (Ougrin, 2011).

Similarly, for the individual who lacks the capacity to say "no," as was Sylvia's plight, there will always be some kind of accompanying cognitions, such as "If I say 'no,' I'll get hurt"; "If I say 'no,' I'll be a bad person"; or "People have the right to do anything they want to me." In other words, it is completely ordinary to find that when there is a damaging skills deficit, there are troublesome cognitions that accompany it. And as for considering problematic cognitions alongside the operant theory of behavioral change, the process by which a maladaptive behavior can be repeatedly reinforced and therefore maintained in a person's repertoire, we again almost always finds problematic cognitions that accompany the reinforced problematic behaviors. If the individual who cuts herself is reinforced by the immediate reduction of a swirl of intense negative emotions, beliefs emerge that cutting is the only way to live and that to refrain from cutting would be to decide to die.

To reiterate more concisely: (1) In the causation of disorders involving severe emotional dysregulation, the transaction between emotional reactivity and sensitivity, on the one hand, and the invalidating environment, on the other hand, is central; (2) conditioned emotional responses, skills deficits, and problematic contingencies conspire toward a life of avoidance, escape, maladaptive behavioral patterns, and constant misery; and (3) cognitions come into being that are compatible with, and accompany, the situational, emotional, and action components of the problem. As a result, cognitions may not be primary in causing the problems (though it may occasionally be the case for some behavioral patterns for some individuals) that bring an individual to DBT, but they have become a piece of the problem, and addressing them is part of the solution.

In keeping with this way of thinking about the role of cognitive mediation in generating problems that patients present in DBT, Linehan (1993a) has recommended that therapists remain continually alert to the emergence of problematic cognitions, never letting them pass by without some intervention, even if minimal. For instance, if a patient were to say, "I'm just not a competent person," the therapist might respond, "Yes, I know, you have the thought that you are not very competent." The patient, recognizing the challenge, might then go on, "But I mean I'm really *not* very competent." The therapist might just leave it at that point, having underlined the problematic thought; or clinical judgment might lead to something like, "Yes, I know that you have a lot of conviction that that thought is true," and so on. At other times, the therapist might just respond to a patient's negative statement "There is no solution to this" with a brief comment such as, "Yeah, I realize you don't believe there is a solution." If the thought is proving to be persistent and damaging, the therapist might further comment, "This thought keeps coming back, and it's paving the road to hell for you."

I was once working with a young woman who was intelligent and quite pretty, but in her family and school environment had come to have the firm belief that she was "fat, ugly, and stupid." It took awhile in the therapy for me to appreciate how constant these thoughts were, how they lurked in the background of every consideration of whether she could improve her life. They seemed to me to have acquired an independent status, a damaging impact, and I began to target them. To get her agreement to target them, she had to at least consider that they were her *thoughts* and not necessarily *facts*. I had to martial some evidence to get her to that point—comments from others, opinions of mine. We took the process of cognitive restructuring further than generally is done in Stage 1 of DBT. I had her track the presence and occurrence of these thoughts on a daily log, tried various ways to challenge them, helped her find the ways that she could challenge them. After weeks of this kind of "over" focus on these thoughts, they became almost like a joke as she would use them consciously, and extremely, as ways to make excuses.

"I'm sorry I was late to session today. After all, I'm fat, ugly, and stupid." I knew then that we had turned the corner. She had begun to recognize thoughts as thoughts.

This work, known as *cognitive restructuring*, involves recognizing and challenging dysfunctional thought content, finding acceptable alternative statements, and persuading the patient of the perspective that thoughts are thoughts, not facts. It is usually done in DBT sessions with immediacy, often with quick "brushstroke" kinds of comments, chipping away. On occasion, as in my example above, the therapist focuses in to do more "reconstructive" work on particular cognitive formations.

Alongside cognitive restructuring, the other thrust of cognitive modification is known as *contingency clarification*. Essentially, this is the avenue for making sure the patient understands the rules of life, mostly unwritten ones between human beings, and the rules of therapy. Because of the distorted nature of the environments from which many of our patients come, and the distorting impact of severe emotional dysregulation, they come into treatment without understanding the "rules of the game," both as they apply to life and to therapy. It is not unusual to find that the patient believes that staying ill is the only way to retain support and make it through life; that there is no way to improve and still garner support. Similarly, it is common to think that speaking up and being assertive will ruin everything. On the other hand, some patients believe that they should say everything, withhold nothing, that it's the only way to be "true" and "real." These and other "contingencies" that deserve clarification, are "if . . . then" statements. The distorted products of this kind of faulty learning are often so thoroughly taken for granted by the patient, and so surprising to the therapist, that they are missed for some time.

DBT therapists need to be on the lookout for erroneous thinking. Not long ago I was in the second year of therapy with a 35-year-old male patient. He had often, humorously, made comments about some of my interventions that he found surprising and helpful. In fact, he started to kid that if we went through a session without one of these "Swenson gems," he didn't know what to do. Correspondingly, he thought of himself as always right when he disagreed with people, except with me. The way he commented about both of these patterns of thought made them sound rather light, as if he had a balanced perspective on them, even with a touch of humor about them. Once I realized how frequently these beliefs surfaced, I began to press him more about them. As it turned out, they were not light at all—they were lynchpins, almost rules, for his functioning. As I challenged these beliefs, he became at first angry, then deeply sad. If I was not great, and if he was not right, then I was "shit" and he was a total failure. These beliefs had been living in the room with us throughout therapy; they were faulty "rules of life" that rescued him from painful feelings of failure and humiliation, and once we saw them for what they were (and "clarified the contingencies"), the tenor of therapy changed in a direction that felt more real, involved more emotions, and became more productive.

The presence of problematic cognitions in the context of emotional dysregulation should be assumed, even if not yet clarified. Evidence of them might seem minor at the time, and yet they are everywhere. The therapist stance includes a readiness to detect problematic cognitions, which might prove to be more pervasive and influential than they seem. In this respect, the therapist's attention to cognitions, searching out damaging ones for treatment, resembles the work of the exterminator who is asked to detect and eliminate insect infestations from barely visible trails.

Having detected the presence of problematic cognitions, the therapist needs the kind of skill to identify them, name them, and in some cases challenge them in a manner that is quick, tactful, and sensitive. This intervention resembles the ability of an artist, a painter, who can apply quick brushstrokes during the process of painting, just enough to highlight or revise a certain spot on the canvas, not so much as to overdo it. For the DBT therapist, the sensitivity might involve first highlighting a valid aspect of a problematic thought content or process, and then moving on to the problem. For instance, in addressing the suspicious individual from the traumatizing environment: "No wonder you are convinced that anyone who talks to you is trying to exploit you. It must be difficult to figure out when the other person actually just means what he or she says." Finding the wisdom in the thought paves the way for an intervention that highlights the invalid component of the thought. Ultimately, the DBT therapist needs to intervene dialectically, highlighting both valid and invalid components in the thought, thereby helping the patient come to a "wise mind" assessment of it.

APPLICATION OF CHANGE PRINCIPLES IN A CASE

Effective problem solving involves the integration of all seven pervasive problem-solving processes in sessions. In the following vignette of part of a DBT therapy session, I illustrate this process of integration. The patient is a young woman in a DBT program, is in the first stage of treatment, and has committed to altogether eliminating her frequent self-cutting behaviors (*targeting*). A salient factor from her childhood history is that her biological parents were incapable of taking care of her, and she was taken from them and placed with one foster family after another. She has a heightened sensitivity to "being left behind," a pattern that emerged through *behavioral chain analyses* early in the treatment, and which is part of the *case conceptualization*. Although her relationship with her roommate has been stable and long-lasting, she never stops thinking that the roommate is about to leave her (*cognitive mediation*). In one particular session following an incident of self-cutting, the therapist and patient elaborated the following behavioral chain:

After a long argument between the patient and her roommate,
→ The roommate angrily stormed out of their apartment.
→ Instantaneously, the patient experienced intense fear, "panic," and a deep sense of shame.
→ Almost simultaneously she thought, "I'll never see her again," "I've destroyed another relationship," and "What's wrong with me?"
→ In the context of those emotions and thoughts, she had a strong urge to cut herself.
→ She tried to think of something to do to tolerate the distress, but could think of nothing, and the intensity of the emotions, thoughts, and urges escalated.
→ She got a knife from the kitchen and made a one-inch cut on her wrist just deep enough to draw blood.
→ She experienced an immediate reduction in her panic and felt more in control of her emotions and thoughts.
→ She texted her roommate that she had cut herself, and the roommate returned to the apartment.
→ The patient was further relieved.

In this session, the patient and therapist are *targeting* a high-priority target behavior, self-cutting, and *monitoring* progress on a diary card. They are engaged in *behavioral chain analysis*, which is feeding into an evolving *case conceptualization* that affects the next interventions. This patient demonstrates a *commitment* to the treatment of the target, bringing the necessary information and collaborating with the therapist to generate understanding and change. We can presume that if the therapist was proceeding without a defined target, or guiding the interventions based on intuition rather than with an evolving case conceptualization through behavioral chain analyses; and/or if the patient's commitment to the target and the process was insufficient; the treatment would hardly stand a chance to succeed. Because these problem-solving processes are in place, the stage is set for considering the chain from the perspective of each of the four behavioral models discussed above. Even in this brief vignette, we can get a glimpse of the role of all four in coming up with change-oriented interventions.

The *classical conditioning* model directs our attention to the role of a *cue* (something about the roommate's angry departure that triggers the patient's intense emotions), the *emotion* (the particular mixture of fear, panic, and shame set off by the cue), and the *escape* (the reduction of the intense emotional pain brought about by self-cutting). The alert therapist will assess the specific nature of the cue as future episodes occur. At some point during treatment, if the specific cue can be identified, the therapist might engage the patient in exposure (to the cue), leading to experience with and expression of the emotion, and the blocking of the escape response (self-cutting).

We find the elements of the *operant conditioning* model in the same brief vignette. The therapist may attend to the stimulus context in which the self-cutting took place, looking for the discriminative stimuli that signaled to her that reinforcement would occur if she were to engage in cutting. Having clearly characterized the cutting behavior, the therapist would want to determine those contingent consequences that reinforced the behavior, such as the relief of painful emotions and the comforting return of the roommate. Spelling out these details will put the therapist in a position to modify the nature of the stimuli that signal the presence of reinforcement, and to consider making changes in the consequences of the self-cutting behavior. Consequently, the next time the patient faces a similar context and a similar choice (to cut or not to cut), the consequences might be aligned in a way that does not reinforce the cutting behavior, but reinforces an adaptive alternative instead. There may be several ways to do this: The therapist could (1) teach, strengthen, and get a commitment from the patient to use skillful alternative behaviors; (2) could ensure that these more adaptive alternatives be followed by reinforcing consequences; (3) could establish a protocol whereby self-cutting does not result in the return of the roommate; and/or (4) could assign the patient to carefully complete a behavioral chain analysis worksheet regarding the cutting episode, which is then presented in the next therapy session. The theory of *skills deficits* will (of course) direct the therapist's attention to the deficits in skills for (1) interacting with the roommate (interpersonal effectiveness skills), (2) managing her own sensitivity and reactivity to the cue so that her emotions do not become so quickly intense and painful (emotion regulation skills and mindfulness skills), (3) regulating the intense emotions in an adaptive manner once they are present (emotion regulation skills and distress tolerance skills), (4) finding ways to increase her tolerance of the intense emotions in order to prevent the need to use self-cutting (distress tolerance skills), and/or (5) using mindfulness skills throughout the process to work toward awareness, balance, attentional control, and wise mind.

The theory of *cognitive mediation* will bring the therapist's attention to all of those beliefs and automatic thoughts that are triggering, or fanning the flames of, intense emotional reactivity and the impulsive loss of control. Whether the cognitions preceded the intense emotions and actions or were triggered by them, they play a role in maintaining the maladaptive behavioral pattern and deserve to be addressed through contingency clarification and cognitive restructuring.

Through the lens of each of the four processes, representing the four behavioral models, the therapist can see how self-cutting is maintained in this patient's repertoire of behaviors, and can see possible ways to reduce that behavior in the future. In all likelihood, all four processes are at work, which can make it difficult to tease out the most important controlling variables. Behavioral assessment, through behavioral chain analyses, can be utilized to figure this out.

Having highlighted the value of teasing out the influences of each of these four processes, it is equally useful to realize that, in truth, there are not really four different processes going on; there is one sequence, a unified wave that flows toward cutting and beyond. The various forces are inextricably intertwined and interdependent in causing the cutting. And in finding the solution(s) to the cutting, each of the four change procedures actually brings about changes in all four story lines. For instance, if the therapist manages to realign the contingencies such that the self-cutting is diminished and some alternative behavior is strengthened, the patient (1) will need to rely on a different skill set, which will then be strengthened; (2) will shift in the nature of beliefs and cognitions in a way that aligns with the new behaviors and contingencies; and (3) the more adaptive behavioral sequence may bring about a greater sense of safety and control, which give the patient a greater capacity to endure exposure to the cues without having to escape. It's important to remember that if the therapist is engaging in one change procedure, bringing one theory to bear, she is actually addressing the story lines of all four stories. This realization can increase the flexibility and the freedom of the therapist to consider drawing from any of the problem-solving principles to change any problem. Successfully assessing the controlling variables and intervening in kind is actually a trial-and-error process between therapist, patient, and consultation team.

CHAPTER 5

The Dialectical Paradigm

I was raised in the state of Oregon, where the lumber industry was huge. Lumberjacks were celebrated, and lumber mills and paper mills stayed "online" 24 hours a day. It was a tough, dangerous industry. Loggers would fell trees upriver and float the logs down to the mill. In early spring, rivers were clogged with logs cut during the fall and winter. Logjams were common, costly, hard to prevent, and difficult to break apart. The most dangerous job in the lumbering industry was held by the log driver, otherwise known as a river pig. His task was to keep the logs flowing by anticipating and preventing jams by breaking up them early in their formation. The log driver, always a man in those days, would run across the tops of the logs as they floated or jammed up in the river, continually risking his life as he could always slip down between two logs into the water. Agility, awareness, and speed were key. One of my cousins married a man who did this job in his 20s. As did all log drivers in that era, he used a specially designed pole known as a *peavey*. It was a long wooden pole with a strategically placed metal spike near the end that could push or pull logs.

It would be difficult to find a better metaphor for the practice of dialectics in DBT. Even with the skilled application of strategies from the acceptance and change paradigms, "logjams" are typical in therapy with individuals with emotional dysregulation. Working with individuals for whom the transaction between a biologically based emotional vulnerability and a pervasively invalidating environment is reflected in intense emotions, high sensitivity, high reactivity, rigid black-and-white thinking, and a tendency toward extremes in actions and relationships, makes for logjams in every aspect of their lives—at home and work, with friends, and in therapy. The therapist equipped with a river driver's agility and quickness, able to understand and use the forces of colliding opposites in a manner that promotes flow, is in a position to:

- Create movement out of impasse.
- Transform rigid and extreme positions into more flexible and realistic ones.
- Highlight opposites as they arise and find the wisdom on each side.
- Facilitate the emergence of synthesis from opposites.
- Maintain a collaborative relationship with the patient when faced with conflict, rigid behavioral patterns, and impasses.

The strategies within DBT's treatment package for addressing logjams are the dialectical strategies. They flow from the three principles of the dialectical paradigm, which are derived from a dialectical worldview and a dialectical way of bringing influence to bear. Particularly suited for "stuck" situations during treatment, the dialectical activity of DBT clinicians is also part of the baseline stance when doing DBT. In this chapter I detail the three dialectical principles—opposites and synthesis, systemic thinking, and flux; discuss the dialectical stance that is part of DBT practice; and illustrate how DBT's nine dialectical strategies flow from the principles.

PRINCIPLES OF THE DIALECTICAL PARADIGM

Opposites and Synthesis

At the core of dialectics is an understanding that reality consists of opposites, and that the tension between opposites is resolved through a process of synthesis. In its simplest form, dialectics begins with a *thesis*, which is a proposition of some sort—for instance: "The sky is blue," "This is a perfect family," or "This patient is doing the best she can." The thesis brings about its opposite, called the *antithesis*—for instance: "No, the sky is actually no color at all," "This family is far from perfect," or "This patient has to try harder and do better." At this point in the process, we have the presence of contradiction, with a thesis and an antithesis.

A possible next move might be to figure out which is more right, the thesis or antithesis. However, to do so would not be dialectical. Another might be to claim that the thesis and antithesis can coexist, side by side, without any need to declare one the winner. This also would not be dialectical. The dialectical approach consists of identifying the valid core of the thesis, the valid core of the antithesis, and then to find a *synthesis* that includes the valid core of each, now in a new proposition. For instance: "The sky itself has no color but appears blue to humans on earth for several reasons"; "This family has the appearance of perfection, but upon closer examination, it is imperfect, as are all families"; or "This patient is doing the best she can, and she has to try harder and do better if she is to change her life." The new proposition, whatever it is, now becomes the new thesis, which will bring about an antithesis, and so on and so forth. In dialectics, nothing stands still; truth evolves as opposing forces arrive at new syntheses. This core concept is woven throughout DBT theory and treatment.

Dialectics arise routinely in the consultation team, as I address in Chapter 15. For instance, one member of the team forcefully disagrees with another in how to interpret a patient's behavior. Or the team leader arouses opposition in team members by being too strict or too lenient about applying DBT. In another example, the team may be divided, some members wanting to spend more time on training exercises whereas others want to preserve all possible time for consulting. Dialectics arise in group skills training settings. For example, patients in a group may want to spend more time sharing in-depth information about themselves, whereas the therapist wants to keep the group focused on learning more skills. Or, one member of the skills group just wants to "sit in" and learn without having to do practice assignments, whereas the therapist insists that everyone in the group practices. And dialectics arise in individual therapy on a routine basis as well.

On my DBT inpatient unit, one of the psychologists was Ed Shearin, who had trained with Marsha Linehan during the beginning years of DBT. Ed had a reserved and very respectful style, a gentle approach, and a playful and savvy mind. He was working with a 19-year-old patient at one point, and the patient wanted to leave the hospital immediately. She encountered him in the hall. "Ed, I want to leave. Today! I want out of here. I'm no longer suicidal; this place is ruining me, and I want to leave today. Would you arrange it?" She was asking on the very day when she had inflicted a serious self-injury with a light bulb, and there was no way Ed would agree to it.

"But just this morning you cut yourself," Ed pointed out. "I want you to get out too, and I'm glad you want out. Let's work on it and get it to happen as soon as we can, safely, but it can't be today."

"It *has* to be today and nothing is stopping me."

"I admire your spirit, but it can't be today."

"I know I have the right to see a judge. I'm going to take you guys to court."

This would be a typical dialectic, or polarization, in inpatient treatment. To recognize it, expect it, stay grounded with it, and work with it is challenging but incredibly helpful. The clarity of the opposing positions, along with the fact that Ed was comfortable with it, made it possible for him to find a creative synthesis.

Ed said to the patient, "Yes, you do have a right to take us to court. You just have to submit what's called a '72-hour notice.' You can get one at the nursing station. If you fill it out, there will be a court hearing within 72 hours, and you will either be committed to the hospital or released. The judge will decide."

"That's what I'm going to do," the patient asserted.

Ed came right back: "OK. as soon as you fill it out, I think you and I should have a session."

"Why? I'll be leaving right after the hearing."

"I'll help you prepare for the hearing," said Ed. "We can work on the skills you will need to make your case as strong as possible. We can even role play."

"I don't get it," she countered. "You want to help me prepare to beat you guys in court?"

"That's right! I want you to be as skillful as you can. That's what this treatment is all about. And I know you're going to need all the skills you can get. It's not easy to make your case against the hospital. And I'll be the one who testifies against you, and I'm really good at it. Let's get started. Whether you win or lose your case right now, I want you to feel that you did your best."

Truth evolves. When opposites face off, the dialectical thinker looks not for winners and losers, but for synthesis, for win–win positions. Ed's patient wanted to leave the hospital. That proposition was probably a synthesis of a prior opposition within her, or between her and the hospital team. And by proposing to leave, she brought about the opposite, namely, that she would not be able to leave immediately. Ed represented the opposition, but as her therapist, he wanted to remain dialectical and find the wisdom on both sides. There was wisdom in the patient's desire to leave. There was wisdom in Ed's insistence that she stay. He found a synthesis of the two sides: He would be the one arguing to keep her in the hospital until she was under better behavioral control, but at the same time he would help her press her case against him as skillfully as possible. The synthesis came not only in his invitation to help her oppose him most effectively, but in his statement that the ultimate goal, presumably for both of them, was to enhance her skills. Had it been my cousin's husband rather than Ed, working with his peavey to solve literal logjams rather than to treat a patient, he may have temporarily aligned himself with the force of one log, pushing against the "opposing" log, in such a way that he freed up both logs to resume flowing down the river. The ideal solution in therapy is to find and articulate the opposing positions, to identify what is valid in each position, and to intervene in a manner that allows for synthesis.

The more clearly we grasp this essential nature of reality, the less surprising it is that we encounter opposition and polarization in treatment. We expect it. Rather than thinking "How could this be? What a surprise! Why is she opposed to what I am saying?," the attitude becomes, "Of course we are on opposite sides of this—how understandable." It is, of course, stressful working with people whose biology and history result in rigid positions that place them in opposition to us. But if we can truly grasp the essential nature of reality, wherein opposites are present on a regular basis, we have a chance to desensitize ourselves to opposition. If we can relax into the awareness of opposition, expect it, perhaps even learn to appreciate it, we stand a better chance of working with it creatively and productively. We model for the patient that opposites need not be feared, but instead can be approached with curiosity and might even serve as the leading edge of growth.

Systemic Thinking

A 45-year-old female patient arrived at my office with a presenting problem of alcoholism. We had worked together for about a month. She was ambivalent about giving up alcohol, and ambivalent about being in therapy. Her 70-year-old mother called me one day to report how much her daughter was drinking. She was concerned, and she asked me for an update on her daughter's treatment. It had been a theme in my patient's life that she experienced her mother as intrusively hovering over her since she was a child, crossing boundaries of autonomy and privacy. I told the mother that I would prefer she either address her concerns directly to her daughter, or to ask her daughter for permission to talk with me. The mother angrily hung up on me. She told her daughter that I was a "controlling idiot" and urged her to stop seeing me. Because my patient was opposed to her mother, the mother's insistence that she stop seeing me actually helped her to decide that I was the right therapist for her and that she would continue in therapy!

The essential feature of systemic thinking is that in a complex system, each element of the system is part of the whole, is therefore interdependent on all other parts, and a change in one results in a change in all others. As a result, if you find that you cannot make a desired change in one element, you can intervene with another element. The alcoholic patient just mentioned was ambivalent about being in therapy. She and her mother were part of the same family system. Whereas my discussions with the daughter had not resulted in her greater commitment to therapy, my intervention with her mother, in which I established a boundary around the mother's involvement with the treatment, increased the daughter's commitment. The fact that we can change the behavior of one person by intervening with another allows us to expand the range of therapeutic possibilities manifoldly.

I was supervising a therapist in a well-established, well-trained DBT consultation team. The therapist was presenting a high-lethality suicidal patient in her supervision. She was very anxious about this patient. I asked her if she was getting sufficient support from her consultation team. She told me that discussion of suicide was limited in her team; there was little room for her to share her fears about the possibility of suicide. As I learned, the team leader, who was also the most senior DBT therapist on the team, had lost a patient to suicide earlier in the year. He was managing his own grief and fear by inhibiting discussion of suicide in team meetings, which limited the help available to my supervisee regarding her suicidal patient, and likely even increased her patient's risk of suicide. As part of my consultation to my supervisee, we held a meeting in which I consulted with her entire team. The highly emotional meeting, in which the team leader shared his grief about losing his patient to suicide, catalyzed a process of healing in the members, which strengthened everyone's capacity to consult with each other about suicidal patients. Everything is connected.

I trained a group of therapists in DBT who went on to develop a thriving DBT-based children's residential program located in a large agency. The morale was high among the therapists, the families of the kids were pleased, and the clinical outcomes were very good. I had not seen the team for months. One of the therapists called me and asked me to a team meeting as a consultant. The atmosphere in the room was constricted, discussions seemed shallow, and morale seemed low. No one could even state clearly why I was asked to consult. The relatively new administrator of the agency was sitting in the room; she attended team meetings to "keep track" of what was going on. We took a break halfway through the meeting. In the men's room, one of the therapists informed me that they could not talk freely with the administrator in the room. Soon after arriving at the agency, the administrator had attended a team meeting. When she heard the therapists freely—and healthily—sharing their thoughts and feelings, she made the statement, "I don't want to hear any more complaining in these meetings. We are professionals. We don't complain." Intimidated (this administrator was the person in charge of the job performance evaluations for all clinicians), the therapists had not directly registered their disagreement. Their incapacity to openly address the "elephant in the room" resulted in the decline of their team, which was in turn hurting the quality of patient care. The tense and nonproductive atmosphere in the team meeting reflected a systemic problem, the solution of which would require change in several levels of the organization and a large number of individuals.

The lesson is that everything matters. Everything affects everything. My conversation with my alcoholic patient's mother led to a stronger therapeutic alliance with my patient. The suicide of a team leader's patient resulted in a prohibition on the discussion of suicide risk in the team many months later, increasing suicide risk of another patient. Hiring a new administrator of a child therapy agency put a stranglehold on the open sharing of emotions and thoughts in a DBT consultation team, negatively affecting the patients' treatment and likely hurting the reputation of the facility. When we try to understand and influence phenomena of importance in program implementation and clinical work, we have to consider factors that are several steps removed from the phenomena.

During my training in psychiatry and psychotherapy, I attended an annual family therapy conference sponsored by a private psychiatric hospital. For several years they invited Carl Whitaker, a renowned and creative family therapist, who would usually interview a family on stage and then discuss the process. He was a master of dialectics in family therapy.

One year, the hospital chose to present the case of a woman in her mid-30s who had been an inpatient there for almost 3 months. They were baffled by her presentation and frustrated by the lack of progress. It was not clear whether she was depressed, psychotic, organically impaired, or willful, but the presenting symptom was that she would not speak. She attended meetings and followed the rules but did not speak to anyone, including her therapist. This behavior was present upon her arrival, and progress in the case was at a complete standstill. The treatment team decided to present her in the context of her family, which consisted of three adult siblings: two brothers and a sister. The four siblings sat on stage in a semicircle, facing Whitaker, in front of about 300 mental health professionals.

Whitaker did not address the patient, seemed not to even look at her as she sat next to her sister, at the end of the semicircle. Instead he started by asking one of the brothers, dressed in a nice suit and looking rather anxious, if he thought he could get anything out of a family therapy session. "Yes, I am here for my sister, and will gladly take part in anything that might help her." Whitaker: "No, that's not what I mean. I mean, could you, yourself, for your own life, get something out of a family session?" The brother: "Look, I meant what I said; I'll do anything if it will help my sister. My own life is fine thank you." Whitaker not only persisted but became suddenly insulting: "I can't believe that everything in your life is just fine. You are a little overweight, for instance, a little fat, and I can't help but think that there might be a layer of fat around your heart. Maybe family therapy could help you trim down and extend your life." The brother turned immediately beet red, clearly embarrassed and furious. He started to raise his voice, and Whitaker quickly backed down and issued a perfunctory apology.

He moved on to brother number two. "What about you? Is there anything from your own life that you might be able to get out of a family therapy session?" Brother number two: "Really, my life is quite good, really no problems. Just like Paul [his brother], I am willing to do whatever to help out my sister." The sisters just listened. Whitaker: "I don't get it. You and your brother don't see anything about your lives that you could improve. For instance, you [brother number two] are thin, tall, kind of stiff, possibly kind of rigid. I wonder if you actually have as much fun as you could. Maybe family therapy could help you loosen up and have more fun." At this point the long-mute patient cracked up! Her laughter quickly became almost uncontrollable. Her sister began laughing too, and both of them were laughing so hard they were crying. Everyone else was quiet and puzzled.

Whitaker asked her, "What are you laughing about? I don't get it." She managed to settle down enough to answer, still almost laughing: "I can't believe what you are saying! What you were saying to our brothers is exactly what we used to say to each of them when they were kids. We used to tease Paul about his weight, and John about how stiff he was. It's just so funny." Her sister was nodding in agreement, still laughing. The brothers looked very uncomfortable. Whitaker noted to them that the two sisters seemed like they had a really nice relationship. The patient spoke immediately: "We used to." Her eyes went down to the floor. "Not any more." Whitaker: "Why not?" Patient: "Ever since my sister had her second child, she has nearly disappeared off the planet. I barely see her or hear from her, she's just gone." The sudden sadness was profound and evoked tears in nearly everyone. Whitaker stayed silent, just allowing her words to be heard. He then made a recommendation. "I know what you should do. Your sister should move into the hospital with you, you should both be patients together as long as it takes for you to rediscover your relationship. I think that's the answer." There was laughter but at the same time an appreciation that he had gotten to the core of something, to a systemic understanding of the symptomatic presentation. As we shall see, his style of intervention, which was successful in getting movement in this logjam, was completely consistent with Linehan's dialectical strategies.

Linehan has acknowledged that some of the well-known family therapists were teachers and models for her in understanding dialectics and building it in to DBT. Carl Whitaker was one of them. These therapists were superb at exercising freedom, using unconventional approaches to break logjams in families. They were masters of the unexpected, using tact, timing, and strategically paradoxical interventions to disrupt the stasis in a dysfunctional system and bring about a new homeostasis. Their interventions were based on the conviction that everything was interrelated, that everyone affected everyone, and that every intervention had systemic ramifications. That is the spirit of this principle in the dialectical paradigm. By thinking in this way, we can widen the scope of our assessments, realizing that an intervention in one place, even several steps removed from the phenomenon of interest, can bring about a change in that phenomenon. We thereby augment the range of interventions in the change and acceptance paradigms.

Early in my career I was treating a 21-year-old man with schizophrenia. Generally excitable and agitated, he experienced feelings of ecstasy, usually based in delusional thinking that could turn instantly into despair. My approach was informed primarily by empathy, direct suggestions, and some interpretations. This was not a DBT treatment. I painstakingly tried to help him make sense of the rapidly changing world inside him and around him. After 2 years of treatment, I needed to terminate with him because I was moving to New York. He had become considerably more grounded and steady over the 2 years. As we approached the ending, I asked him if he thought he had gotten better. "Oh, yeah! Charlie, I'm living on the ground now, not in the air!" I asked if he had any ideas of what had helped him. I had my own ideas of how he was helped by the consistency of our relationship, and some of the growing understanding of his inner world due to interpretive work. Instead, answering quickly, he said, "Remember that shoe you used to wear, the one that had the hole in the bottom? That's what helped me the most." Stunned and puzzled, I asked why that had helped him. He answered, "I knew you and I were together." I asked him if I had ruined things when I purchased new shoes. Again he answered quickly, making it clear that these were well-formed assumptions of his: "No, by the time you got new shoes, I already knew we were alike." We need reminders that our usual hypotheses about cause and effect may make sense but are sometimes too linear, excluding the wider possibilities that come to us from systemic thinking. Linehan includes a dialectical strategy, *dialectical assessment*, the essence of which is to keep us asking the question, "What am I leaving out of my understanding of this problem?"

Flux

The third principle of a dialectical worldview overlaps considerably with the acceptance principle of *impermanence*. At every second, everything has changed from the previous second: every molecule, every structure, every relationship, and every idea. It can be disconcerting, for some people even frightening, to accept the radical truth of this principle: Literally nothing stays the same. After all, what is there left to hold onto, what can we count on, what can we predict? If we are to be in synch with reality, we need to be aware that the past is gone, and that whatever we think is coming is just a fantasy. All that is, is present right now. Reality is a massive mixture of constantly interacting diverse ingredients (compare "Brownian motion" in physics), forever moving and changing.

To remember that everything is changing every second stands in direct opposition to the common assumption when we experience things as "stuck": that nothing is changing at all. When we treat individuals with rigid behavioral patterns, we tend to get mired, unable to move forward or backward, unable to bring about discernible change, sometimes targeting a particular behavioral pattern for months at a time with little evidence of movement. We can grow frustrated, hopeless, and tense. When our minds focus on an increasingly narrow perspective in which change is missing, the flexibility of our thinking can diminish, and therapeutic burnout looms on the horizon (for both therapist and patient!). We come to believe our static perception. To invoke this dialectical assumption, reminding ourselves that actually everything, at every level, at every moment, is changing, can shake up our perspective and provide an antidote to this paralysis, leading to hope and movement. Even if we do "nothing," change is coming. (In fact, sometimes *especially* if we do nothing, change comes into view.)

Once I was treating a woman who relentlessly picked her skin. For a time her skin-picking behavior was at the top of our hierarchy of treatment targets. At the end of every day, she would record on her diary card the number of times she had picked her skin, the depth of the picking, and whether it brought relief. In every weekly session we would review her diary card, and in order to target the relentless picking behavior, we would carry out a careful behavioral chain analysis. It grew tedious, as we never seemed to learn anything new, never could find a new angle or develop a working solution. It is more difficult to conduct behavioral chain analyses on a behavior that is happening almost constantly than on a behavior that happens intermittently.

It was early in my DBT career, and I was in a weekly supervision with Marsha Linehan. In one supervision session I complained to Marsha that my repeated behavioral chain analysis of skin-picking behavior was proving completely useless, and that it was demoralizing for me and the patient. "Marsha, it is the same every week, in every detail. Nothing is changing. Maybe we need to leave it alone!" Marsha: "Charlie, you could do that, but it wouldn't be DBT any more. In DBT we keep targeting the highest-priority behavior until we change it. We don't move on just because it's frustrating. And let me say this about nothing changing: *It's just not true! Every second, every molecule in your brain and body, and every molecule in her brain and body, have changed. Every cell, every idea, everything. Nothing is ever the same. Remember that, and just let yourself relax, go back in, do another behavioral chain analysis. Something is missing; something is left out. Just keep looking.*"

I was disappointed at first, feeling trapped with an unmoving and apparently immoveable situation. But I did believe that it was true that everything was changing. I just couldn't see it or feel it. During the sessions that followed, I just kept thinking, "Nothing is the same, everything is changing, what am I missing?" It couldn't be the same. During my next behavioral chain analysis of the skin-picking behavior, I paid closer attention to every microscopic link in the chain, tried to imagine what we were missing. And lo and behold, I did indeed think of something I had never asked her about the picking. I asked her what she did with the flakes of skin that she stripped from her body? She was mortified. Usually very reserved and polite, her face grew red and she nearly sputtered: "I have been willing to talk about everything you have asked, but I will not talk about this!" She repeated her refusal, indignant, threatening to leave the session. I was caught in a dialectic, as I told her: "I'm not sure what to do, because obviously you want me to retract the question, but on the other hand, it seems like whatever it's about is very important. You can't talk about it, and I can't see just leaving it behind." After three sessions during which we were deadlocked in a struggle about my question, I gave her a multiple-choice test about what she did with the flakes of skin. Because one of the options was far more humiliating than what she did, which was to eat the skin, she told me the truth with great embarrassment. From that time on, her skin picking gradually came under better control and her therapy shifted to the treatment of unbearable shame in her life. The belief in flux can be an antidote to impatience and hopelessness, and it can result in opening up our "eyes" to new possibilities.

Sometimes in therapy when nothing seems to be changing, and no intervention seems to make a difference, I invoke a metaphor in my own mind as a remedy. I imagine myself to be standing on one side of a thick stone wall that is too high to scale and too wide to go around. I want to get to the other side, but there is no obvious way to do it. I am still just faced with a totally impermeable stone wall. Then I relax. I realize that if I continue to stand there, continue to search for the way through or around the wall, continue to push the wall here and there with my fingers, continue to look at the wall from different angles, something will change. Maybe I will see a crack I never saw before, push in a way that is different from any prior push, or maybe there will be a subtle change in the wall, some shifting or crumbling. The wall isn't as solid as we think, and it *is* changing. This principle can help us stay the course when there appears to be no way to proceed, help to renew our attention and curiosity, and help us stay focused and hopeful in the face of hopelessness and restlessness.

THE DIALECTICAL STANCE OF DBT THERAPISTS

Standing on the ground defined by the three principles, DBT therapists can work with enormous mobility and flexibility to prevent and address logjams and rigidity. Dialectics provides a way of working that augments problem solving and helps to keep things flowing or to get back on track. It does not provide a destination. Dialectical interventions are not ends in themselves; they are means. What are some of the practical implications for therapists adopting the principles of the dialectical paradigm?

For one thing, we keep moving. Understanding that everything is interrelated, that everything is changing all the time, that oppositions arise, and that the truth is constructed over time through the synthesis of opposites, we keep moving. Even if the therapeutic work at the moment appears and feels stuck, we keep trying this, trying that, continuing to search for what is left out, pushing for change and accepting things as they are. In our household, my children once had a toy that was a 2-foot-tall replica of R2-D2 from *Star Wars*. When turned on, R2-D2 started marching forward in a straight line, shuffling his plastic legs like a soldier marching in formation. When he bumped into something, he would bounce back a little, and then march forward again. He might bump into the wall, or some immovable object, again and again, but each time he bounced backward, it would be at a slightly different angle. Over time, he might "get stuck" for a minute or two, hitting the same wall or fixed object, until he rotated sufficiently that he would move past the wall, on to another obstacle. Life for R2-D2 involved constant movement and one obstacle after another. He never would stop (until we switched him off!). Similarly, as DBT therapists we continue to move, hitting obstacles (oppositions), bouncing back, rotating (using different strategies or variations of the same ones), again and again without visible progress, until things shift sufficiently to bring clinical change. Using dialectics involves trial and error, buoyed by the belief that everything is interrelated, that everything is moving, and that syntheses between opposites can always be found.

Whereas the oppositions that arise in the course of treatment can involve almost anything, certain themes are familiar to DBT therapists. First, and most fundamental to the philosophy of DBT, is the opposition between acceptance and change. Starting with an attitude of acceptance, we push for behavioral change in the direction defined by the treatment targets. Pushing for change, we eventually "run into a wall." We bounce back (assess the situation), then move forward, possibly with a different change strategy, or with the same change strategy but applied somewhat differently. We may arrive at the impression that the push for change, regardless of which strategy, is not working. Then we shift to acceptance, using a validation strategy and a reciprocal tone. We let go of change and offer acceptance. The patient feels better understood. Then we may shift back to change strategies. We continue to move: R2-D2 doing psychotherapy! We may need to find just the right synthesis of pushing for change in the context of acceptance, and we will undoubtedly arrive there through trial and error. We might be shifting rapidly between acceptance and change interventions, so much so that they form one intervention. Or, as we saw in the example of Ed Shearin and the suicidal patient wanting to leave the hospital, we may find a way to ally with both sides, opposed to each other, at the same time. Dialectical work relies on improvisation, through which we discover creative syntheses of acceptance and change strategies.

Early in the days of my inpatient DBT program, I agreed to do therapy with a 15-year-old girl. Energetic and stubborn, she had very low tolerance for frustration, was highly impulsive, and acted as if she were determined to destroy her own life. Because she was on a constant supervision status, a nursing staff member escorted her to my office. She came in and immediately proceeded to my bookcases. Without speaking, she started throwing my books on the floor, row after row. I asked her to stop; she continued. I told her to stop; she continued. I told her she would have to go back to the unit; she said she couldn't wait. I called the nursing station and they sent a staff member back to my office to get her. She stopped throwing the books. We stood there. I said, "I guess that was the shortest therapy in history." She said, "Thank God!" I said, "Maybe we aren't such a good match to work together in therapy." She said, "You can say that again!" I said, "Since therapy isn't a good way for us to work together, I guess we need to find what kind of relationship we can have that will help you." She was uncharacteristically speechless and puzzled. "What are you talking about?" I suggested that our relationship would have to be based on something else. "What would you like to do?" She was quick to respond: "I want to go outside; I haven't been allowed out for months!" I suggested that we could take walks outside if she would not run away. She agreed to it. I knew she might run, but given the current course, I thought it was worth a chance.

We took a walk outside on the beautiful grounds of the hospital. Hospital staff had homes on the grounds. After walking several hundred yards, mostly in silence except for her expressions of joy about seeing the outside world, we came across a dog pen with a black labrador retriever in it. She started talking to the dog: "Oh, no, you're in the hospital! How sad! What's the matter? Do you miss your mommy?" She went on talking to the dog. We talked about the dog. Little did she know it was actually my family's dog, since we lived on the hospital grounds. I told her. She was obviously pleased. She started kidding me: "What, you don't have enough patients in the hospital that you have to put your dog in the hospital too?!" There was a smile. It was the beginning of a series of walks and talks between us, a therapeutic relationship between us, but not to be called *therapy*.

Our walks, our talks with the dog and about the dog, represented a synthesis between maintaining a therapeutic relationship, on the one hand, and redefining its terms in a way that was acceptable to her. This was an example of DBT's dialectical strategy, *allowing natural change*, whereby the synthesis between two opposing positions is found by allowing change, following the direction in which pressure is being applied.

Although the dialectic between acceptance and change is central to DBT, the therapist balances other opposing positions as well. For instance, she balances centeredness and flexibility. The need for this kind of balance can come into play when the therapist is trying to hold the patient to one of the expectations of treatment, such as the daily completion of a diary card. When the patient objects to completing it, it can become one of the many stalemates in treatment. The therapist orients the patient to the rationale and firmly insists on its completion. "I need you to complete the diary card so that I can see how you are doing every day on your target behaviors and your skills." The patient may refuse, or only complete part of the diary card. Therapist and patient may become stuck, facing off against each other. Both sides can get rather rigid about it. In fact, the work done toward finding the synthesis can be valuable, and should not be rushed. As Linehan has put it in her supervision of therapists, "diary card therapy" might be valuable since "there are so many 'diary cards' in life, tasks we have to complete even though they are not particularly pleasurable." One possible synthesis regarding the diary card involves shifting focus away from the form of the card and the details of the expectations, and instead focusing on the functions of the card. If we emphasize the functions of self-monitoring and communication of details to the therapist, we can be more flexible about the rules and the form of a diary card review. In one case, when I was working with someone who had significant learning disabilities and found the card to be too dense with cognition and numbers, we created a new card that was less dense, was more visually appealing, and allowed for ratings on a 1–3 scale rather than on a 0–5 scale. The patient was then willing, even proud, to do it. The better that therapists understand the real principles and functions of DBT, the more they can be flexible in negotiating the trappings.

DBT therapists balance nurturance, on the one hand, with challenging patients to change their behavior on the other, moving easily and quickly between the two to find the balance that allows the therapy to continue to flow toward the targets. I was seeing a young man who had several problems with sleep, eating, and hoarding in addition to suicidal behaviors. I wanted him to keep a record of his eating and sleeping patterns for a more accurate assessment, but he found it burdensome and refused. Yet he insisted on having the right to send me lengthy e-mails between sessions and expected a response from me. The request was actually a positive development for him, since he had almost no relationships in his life, but it was beyond my usual personal limits regarding e-mail correspondence. I told him that I would stretch my limits and accept his e-mails, doing the best I could to respond in a timely way (nurturance). He was visibly pleased. I then told him that if I was going to stretch my limits, I wanted him to stretch his limits and to keep a record of his eating and sleeping. He agreed immediately.

In another example, the therapist keeps a dialectical balance between a focus on the facts and consequences of the patient's deficits, on the one hand, and a focus on the patient's capabilities, on the other. All of us, and all of our patients, have both deficits and capabilities, and we attend to both in treatment. In treating one young woman who was transitioning from female to male, having begun hormonal treatments and planning to have sex-change surgery, I met with her rather distraught family. Her parents were confused, upset, and unsupportive. She was asking for their approval, but was doing so in a way that was not so skillful, consisting mainly of chastising them for their backward attitudes. Anytime I suggested that I might help her improve her skills in talking with them, she grew defensive and argumentative. I shifted my focus from her deficits in communicating with her parents to the extraordinary courage and fortitude (capabilities) she had shown in continuing on the difficult path she was on with little support. I noted that her family members could probably learn a lot from her if only they could see things from her perspective. She then acknowledged that she was not being very skillful when she talked with them. That's when she asked if I could coach her in her communication skills, which led eventually to family meetings.

To accurately recognize opposing positions, to find the validity on both sides, and to shift back and forth in search of synthesis requires several therapist qualities. First, we need to stay alert, "awake," agile, and responsive. Second, we need to maintain speed, movement, and flow, especially in the face of stalemates, impasses, and conflicts. Third, when we take positions in therapy, whether in concert with a patient or on the opposing side, it is valuable if we can take those positions with certainty, strength, and conviction in the moment, while at the same time being willing to listen to, and see the wisdom in, the other side. For instance, DBT therapists will typically hold patients to the expectations of treatment rather than treating them as fragile, but then will come to the patients' aid, supportively coaching them in trying to meet those expectations that are difficult for them. Finally, DBT therapists work hard to keep the relationship intact, preserving it through inevitable challenges.

THE DIALECTICAL STRATEGIES

Linehan has named and described nine dialectical strategies. Each one describes a particular way to deal with the problem of logjams in therapy characterized by polarization, rigidity, or stasis. I do not describe the strategies here; they are described and illustrated with clinical examples in her DBT treatment manual (Linehan, 1993a). Instead I consider how the dialectical strategies flow from the principles discussed above. My emphasis is on elucidating the essential "formula" for dialectical strategies, such that a therapist might even improvise and create new ones that fit the situation. By keeping our minds on the principles, while applying dialectical strategies, we will "be dialectical" in treatment, alongside "being behavioral" and "being mindful." Being dialectical affects the conduct of DBT more pervasively, so that we are not only resolving logjams, we are breaking up logjams almost before they happen through systemic thinking; speed, movement, and flow; and the awareness and synthesis of opposites.

The most straightforward dialectical strategy is known as *balancing treatment strategies*. All three dialectical principles come into play. The therapist faces an impasse in the patient who is stuck between two opposing positions, or in the therapy relationship, even paralyzed by opposing positions. He tries one or more problem-solving strategies, resulting in no discernible movement. He shifts over to the use of validation and an acceptance-oriented communication style, but this too leads to no change. Pushing for change may set off too much anxiety, fear, shame, or anger. Shifting over to acceptance may set off hopelessness or despair. *Balancing treatment strategies* refers primarily to the acceleration of the pivot between problem solving (change) and acceptance, or the simultaneous use of change and acceptance strategies. For instance, when I was the unit chief on a DBT inpatient program, a 23-year-old female patient asked to speak with me. She complained that her treatment team was extraordinarily rigid in their decision making, refusing to increase her privilege level for weeks. It was her impression that she was engaging in all aspects of treatment, but that they didn't like her "in-your-face" confrontational attitude. She felt she was being punished and had tried everything she knew how to do. Although I was not her therapist, I consulted with her about how she might more effectively deal with the team. I suggested that she might be violating their personal limits by her forceful approach and harsh language, and that she might consider toning it down. She was furious with me for suggesting that she was "doing something wrong." Responding to her tone and to her flat-out rejection of my suggestions, I probably became a bit defensive. As we went back and forth, it felt as if we were both digging in our heels and making no progress. I imagined that this was the nature of her interaction with the team.

While I had begun with the intention of validating her disappointment and anger with the team, I realized that I had rather quickly pushed for her to change her attitude and her approach, to them and then to me. I took a minute to reflect, searching for my "wise mind" response. I suddenly and simply "let go" of trying to change her, and asked if she could give me more detail about the team's approach and how it affected her. My tone was warmer, more interested in her perspective, and I was able to validate several thoughts and emotions. She elaborated on her complaints, I validated her thoughts and feelings, and she then showed some understanding of her team's point of view. As things "softened" between us, I continued to validate her while returning to the question of what she could do differently. By this point she was able to consider making some changes without feeling so threatened or defensive. This shift in her was facilitated by *my* shifting rather quickly between 100% acceptance and then 100% change. Each instance of *balancing treatment strategies* looks different from all others, but each contains this trial-and-error effort to find the most effective balance between genuine acceptance and insistence on change to kindle movement toward behavioral targets and a life worth living.

The therapist uses *entering the paradox* when she recognizes that the patient is in a position, in life or in treatment, where two sides of a contradiction are simultaneously true. Examples abound. In life: To be more fully present requires having attended to the future; to plan the best vacation requires being fully in the present moment; and to be really independent is benefited by a capacity for healthy dependency. In treatment: If we repeatedly rescue our patients, we may lose the opportunity to help them save themselves; and even though someone's problems may have been caused by others, the patient will need to solve them herself. None of these contradictions is difficult to understand, but if the therapist highlights the truth of both sides in the moment, in brief and without explanation, the patient may experience disbelief and confusion while vaguely recognizing the truth in what the therapist is saying. As Linehan (1993a) mentions in the treatment manual, the therapist should refrain from the urge to explain to the confused patient that the paradox "makes sense." The goal is not to educate; the goal is to derail the patient from a stuck position. This approach to therapy is an echo of the earlier innovative work by Milton Erickson, who was a master of paradoxical interventions (Haley, 1973). The therapeutic style for this strategy is to be pithy, brief, matter-of-fact, stating truths that appear to contradict each other. It might be possible to break up the logjam of the moment by purposefully destabilizing the paralyzing homeostasis. For instance, the therapist might say:

"Your behavior makes total sense, and it has to change."
"If I didn't care so much for you, I would try to save you."
"You have the right to kill yourself, and I have the right to stop you."
"If you want to get better at truly being with others, you have to spend more time truly being alone."

Two other dialectical strategies start with the recognition that the patient is engaged in a maladaptive position, almost inviting the therapist to challenge it. The patient holds the maladaptive position; the therapist holds the adaptive position. Both parties dig in their heels in opposition. Suddenly the therapist "leapfrogs" past the patient's maladaptive position, taking a stance that is even more maladaptive than the patient's. If done effectively, the patient is momentarily surprised and thrown off balance, again allowing for the possibility of repositioning and movement. One of these two strategies is the *devil's advocate*, in which the therapist argues the patient's maladaptive position more forcefully than he has (e.g., "Why would you ever want to give up self-cutting behaviors that have been your main solution to distress?"). If done effectively, the therapist's argument catapults the patient toward a more adaptive stance ("But I really have to give up self-cutting behaviors—they are ruining my life!"). The other dialectical strategy in which the therapist proposes a more maladaptive behavior than the patient is called *extending*. The therapist starts with the patient's maladaptive, usually emotionally driven statement (e.g., "I'm quitting therapy; I'm fed up with you"). Rather than arguing against it, he extends it beyond where the patient meant to go (e.g., "So let's find you a therapist who can work better with you; I have a list of possible referrals in my files"), with the hopes that the patient will let go of the argument and articulate the emotion that drives the maladaptive urge (e.g., "You know that I don't really want a different therapist; I'm just really angry at you!"). The therapist uses the understanding of opposition in order to create surprise and prompt movement. It is characteristic of these two strategies, as is the case with all of them, that the therapist has to have (1) an intuitive feel of the current state of things in the patient and in the therapy relationship, and (2) good timing and delivery. Otherwise, all of these interventions fall flat.

Again, starting from the recognition that a stalemate involves the nondialectical balance between two opposing positions, the dialectical strategies of *making lemonade out of lemons* and *eliciting wise mind* are two different ways for therapists to reframe the stalemate. *Making lemonade out of lemons* brings attention to the opportunity that exists within the current crisis. For instance, "I know you hate doing the diary card; it's understandable, almost no one likes it. But your refusal to do it is just perfect for our work, since life presents so many situations like this, where you have to do stuff that is tedious, even troubling, and that makes little sense. You should continue to refuse to do it until it makes sense to you."

The therapist usually applies *eliciting wise mind* when the patient is driven to dysfunctional behavior by "emotion mind." The therapist asks, "If you were in wise mind, what would you say about this situation?" This question allows the patient to maintain the emotion-mind position with all necessary force, and at the same time to identify what a wise mind position would be. Metaphorically, it involves splitting the patient's position into two coexisting, opposing stances.

A 47-year-old female patient of mine was very discouraged about the highly invalidating conditions at her workplace. She could not afford to leave the job, had been unable to find another job with benefits, and felt that she could not stand one more day of the oppressive atmosphere. During the session, her mood grew darker and her sense of urgency intensified. With only a few minutes left in the session, she told me she was quitting the job the next day. She had gotten to this point in the past, but not to this degree.

I asked her, "If you were to quit tomorrow, would that decision be coming from rational mind, emotion mind, or wise mind?" It was not so clear to her, since it struck her as both rational and wise to leave her job, and she felt very emotional and pressured. As I led her through a more thoughtful evaluation of the contribution of the three states of mind, she quickly realized that while it was rational for her to leave her job, and would be wise to find another one, she realized that the urgency was driven by emotion mind. She agreed to work with me toward a wise transition in her life, as well as a wise approach to tolerating her daily work life.

Metaphors provide extraordinary utility in DBT as constructions that can creatively represent polarized situations and systemic thinking, and that can allow for movement in an otherwise stuck situation. They allow dialogue, which may have ground to a halt, to continue on a new plane, within the framework of the metaphor. More ambitiously, they open the possibility of representing opposite positions and finding a way to move toward synthesis. The variety of metaphors is infinite. Some metaphors can be invoked for a moment and then left behind; others may become the framework for an extended piece of work, providing a convenient reference point to which therapist and patient return for weeks or months. Metaphors are not simply another strategy; they are integral to the teaching and practice of DBT. Linehan's (1993a) therapy manual is replete with metaphors in chapter after chapter. Metaphors have been borrowed and adapted among teachers and therapists in the DBT treatment community many times over. Next I give an example of using a metaphor that I first heard from Linehan and that I have adapted to several situations with several patients. It is especially useful for addressing the patient who is maintaining a nonproductive, even self-destructive, stance over time, in spite of ordinary problem solving and validation. The patient is stuck, and the therapist is frustrated.

A bright and capable college student was not progressing at school. She was not doing homework, and she was skipping many classes, watching lots of television, playing videogames every night, and smoking marijuana every day. She acted as if she didn't care, and even though she appeared to appreciate my interventions to help her change, nothing was changing. We had the following dialogue:

THERAPIST: The way I see it, you are in prison. It's a prison of your own making. It's made up of pot, videogames, television, and neglect of your schoolwork, even though you want to graduate. And when we meet each week, it's as if I'm visiting you in prison, and I'm listening to you and giving suggestions, and being a friend, and comforting you, helping you survive prison. But there's another way to visit someone in prison, whereby I try to help the person break out. I bring plans of the infrastructure of the prison, I bring spoons and knives and other tools, I make sure the getaway car is ready, and we plan to get you out. That's what I prefer to do at this point in my career. I want you to think about whether you want me to visit you like a comforting friend, accepting that you have a long sentence, or whether you want help breaking out.

PATIENT: Are you saying you are stopping with me?

THERAPIST: No, I'm telling you that I am realizing that I want to help you break out of your prison. I want to know if you want a partner like that. If you decide you don't want to break out, I have to decide whether I keep doing the comfort work or whether we find someone else to do it, someone who is more suited to that kind of work.

This dialogue helped me to say some of the same things I had been saying to her, but in a different way and with an added element of suspense that created new movement in her. It reframed our work together, and by the next week she had decided she wanted to "break out of jail." We set to work on that task.

Earlier I mentioned the strategy of *allowing natural change*. This strategy flows from an understanding that standstills result from tension between opposites, and an awareness that things are always in flux. Stalemates, especially those regarding conditions and ground rules in the therapy relationship, can be handled by allowing natural change rather than by holding all conditions in place. When meeting for several months with a college student, I began to notice that our sessions usually went about 10 to 15 minutes longer than my usual 50-minute time frame. When 50 minutes were up, I usually found that we were in the middle of an important discussion. For some reason, it seemed to take us 50 minutes to get to a crucial point. When I realized it, I felt I was violating the limits that I had set and was a bit embarrassed about it. I brought it up to the patient: "Have you noticed that we usually go longer than the 50 minutes I told you we would meet for?" Patient: "Of course, I've noticed all along." Me: "Why didn't you say something?" Patient: "I was afraid you would take it away, and I feel like I need it." Me: "I don't know why, but maybe there is some kind of wisdom in our meeting a little longer.

How would you feel if we just agree to 1-hour sessions, and let's see if that works." Patient: "That's good, I would like that." I actually feared that our sessions might then need to be 70 minutes, as if the underlying constant was our tendency to go beyond our designated time, regardless of what it was. In fact, it seemed to work perfectly well over time to meet for 60 minutes.

Finally, there is a dialectical strategy, *dialectical assessment*, which is applied very broadly. It simply means that when we face an impasse, we assume that we are leaving something out, and we open our minds to search for it. I gave an example earlier about the treatment of a patient who engaged in skin-picking behavior. As you may recall, my supervisor, Marsha Linehan, insisted that I continue to assess the behavior with behavioral chain analyses, and that I should assume that I was missing something. By framing what I was doing in that manner, as dialectical assessment, I found that my mind relaxed, opened up, and I came up with a new intervention that broke the logjam.

CREATING NEW DIALECTICAL STRATEGIES

As we consider later in the book, there is no reason to limit one's use of dialectical strategies to nine as described by Linehan. Two new ones, along with the rationale for their development, are presented there. There is something of a formula for creating strategies when we need them, based on the principles of opposition and synthesis, systemic and transactional thinking, and flux. This is an area in which a therapist can be creative and flexible when the usual change and acceptance strategies fail to generate movement.

CONCLUDING COMMENTS

Finally, having given so many examples that sound "out of the box," I feel compelled to make it very clear that a dialectical position or its resulting dialectical intervention is not tricky, contrived, or gimmicky. It flows naturally out of "beginner's mind," a stance in which the therapist is pushing very hard for change; has applied acceptance, validation, and compassion; remains terribly stuck; and lets her mind open up to more options. These interventions come naturally out of being fully engaged, paying attention, searching for what is missing, and genuinely trying to hold onto the wisdom of both sides of a dialectic. They come from truly believing that no one person holds the truth; that the truth evolves from opposing vectors in a reality where everything is interrelated and everything is always changing. And they come from a trial-and-error approach in which everything, within ethical limits and within the essential principles of DBT, is fair game when straightforward interventions are not working. All is fair in love and in DBT, as long as we are treating the targets that lead toward a life worth living for the patient.

CHAPTER 6

The DBT Tree

The Structural Anatomy of DBT

T o this point we have explored the "physiology" of DBT; that is, how it works and flows. In doing so, I have argued that a deep working grasp of the underlying principles of the treatment facilitates flexibility, fluidity, and creativity without sacrificing precision and rigor. Working from principles helps us to navigate challenges in treatment without losing momentum. Some of the value added to the treatment by knowing and using the principles results from keeping the "big picture" in mind: a bird's-eye view of how the treatment flows, and augments the catalogue-like awareness of strategies, skills, and protocols.

Having in mind the big picture of the *frame* of the treatment—what we might call the *anatomy* of DBT—helps as well. It benefits the team that designs and implements a DBT program, the therapists who carry out the treatment, and the consultant who assesses the health of a program in order to make recommendations for improvement. For the individual therapist to understand the desirable anatomy of the treatment frame is invaluable. It helps her in diagnosing "frame problems" that might impact therapy, in catalyzing her efforts to strengthen and correct the frame, and to understand her patients' responses to the overall treatment.

A number of metaphors have helped in the teaching and practice of DBT. As I describe in Chapter 7, on targeting, the "DBT House of Treatment" illustrates the flow of DBT from beginning to end through several stages, each with its central goal and each with its many specific targets.

I created the metaphor of the "DBT Tree" to illustrate the relationship of the various structural elements of the treatment to each other and to the treatment as a whole. These elements include the three sets of principles; the biosocial theory; the ultimate goal of a life worth living; the goals, stages, and targets; the functions and modes; the various sets of agreements made by patients, therapists, and teams; the sets of assumptions about patients and about therapy; and the entire collection of strategies used in DBT (which includes the skills). The DBT Tree, illustrated in Figure 6.1, functions as a guide in several ways:

- To understand DBT, it depicts this huge, multifaceted treatment in a manner that allows us to see all of the parts and their interrelationships.
- To implement DBT, the tree serves as a blueprint of a comprehensive DBT program, diagramming all essential ingredients, allow-

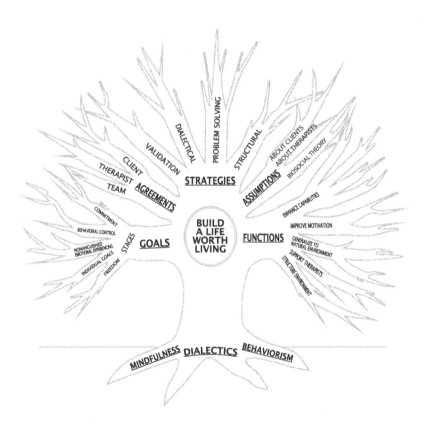

FIGURE 6.1. The DBT Tree.

ing the implementation team to consider the presence and strength of all parts of the treatment and their relationship to each other.

- To adapt DBT to a different population or context, the implementation team can systematically consider which aspects of the original model program to preserve (as much as possible!) and which to modify.
- To consult with an existing DBT program, the DBT Tree serves as a mechanism for systematically assessing the roots, the trunk, and all branches, large and small, locating strengths and weaknesses, leading to a plan for strengthening the program.

FACTORS IN THE CONTEXT OF THE DBT TREE

In using the metaphor of a tree to represent the elements of a DBT program, we immediately realize that the tree grows within an environment. The nature, viability, and strength of the tree will be both facilitated and constrained by three environmental elements: the *soil* in which the roots grow, the *vegetation* surrounding the tree, and the *climate*. Each of these elements has its counterpart in the context in which a DBT program grows. Just as the constitution of the soil determines the availability of nutritional ingredients for the tree's development, the intellectual and organizational context in which a DBT program grows will nourish or deprive the program of needed "nutrients." Just as the nature of surrounding vegetation strengthens or limits the possibilities for a particular tree to thrive, the nature of surrounding programs and organizations will strengthen or limit the likelihood that a particular DBT program will thrive there. And just as the climatic variables of sunshine, wind, rain, and temperature will select for some types of trees over others, the resources available in a given programmatic context will determine whether DBT programs get enough of what they need to take root, grow, and survive.

The Soil: Acceptance, Change, and Dialectics

Let's consider the role of the "soil" in more detail. A DBT program needs three types of nutrients from its organizational soil, corresponding to the three underlying paradigms of DBT. It needs those nutrients that support mindfulness by promoting acceptance, behaviorism by pushing for behavioral change, and dialectics by advancing the principles in the worldview of dialectics. The administrator of a new DBT program, or the individual assessing the strength of an established program, would be wise to "sample the soil" in which that program grows, asking whether it includes the nutrients to support mindfulness, behaviorism, and dialectics. If imbalances or deficiencies are found, there may be ways to fortify or rebalance the soil to get the right mixture.

I first implemented DBT on an inpatient unit in a large psychiatric hospital that had grown out of a long tradition of providing a compassionate "retreat" for those with mental illness. Beautiful and pastoral, the hospital was also rich in biological and psychoanalytic traditions. Research, with its emphasis on objectivity, played an important role, as did the effort to understand people in depth and empathize with them. In this respect, the soil included some nutrients to support the roots of acceptance in DBT. Furthermore, and not entirely by coincidence, several members of the original DBT implementation team had practiced various forms of meditation for years. The "mindfulness titer" of the soil was rich enough to support the roots of the acceptance paradigm.

However, the soil was deficient in the nutrients that would support the behavioral roots of DBT. In fact, there were some "anti-behavioral" elements. Behaviorism was rarely studied or taught in a systematic way, and opinion leaders often made comments suggesting that behavioral therapy was simplistic and superficial compared to the psychoanalytic tradition. Once the members of the implementation team understood that DBT, at its core, was a CBT, they realized that in growing a DBT program, they would need to enhance the behavioral nutrients of the soil. For the following year, those seven individuals arranged for cognitive-behavioral training with faculty members in a nearby city. During the weekly drives, team members began to design the DBT inpatient program. Once the DBT program was under way, clinicians continued to find ways to supplement the behavioral elements in the soil through reading and participating in study groups and outside training experiences. Still, even with all of that, the local nutritional deficiency created an ongoing vulnerability in the DBT program, in which the clinical reflexes remained more psychoanalytic than would have been ideal for DBT.

It's not so easy to determine whether the soil in which a program grows contains nutrients that support the dialectical roots of DBT. Whereas one can easily identify traditions that include mindfulness, empathy, or compassion, and those that nurture a cognitive-behavioral framework, those traditions supporting dialectical thinking and practice are less likely to be clearly evident. Still, deep familiarity with a particular organizational context may make it possible to see that the soil may or may not support flexible, creative, "out-of-the-box" thinking or tolerate and value differences and conflict. Rigid, hierarchical systems that prescribe the "right way" to think and to act, and that show little tolerance for opposing positions, are not as likely to nurture systemic thinking and dialectical processes.

The hospital context in which we developed our inpatient DBT program had elements that facilitated dialectical thinking and other elements that constrained it. The organization was heavily influenced by a medical model with typical organizational hierarchies. Decision making was often "top-down"; deviation and unconventionality could be subject to suppression and disapproval. At the same time, it was an academic center with highly creative faculty and programs, valuing innovation. As a relatively large and complex institution, it contained a number of "micro-environments" that supported improvisation and embraced the wisdom of valuing both sides of a conflict. One factor that allowed for the improbable growth of a DBT program in a hospital in which psychoanalysis prevailed was the location of the program within a service (one of the micro-environments) that was directed by a creative administrator who embraced a variety of competing models. He valued the DBT program and served as a buffer between the program and the prevailing organizational dynamics.

When I consult on the initial design of a DBT program, I typically use the DBT Tree as an architectural template, and in doing so, I quickly raise the question about the nature of the organizational soil, trying to anticipate the strengths and deficiencies of the nutrients, and sometimes prompt the implementation team to brainstorm possibilities for enhancing the soil mix. In spite of the best intentions of a creative implementation team, a serious deficiency of nutrients supporting mindfulness, behaviorism, or dialectics will cause a deviation from the ideal balance for DBT.

The Vegetation Surrounding the Tree: Programs and Philosophies in the Environment

As critical as analyzing and correcting the soil mix, it is also worthwhile to consider the influence of surrounding forms of "vegetation," by which I refer to the other treatment philosophies and programs sharing the same resource pool. During the 1990s, when DBT programs began to take root across the United States and in other Western countries, it was interesting to notice where they seemed to thrive and where they didn't. In the northeastern United States, where I was located and where I did considerable training and consultation, DBT programs quickly flourished in community mental health settings that were relatively rural yet also had some community-oriented resources. Large parts of the states of Maine, New Hampshire, Vermont, and Connecticut, and the Canadian province of New Brunswick, served as hosts to early DBT developments. Major state-funded implementation projects occurred across New Hampshire and Connecticut, as well as in the Midwest. In contrast, there was a notable absence of early program development in New York City or other major urban centers. Through my work consulting in urban centers, it appeared that there was less "room" for DBT programs to grow and thrive. Mental health programming was heavily influenced by major academic medical centers peopled by passionate treatment developers and researchers who favored their preferred models of care, such as psychoanalysis, biological psychiatry, or various trauma-informed treatments. When DBT practitioners developed small programs within psychoanalytically oriented environments, implementers often fought for space, resources, and respect. It was difficult to "grow DBT" in an environment where it was viewed merely as a circumscribed protocol offering skills specifically to those with self-injurious behaviors, rather than being seen as a comprehensive model of psychotherapy for a group of complex disorders. As DBT eventually won respectability based on the steady growth of the evidence base in randomized controlled trials, and through championing by local DBT clinicians, these centers changed their attitude and DBT grew in stature and application.

In contrast, when DBT was introduced as a new sibling of the cognitive-behavioral family in contexts already rich in behaviorally oriented treatments, DBT could thrive, and significant cross-fertilization of programming and resources between DBT and CBT took place. A new model needs space and time to grow. It requires mutual cross-fertilization between this new approach and existing programs in the surrounding environment. The lesson for those implementing DBT is to consider the competing "vegetation" in the chosen context, and to build bridges with other organizations, programs, and models in the area.

The Climate: Resources for the DBT Tree

Along with soil and vegetation, likewise climate determines the strength of a tree. By *climate* in the natural environment I refer to certain kinds of resources: rain, sun, wind, and temperature. Corresponding resources in the atmosphere of a DBT program would include money, time, personnel, materials, space, and so on. If a DBT program is situated in a mental health center in a state or province that has committed itself philosophically and financially to regional DBT development, and if the executive and clinical leadership of the mental health center supports DBT implementation, the program more often thrives. There is sufficient rain and sufficient sun. If a hospital or mental health system sends several individuals for DBT training, but then fails to understand the need for ongoing allocation of resources to support the project, it can be likened to transplanting a sapling during the summer but then failing to provide the needed daily watering.

I once consulted with a public sector agency in a bordering state that had sent a very talented young clinician to a DBT intensive training. That agency decided it lacked the resources to send more than one clinician, so the sole clinician joined three clinicians from a program in a neighboring county in order to constitute a "DBT team" for the training. She brought her new knowledge and passion for implementing DBT back to her agency, started a DBT skills group, coached the patients by phone to use their skills, and did her best to interest other therapists in DBT. Although pleased to have DBT established in his agency, the medical director refused to support assigning another clinician to the DBT project. The DBT-trained individual worked hard for the following year, but her energy began to flag as she endeavored to establish an enduring program. Despite the tremendous efforts of this one dedicated clinician to compensate for the deficiency of resources, the result was a tree with areas of strength, where resources were available, and areas of weakness, where they were not. Aware of her own impending burnout, she invited me for a clinical and programmatic consultation. Skillfully, she arranged for the medical director to have lunch with me (she paid for it herself!). As it turned out, this intervention led to an infusion of resources that allowed the small program to flourish, with her as the in-house DBT champion, and garner several willing followers. As important as the nutrients in the soil, and the impact of surrounding vegetation, the program lives or dies, thrives or shrinks, based on the climatic resources that "fall from the administrative skies." The lesson for those implementing DBT programs is that the initial design should take into account the contextual factors corresponding to the soil, surrounding vegetation, and climatic resources in defining the scope and projected growth of the implementation. Correctly assessing the contextual reality in advance will lead to a realistic and successful startup, even if smaller than desired, rather than suffering through the headaches that occur when a more ambitious startup lacks necessary resources.

THE BRANCHES OF THE TREE

As I have already mentioned, the three major root systems of the DBT Tree represent the three paradigms and their associated principles. The trunk represents the ultimate goal of DBT: a life worth living. Extending from the trunk are five large branches; four of them (two on each side) represent the structuring of the treatment, and the fifth (a particularly large one at the top), represents all of the treatment strategies of DBT. To grasp all of DBT is to intimately know the many details inherent in the roots, the trunk, and the five branches. Most DBT workshops, whether short or long, are structured around an agenda that coincides with what is represented by the roots, the trunk, and the five branches of the DBT tree.

The first chapter was devoted to the life-worth-living conversation. The trunk represents this ultimate goal of the treatment. Whether the particular DBT adaptation is designed to treat self-harming behaviors, suicide attempts, eating disorders, substance use disorders, dissociative disorders, antisocial disorders, or others, they all still converge around the central goal of helping to build each individual patient's version of a life worth living. Whereas the roots and the trunk remain the same, the branches of the tree may adopt different configurations depending on the population to which DBT is applied, and the treatment context in which it takes place.

Emerging from the trunk are four large branches, two on each side, that represent the way the treatment is structured. Represented in the order in which I discuss them, these are the *Goals Branch*, the *Functions Branch*, the *Assumptions and Theory Branch*, and the *Agreements Branch*. These individual branches have features in common. Each branch represents a major and necessary structural element of DBT. Each branch is at its largest when it departs from the trunk, then extends to increasingly fine-tuned branches. The large part of each branch, closest to the trunk, represents an element in DBT that is relatively the same from program to program; it represents a necessary ingredient of a DBT structure. The finer and finer branches represent elements of a DBT program that might be adapted to the particular context and particular patient population. In other words, these finer branches represent aspects of DBT that may be modified to fit the circumstances of each program. Next, I describe each major branch in more detail to show how this process unfolds.

The Goals Branch

It makes most sense to look first at the large branch that represents the goals, stages, and targets of the DBT program for each patient. Let's call it the *Goals Branch*. Extending out from the large Goals Branch closest to the trunk, we find a few branches, each of which represents one overarching goal of treatment. Each of those overarching goals will be the focus of one stage of treatment. DBT seeks to actualize the patient's "life worth living" through a sequence of stages, each one with a goal. In standard outpatient DBT, there are five overarching goals, which means there are five stages, and on the accompanying picture of the tree there are five branches representing them.

Keep in mind that in some adaptations of DBT there are likely to be a different number of overarching goals to fit the circumstances. For instance, in short-term inpatient DBT there might be just three stages, each with a goal: (1) *getting in*, which involves successfully entering the program and making a commitment to treatment; (2) *getting in control*, which involves stabilizing serious symptoms and achieving the needed degree of behavioral control; and (3) *getting out*, which involves the development and execution of a successful discharge plan. Note that even though the short-term inpatient application of DBT will have a number of variations from the standard outpatient tree on every branch, the five major branches will be the same: Goals, Functions, Agreements, Assumptions, and Strategies. The variations appear on the finer branches.

Let's consider the five branches of the Goals Branch in standard outpatient DBT.

- The first branch represents the initial stage of treatment, known as *pretreatment*, and corresponds to the goal of entering treatment, becoming oriented, making agreements, and committing to the treatment plan.
- The second branch represents the next stage of treatment, known as *Stage 1*, and focuses on replacing chaotic and destructive behavioral patterns with greater stability and control.
- The third branch represents the next stage of treatment, known as *Stage 2*, and works on replacing emotional anguish with reduced suffering and improved emotional processing.
- The fourth branch represents the next stage of treatment, known as *Stage 3*, and addresses individual life goals and increasing self-respect.
- The fifth branch represents the final stage of treatment, known as *Stage 4*, and aims to establish a sense of freedom, meaning, and sustained joy.

Having identified the five stages with the five overarching goals around which DBT is structured, we can now consider the finer branches extending out from each of the five goals. The work on each of the five overarching goals takes place through accomplishing a sequential series of treatment targets. For instance, the goal of Stage 1 in DBT is to replace disorder and dyscontrol with more stability and regulation. The treatment targets leading to that goal, represented by the four fine branches extending out from the Stage 1 branch are to (1) decrease life-threatening behaviors, (2) decrease therapy-interfering behaviors, (3) decrease severe quality-of-life-interfering behaviors, and (4) increase behavioral skills. Sometimes even finer branches extend out from a given treatment target branch, representing "subtargets" on the way to accomplishing that treatment target. For instance, when the therapist works with the patient to decrease substance use, a severe quality-of-life-interfering behavior, the task is broken down into several sequential subtargets on the way to eliminating the target of substance use. In Chapter 7, on targeting, we consider the ways in which the DBT therapist uses the prioritized list of treatment targets to structure the agenda of therapy with a given patient; and how the director of a DBT program uses the goals, stages, and targets to structure a coherent, effective, and motivating agenda for the entire program.

When a clinician designs and implements a new DBT program to apply the treatment to a clinical population or treatment context that is different from the original programs, she can use the tree as a template. She considers each of the five major branches of the original DBT Tree and asks, "What modifications do I need to consider for each branch?" When considering the Goals Branch, she asks, "Do I expect my patients to proceed through the five overarching stages and goals in the standard model, or do I need to consider a modification?" For each of the overarching goals, she then needs to ask, "Do I expect my patients to proceed through the same specific treatment targets as outlined in the standard model, or rather consider modifying the targets because of our population or our treatment context?" And in defining the treatment targets, she may need to ask herself, "Are the treatment targets specific enough, or do I need to spell out more specific subtargets for any of these targets?" The visual representation provided by the tree helps to focus on the question of what modifications will be required. For instance, when I represented acute inpatient DBT as a tree, there were three overarching goals rather than five, three corresponding stages of treatment, and for each goal or stage I specified the treatment targets for that goal or stage. The template of the tree helps us to systematically consider the range of options and choices when adapting DBT.

The Functions Branch

If we move to the other side of the tree as pictured, we see another large primary branch extending out from the trunk representing the functions of DBT. Much as the Goals Branch quickly subdivided into the five major goals of a standard DBT program, the Functions Branch quickly subdivides into the five major functions that we find in a standard and comprehensive DBT program. These five functions are to . . .

1. Enhance patient capabilities.
2. Improve patient motivation.
3. Generalize the patient's capabilities to the natural environment.
4. Increase the capabilities and improve the motivation of therapists.
5. Structure the treatment environment.

These five functions apply to all comprehensive DBT programs, in whatever contexts and with whatever patient populations. These five basic and specific functions are depicted as the parts of the Functions Branch most proximal to the trunk, the parts that remain most constant across different program implementations. Each of these five functions then subdivides further into the *modes* of the treatment program through which those functions are accomplished. The modes might be considered the concrete vehicles that "carry" those functions. The typical modes of the original standard outpatient DBT program were (1) skills training (to enhance patient capabilities), (2) individual psychotherapy (to improve patient motivation), (3) telephone coaching calls between patient and therapist (to generalize the patient's enhanced capabilities to the natural environment), (4) DBT consultation team meetings (to generalize capabilities and improve motivation in the therapists), and (5) the DBT director and case manager (to structure the treatment environment).

In parallel with our discussion of the Goals Branch, these smaller branches representing the modes of treatment, each extending out from a larger branch representing functions, are likely to vary depending on the type of DBT program. For instance, whereas the primary mode in standard outpatient DBT, subserving the function of motivating the patient, is individual psychotherapy, with inpatient and other milieu-based DBT programs, the function of motivation may be targeted in group therapy meetings, community meetings, one-to-one check-ins in the milieu, and possibly peer-to-peer programming (where patients motivate each other, as occurs in 12-step programs). In another example, in standard outpatient DBT the primary mode for generalizing patients' capabilities is the coaching telephone call, but in community mental health systems, the case manager or outreach counselor may "carry" the function of generalization through *in vivo* coaching of the patient in the community. Understanding this way of modifying the outer branches of the tree—in this case, considering which modes would be the most effective in "carrying" certain predefined functions—affords the implementation team a range of creativity in adapting the essential ingredients of DBT to varying conditions.

When a program lacks the conditions or resources to be truly comprehensive, program leaders might choose to limit the number of branches, and therefore the number of treatment functions, that extends out from the Functions Branch. Rather than doing a comprehensive implementation, the program leaders choose to do a selective implementation of DBT. For instance, an inpatient program with limited resources for DBT might select the functions of enhancing capabilities (skills training), generalizing skills to the inpatient environment (skills coaching by frontline clinical staff), structuring the inpatient environment (schedules, privilege systems, contingency plans), and supporting the inpatient staff (consultation team meetings). For anyone designing a DBT program, the Functions Branch takes center stage because it represents the program's level of comprehensiveness and the nature of the modes, answering the pragmatic question, What kind of treatment is this and how comprehensive is it?

The Assumptions and Theory Branch

The next branch to consider, thinner than the prior two but of crucial importance, is the one that includes the working theory and assumptions in DBT. These two aspects of DBT are located on the same branch because they are comprised of the hypotheses and assumptions that guide the DBT clinician. Ultimately, both the theory and the assumptions should be subjected to testing and validation through research, but for now, the Assumptions Branch represents what you might call the "working philosophy" of DBT. This branch quickly subdivides into two branches: one representing DBT's biosocial theory, the other representing the assumptions made in DBT. Because Linehan (1993a, pp. 106–118) has detailed a set of assumptions about patients and a set of assumptions about therapy, the assumptions sub-branch itself divides in two. Nearly all adaptations of DBT include the biosocial theory, as originally outlined by Linehan (1993a, pp. 42–65), and the original assumptions about therapy and patients. However, in certain cases where DBT is conducted with a nonstandard population or in a nonstandard treatment context, program implementers may modify an assumption, or more commonly, add one or two assumptions appropriate to the specific situation. For instance, some inpatient DBT programs have added assumptions appropriate to inpatient care, such as the assumption that inpatient life, with locked doors and round-the-clock circumstances, is stressful; or another one stating that any skills acquired on an inpatient program must be generalized to outpatient life. Specialized DBT programs for individuals with substance use disorders, eating disorders, antisocial disorders, or with cognitive limitations, might add one or two specialized assumptions. These are best derived after using standard DBT treatment long enough to realize which modifications make sense.

The other sub-branch of the Assumptions Branch represents the biosocial theory. It quickly subdivides into three smaller branches representing the central factors of the theory: (1) the biologically based emotional vulnerabilities; (2) the invalidating environment; and (3) the severe, chronic emotional dysregulation, which is the product of the transaction between the first two. Each of these three branches undergoes further subdivisions to represent, respectively, features of emotional vulnerabilities, characteristics of invalidating environments, and features of severe emotional dysregulation. Although DBT's biosocial theory, as originally formulated, is central to nearly all adaptations of DBT and is currently subject to considerable research verification, there are occasions when the theory may require modification to fit a population with different characteristics. For instance, in formulating the factors that cause and maintain the behavioral patterns in individuals with antisocial personality traits, forensic DBT experts have suggested that the fine branch representing "increased emotional sensitivity" may need to be replaced by "reduced emotional sensitivity."

As we proceed to consider the details of the numerous branches, large and small, we can begin to notice that changes in any one branch may result in changes in several other branches. To revise the "emotional sensitivity branch" to the "reduced emotional sensitivity branch" changes the biosocial theory, which could possibly result in modifications to the branches representing assumptions, targets, and strategies. It is a reminder that systemic thinking, in which a change in any one part results in changes in other parts of a system, applies to implementation as much as it does to therapy.

The Agreements Branch

The fourth branch to consider is the one representing the agreements made in a DBT program. This branch quickly subdivides into three smaller branches in standard outpatient DBT, representing three sets of agreements: (1) those made by the patient; (2) those made by the therapist; and (3) those made by members of the DBT consultation team.

The agreements made by patients, across various DBT programs, include certain predictable types: a "duration agreement" regarding the agreed-upon length of treatment, an "attendance agreement" specifying the expectations regarding attendance at various treatment meetings; "treatment target agreements" specifying that in order to be in the DBT program, patients must target suicidal behaviors and behaviors that interfere with treatment; a "skills training agreement" stipulating the necessity of taking part in the skills training program; and a "research and payment agreement" stipulating the patient's obligations with regards to research measures and payment. In certain adaptations of DBT, standard agreements may be modified, or specialized agreements appropriate to that context may be added. For instance, when DBT was adapted for teenagers and their families, the "duration agreement" was modified to a shorter time period (16 weeks rather than 1 year), based on the assessment that teens may experience 1 year of treatment as eternity and will be very unlikely to commit to it. In DBT for residential programs that have a daily schedule of groups and activities beyond the usual skills training program in standard DBT, agreements might be made regarding attendance at other meetings. In DBT programs for substance use disorders, there are often agreements regarding random urine screening for substances and the use of "replacement drugs" during treatment. As mentioned when discussing the Assumptions Branch, implementation teams are advised to try the standard model, using the standard assumptions and agreements, and in response to implementation experience consider modifying and adding agreements as indicated. In implementation, one wants to remain as close as possible to the model that has been demonstrated by research to be effective, and yet make sensible modifications that enhance the fit with the new circumstances (Koerner, Dimeff, & Swenson, 2007).

In parallel with the branch representing patient agreements in DBT are two other agreement branches: those representing therapist agreements and those representing therapist consultation team agreements. Linehan (1993a, pp. 112–118) initially listed six agreements in each category. Much like discussing modifications to the patient agreements, program leaders must review each agreement in these categories to see how it fits in each individualized program. In the case of therapist agreements, we can expect that adapted programming will include revisions and/or add-ons suited to the context. In the case of therapist consultation team agreements, I have not yet encountered a DBT program of any type that modifies the six team agreements originally laid down. They have stood the test of time, as they are remarkably effective at creating a healthy team atmosphere.

The Strategies Branch

Given that DBT includes upward of 80 strategies, the fifth and final branch for us to consider, depicted as extending out from the top of the trunk, represents the targets and is known as the Strategies Branch. The other four branches represent the framing of the treatment (goals, stages, targets, functions, modes, assumptions, biosocial theory, and agreements). This branch represents the "doing" of it. The Strategies Branch, most appropriately depicted as the one arising out of the top of the trunk, quickly subdivides into five branches, each still rather large: change-based strategies, acceptance-based strategies, dialectical strategies, structural strategies, and special treatment strategies. The acceptance-based strategies sit to the left of the other groups, representing their intimate relationship to the tree roots of the acceptance paradigm, which are to the left of the other sets of roots. Similarly, the change-based strategies lie to the right, just as the behavioral principles are represented as the rightmost root system. The dialectical strategies, somewhere in the middle, parallel the position of the dialectical principles as the root system in the middle. Also found relatively in the center of the categories of strategies are the structural and special strategies categories, oriented neither toward acceptance nor change.

The acceptance-based strategies branch quickly subdivides into three smaller branches, representing (respectively) the validation strategies, reciprocal communication strategies (one type of stylistic communication strategy), and environmental intervention strategies (one type of case management strategy). All of these strategy groups share the focus of accepting the patient as he or she is in the moment. The change-based strategies branch quickly subdivides into three smaller branches, representing (respectively) the problem-solving strategies, the irreverent communication strategies (one type of stylistic communication strategy), and the consultation-with-the-patient strategies (one type of case management strategy). All of these strategy groups share the focus of pushing for behavioral change. The dialectical strategies branch subdivides to fine branches representing the nine dialectical strategies described by Linehan (1993a, pp. 201–219). Structural strategies focus on how the DBT therapist structures therapy sessions throughout the entire treatment. The structural strategies branch quickly subdivides into five smaller branches representing (1) contracting strategies, (2) session-beginning strategies, (3) targeting strategies, (4) session-ending strategies, and (5) terminating strategies. Each of these five structural strategies extends to finer branches representing the steps and strategies for their application. Special treatment strategies address specific problems and issues in treatment with patients who have severe and chronic emotional dysregulation. The special treatment strategies branch quickly subdivides into six smaller branches representing strategies for addressing (1) patient crises, (2) suicidal behaviors, (3) patient therapy-interfering behaviors, (4) telephone calls, (5) ancillary treatments, and (6) patient–therapist relationship issues. And of course each of these six further subdivides into the particular steps and strategies to accomplish each of them.

Like other branches, the larger strategy branches closer to the trunk are relatively invariant across programs; that is, all DBT programs use acceptance, change, dialectical, structural, and special treatment strategy groups. But extending out each of these branches, the presence and prominence of particular strategy groups and strategies vary depending on the program. For instance, when McCann and colleagues adapted DBT for use in their secure forensic facility, they added strategies and skills that were useful in the treatment of individuals with antisocial disorders (McCann, Ball, & Ivanoff, 2000). When Brown (2016) adapted DBT for individuals with developmental disabilities and cognitive deficits, she added a 10-set "skills system" and a range of treatment strategies to adapt DBT to the unique characteristics of the patient population.

APPLICATION: MODIFYING DBT FOR TREATMENT OF SUBSTANCE USE DISORDERS

Having presented the DBT Tree piece by piece, from roots to trunk to all five branches, I now demonstrate the usefulness of the metaphor by illustrating the modifications that were made to standard DBT when it was adapted for use with individuals with substance use disorders. In this demonstration, I scan the entire tree, from bottom to top, considering where modifications are needed, realizing that the same process could be used to envision modifications of standard DBT for any population other than Linehan's original target population. Beginning at the roots, we find, as usual, that the elements remain the same. In DBT for substance use disorders (DBT-SUDs), we use the same principles of acceptance, change, and dialectics that we use in standard DBT. In fact, the Serenity Prayer, a foundation of Alcoholics Anonymous and other 12-step programs, captures the three paradigms perfectly: "Grant me the serenity to accept what I cannot change, the courage to change what I can, and the wisdom to know the difference." The roots then converge into the trunk, which represents the ultimate aim of DBT: to build a life worth living. Again we find no difference between standard DBT and DBT-SUDs. The individual with a substance use disorder along with chronic and severe emotional dysregulation works with the therapist to envision and build a life worth living, aligned with a hopeful view of the future consistent with his or her values. Because of the damaging role of substance use in these patients' lives, therapists working with this population can emphasize the added point of attempting to build a life worth living *without relying on substances*.

We begin to find the significant modifications as we consider the major branches of the tree. As we shall see, the theme is, on branch after branch, that those factors represented as most proximal to the trunk on the DBT-SUDs Tree are likely to be very similar, if not identical, to the factors proximal to the trunk in standard DBT. More modifications are found as we move out from the trunk to the secondary and tertiary branches. Starting with the Goals Branch (see Figure 6.2), we find that the major goals of the treatment, worked on sequentially through the various stages, are the same as they are in standard DBT. Both treatments, if done comprehensively, move sequentially through (1) getting a commitment (pretreatment); (2) establishing behavioral control (Stage 1); (3) acquiring the capacity for nonanguished emotional experiencing (Stage 2); (4) pursuing individual goals and self-respect (Stage 3); and (5) increasing the experience of freedom, meaning, and joy (Stage 4).

Having established that no modification is required in naming the five goals and stages, the challenge arises as we decide, in the step-by-step treatment agenda, where to target substance-use-related behaviors: in the pretreatment stage in which orientation, agreement, and commitment take place?; in Stage 1, in which behavioral dyscontrol is addressed?; in Stage 2, in which ongoing suffering is addressed?; in Stage 3, in which problems in living are addressed?; or in Stage 4, in which problems with freedom, meaning, and joy are addressed? Having this framework to begin helps to organize the questions and figure out the answers. Substance use disorders would be addressed in pretreatment insofar as there would be an orientation about the treatment of substance use disorders in the program, agreements about the expectations of substance-related behavioral patterns and the targeting of those patterns, and a focus on obtaining the strongest possible commitment to reducing or abstaining from using substances. Beyond pretreatment, substance use disorders will most commonly be targeted in Stage 1, where the program helps each patient establish more stability, control, and connection to replace instability, impulsivity, and chaos.

Still, since Stage 1 typically consists of work on four target categories—life-threatening behaviors, therapy-interfering behaviors, severe quality-of-life-interfering behaviors, and the enhancement of skills—the question remains where to target substance use behaviors among these four. Obvi-

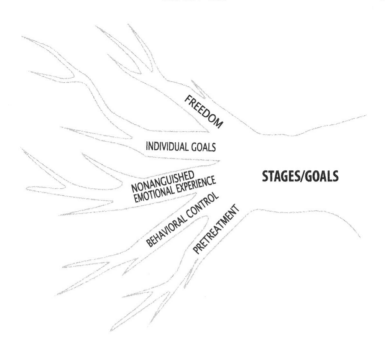

FIGURE 6.2. Goals, stages, and targets as modified for DBT for substance use disorders.

ously, if substance use behaviors belonged to an imminent life-threatening pattern, they would be targeted under the first target category, reducing life-threatening behaviors. Although chronic substance use is a destructive pattern that will erode life and could eventually result in life-threatening behaviors, it is the exception rather than the rule that the substance use itself is imminently life-threatening. If substance use behaviors were part of a pattern of therapy-interfering behaviors, they would be targeted under the second target category of reducing therapy-interfering behaviors. This often is the case when patients routinely miss sessions because they arrive intoxicated and are unable to make good use of treatment, call for coaching while intoxicated and therefore cannot appropriately use coaching, or fail to learn skills because they rely on the substances to enhance their capabilities (as they see it).

But most commonly, it turns out that the targeting of substance use behaviors takes place in the third target category of reducing severe, quality-of-life-interfering behaviors—those behavioral patterns that positively erode the possibility of solving life problems, ensuring a spiraling path toward the destruction of hopes and dreams. Typically, the targeting of substance use behaviors in those who agree to target them takes place as the highest priority in the treatment of quality-of-life-interfering behaviors.

Having determined where—that is, in which stage and as part of which category of treatment targets—to locate the treatment of substance use behaviors, we still need to specify the substance-use subtarget behaviors that will comprise our agenda when we are trying to help the patient eliminate or reduce substance use. It is not enough to simply "reduce substance use"; this wording provides an overly general goal. We can use a strategy to determine the specific subtargets of substance use, and just as that same strategy can be used when breaking down the specific component behaviors to be treated with other disorders, such as eating disorders, antisocial disorders, and so on. In fact, I apply that strategy to define the treatment agenda for binge eating disorder in the next chapter.

We begin by specifying the primary behavior to be reduced. In the case of substance use disorders, the primary subtarget is to "reduce or eliminate using." Now imagine that the patient has stopped using her primary substance. She would then probably face the physical distress of withdrawal or the emergence of physical pain that has been suppressed by the substance. Therefore, the next subtarget is to "decrease physical distress." Taking it a step further, if substance use has been eliminated and physical distress has been reduced or is better tolerated, the patient will continue to encounter urges and cravings to use the substance. So, "reducing urges and cravings" becomes the subtarget behavior that follows "decreasing physical distress." If any of these are ignored or are taken for granted, the patient risks resuming active substance use. Once the individual stops using, has decreased physical distress, and can readily tolerate urges and cravings, several other substance-related subtargets show up in the foreground, such as reducing the option to use substances. Within DBT-SUDs, this step-by-step treatment of subtargets in substance use is called "the path to clear mind":

- Decrease substance use.
- Decrease physical distress associated with substance use.
- Decrease urges, cravings, and temptations to use substances.
- Decrease the option to use drugs.
- Decrease contact with cues for drug use.
- Increase reinforcement for "clear mind" behaviors.
- Clear mind (a state of mind resulting from the reinforcement and consolidation of clear mind behaviors).

To review how all of this is represented on the tree: The subtargets within the path to clear mind are most commonly represented as fine branches extending out from the branch, as part of Stage 1, representing the decrease in quality-of-life-interfering behaviors. Whereas it is cumbersome to spell out all these components sequentially in words, the picture of the tree with its primary, secondary, and tertiary branches is worth a thousand words.

When we move on to the Functions Branch of the DBT-SUDs Tree (see Figure 6.3), again we find essentially no modifications in the branches of the five functions most proximal to the trunk. But as we extend out from each function to the finer branches representing modes that "carry" those functions, we find modifications and additions. For instance, as we move from "enhancing capabilities," where we find the typical modes

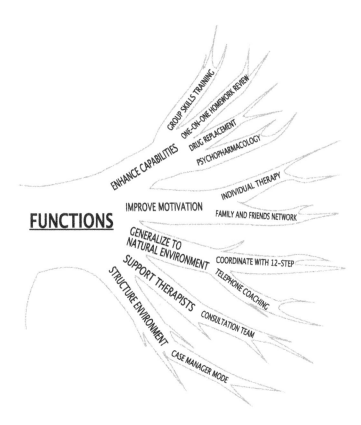

FIGURE 6.3. Functions and modes as modified for DBT for substance use disorders.

of skills training and psychopharmacology, we may find modifications of the skills training mode to address certain typical features of those who abuse substances. When Linehan in a personal report discovered the extremely high rate of social anxiety disorders among individuals with substance use disorders, which made it a challenge for them to share their homework in a group, she created a one-on-one mode for homework practice review, while keeping the group setting for teaching new skills. Furthermore, a "drug replacement mode," such as the use of methadone and other chemical agents to replace the use of heroin, was added to the function of enhancing capabilities. In addition, several substance-abuse-specific skills were added to the manual and are represented by fine-tuned additions to the skill set out of the group skills training mode.

Enhancing capabilities is not the only function with modifications for the treatment of substance abuse. The function that involves structuring the treatment, which usually is carried out by a DBT program director, is often augmented by another mode: case management. The case manager helps the patient to structure a functional life. Additionally, the treatment structure may include yet another mode, random drug testing, which is used to monitor progress. A third function, the generalization of skills to the natural environment, which is usually enacted through telephone coaching, is sometimes furthered by collaborating with 12-step programs such as Alcoholics Anonymous and Narcotics Anonymous through which the patient has a sponsor to turn to for support during the week. Finally, extending out from the branch representing the function of improving the patient's motivation, which is usually carried out through the mode of individual therapy, Linehan (Dimeff & Koerner, 2007, pp. 160–161) added several attachment strategies: a specific orientation to the patient regarding the attachment problem, increased contact early in therapy in order to strengthen the engagement, actively pursuing patients when they get "lost" from treatment, and building connections with important family members and friends early in treatment. Obviously some of these added attachment strategies also served another function: structuring the treatment environment.

The modifications of the Agreements Branch and the Assumptions and Theory Branch when adapting DBT to substance use disorders are relatively minor, and mainly involve adding whatever assumptions, agreements, and elements of theory that are indicated for targeting substance abuse behaviors. But the modifications of the final major branch, the Strategies Branch, are significant and numerous, identified and illustrated in Figure 6.4. I refer the reader to Dimeff and Koerner (2007) to read about the modifications of strategies for DBT-SUDs in more detail. Here are the strategies:

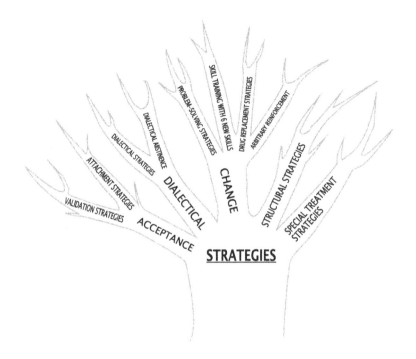

FIGURE 6.4. Strategies as modified for DBT for substance use disorders.

1. Attachment to address the typical deficiency in the strength of attachment from the substance-using patient toward the therapist (there are several of these).
2. Arbitrary reinforcement strategies to reinforce abstinence.
3. Drug replacement strategies to reduce relapse to use of the primary substance.
4. Skills training, including the teaching of each DBT skill as applied to substance use behaviors and six additional skills added to the manual for DBT-SUDs.
5. Dialectical abstinence, referring to the modification of commitment strategies for the treatment of substance use disorders.

CONCLUDING COMMENTS

In concluding this chapter, I am aware that this way of organizing the entire treatment package of DBT may not be to everyone's liking. For purposes of understanding DBT, however, highlighting the interrelationships of all parts, creating a blueprint for program implementation, and orienting people to this complicated treatment within 30 minutes can be invaluable. Like taking inventory with any checklist, or like doing a mental status exam of the various domains of mental functioning, therapists are able to identify areas of strength, weakness, and deficiency, and to consider ways to strengthen the program. I refer back to the tree metaphor later in the book, especially when considering issues of DBT implementation and case conceptualization.

CHAPTER 7

Goals, Stages, Targets, and Target Priorities

Linehan's answer to the substantial degree of chaos, crisis, and comorbidity characteristic of individuals with severe emotional dysregulation was to establish a clear, prioritized, sequenced, specific list of behavioral treatment targets, known in short as the "target priority list." In the initial sessions, therapist and patient collaborate to tailor a target priority list that will serve as the treatment agenda. It is done with reference to the target priority list template in the manual (Linehan, 1993a), which represents a distillation of years of treatment development and practice. It is organized around the individual patient's unique preferences, life-worth-living goals, and the obstacles to those goals. And it is applied with a substantial dose of common sense, so that the list is realistic and useful session after session for weeks, months, maybe even years. The target list should be built to last. It needs to hold its form under pressure and over time, and to be flexible enough to undergo revisions as new information comes to light. It serves as the temporal framework of DBT, the sequential blueprint for treatment, as crucial to effective treatment as the spine is to human functioning. Without it, the course of treatment can drift over time, even within a given session, driven by emotional priorities rather than behavioral goals.

As valuable as it is, the process of targeting can interfere with treatment if it is done by rote, too rigidly or severely, prioritizing the form of targeting over the function. In this chapter, I provide a deep and broad perspective on this crucial structure and practice in DBT, to enable therapists to make order out of chaos, provide a sequential treatment agenda in the midst of pressing concerns, while simultaneously strengthening collaboration with the patient. After taking a closer look at the nature of the standard target priority list template, I examine how the therapist does the following:

1. Moves from assessment of the patient to the collaborative development of the target priority list for that treatment.
2. Uses the target priority list to set the session agenda at the beginning of each session.
3. Provides structure in the nonindividual therapy modes of DBT (e.g., skills training group, telephone coaching calls, case management interventions) by providing a unique target priority list for the mode-specific agenda, and linking the mode-specific list to the "master target list" created and used in individual therapy.
4. Utilizes, as the leader of a DBT program, the target priority list template to structure and maintain a viable, comprehensive, DBT program.
5. Modifies, in a systematic way, the standard target priority template for the adaptation of DBT to a nonstandard patient population or treatment context in a way that preserves the essential elements of the standard format while tailoring it to the particular circumstance.

THE TARGET PRIORITY LIST TEMPLATE

The target priority list template was discussed in the context of the DBT Tree (see Chapter 6). To briefly review, there are five stages of treatment, and each stage is organized around an overarching goal. To accomplish the overarching goal, the therapist undertakes a step-by-step process to complete one or more specifically defined behavioral targets. At any given point in treatment, the therapist and patient do the work of a particular stage, working on one overarching goal; and at any given moment in a therapy session, the therapist and patient focus on a particular target within that stage. Having a clear and detailed target list keeps the therapist focused on one target behavior at a time. For ease of reference as we discuss the widely known template, it is repeated in the following box. Note that the overarching goal of each stage is indicated in parentheses.

DBT Target Priority List Template

Pervasive target throughout all stages (dialectical synthesis)
Dialectical analyses
Dialectical lifestyle ("middle path")

Pretreatment stage (orientation, agreement, and commitment)
Target: Increase commitment to treatment plan.

Stage 1 (severe behavioral dyscontrol → behavioral control)

Target 1: Decrease suicidal and other life-threatening behaviors.
- Suicide and life-threatening crisis behaviors
- Deliberate self-harm acts, severe aggressive acts
- Significant increase in suicidal and aggressive ideation and communications
- Suicide/homicide-related expectancies and beliefs
- Suicide/homicide-related affects

Target 2: Decrease therapy-interfering behaviors of the patient.
- Nonattending behaviors
- Noncollaborative behaviors
- Noncompliant behaviors
- Behaviors that interfere with other patients
- Behaviors that burn out therapists
  - Pushing therapist's limits
  - Decreasing therapist's motivation to treat

Decrease therapy-interfering behaviors of the therapist.
- Behaviors that unbalance therapy
- Disrespectful behaviors

How to prioritize among therapy-interfering behaviors:
1. Client or therapist behaviors likely to destroy therapy
2. Immediately interfering behaviors of therapist or client
3. Client or therapist behaviors functionally related to suicidal behaviors
4. Client therapy-interfering behaviors similar to problem behaviors outside of therapy
5. Lack of progress in therapy

Target 3: Decrease quality-of-life-interfering behaviors.
- Substance abuse
- High-risk or unprotected sex
- Extreme financial difficulties

- Criminal behaviors
- Seriously dysfunctional interpersonal behaviors
- Employment- or school-related behaviors
- Illness-related dysfunctional behaviors
- Etc.

How to prioritize among quality-of-life-interfering behaviors:
1. Behaviors causing immediate crisis
2. Easy-to-change behaviors over difficult-to-change
   a. Quick reinforcement of active problem solving
   b. Strengthen motivation to take on harder problems
3. Behaviors functionally related to higher-order targets (self-injury, suicide, therapy interfering)

Target 4: Increase behavioral skills.
- Distress tolerance skills
- Emotion regulation skills
- Interpersonal effectiveness skills
- Core mindfulness skills
- Self-management skills

Stage 2 (quiet desperation → nonanguished emotional experiencing)

Target 5: Reduce quiet desperation.
- Reduce residual psychiatric disorders (mood disorders, anxiety disorders, impulse control disorders, etc.).
- Reduce sequelae of childhood invalidation.
- Reduce unwanted outsider status (shame, sensitivity, anger, loneliness).
- Reduce inhibited grieving/emptiness/boredom.

While pursuing
- Nonanguished emotional experiencing
- Connection to the environment
- Sense of essential "goodness"
- Sense of personal validity

Stage 3 (problems in living → ordinary happiness and unhappiness)

Target 6: Increase self-respect.
Target 7: Decrease individual problems in living.

Stage 4 (incompleteness → freedom)

Target 8: Increase freedom.
- Expanded awareness
- Peak experiences and flow
- Spiritual fulfillment

"HOUSE OF TREATMENT" METAPHOR

Like the DBT Tree, there is yet another very useful metaphor, developed by Linehan, regarding the structuring of DBT around the target priority template. This template provides the therapist with the necessary level of detail and order to set up the target list with the patient and to set the session agenda. The House of Treatment metaphor has proven useful for therapists, patients, and family members of patients in envisioning the flow of treatment from beginning to end, from stage to stage. While on a 1-year sabbatical in 1990–1991, during which she was writing the first edition of her treatment manual and skills training book, Linehan spent 3 months on the campus of our hospital, the New York Hospital–Cornell Medical Center in White Plains, New York. She served as a consultant to our inpatient DBT program, which was still in its early stages of development. She lived on the grounds, directly across from my family's residence, and each day she came to our program. She met with staff and patients, reviewed and gave feedback about our program, interviewed patients to show us how to do various strategies, and sometimes assisted in teaching our skills training sessions. During one of those sessions, a patient asked if Marsha could provide an overview of the entire treatment process. She responded by drawing the "DBT House of Treatment" on the blackboard. For her it seemed like a "quick-and-dirty" illustration to answer the question; for me, and eventually for our program, it became a standard tool for orientation to DBT, and we wove it into our assessment process. As a metaphor, it serves as a model vehicle for envisioning the entirety of the treatment protocol; for discussing different perspectives regarding goals, stages, and targets; and for expertly showing how to collaborate with particular patients to "find themselves" in the target hierarchy. I have taught this metaphor, in the way we developed it, to generations of DBT therapists and program developers, and they have found it useful every time. Look at Figure 7.1 as I explain the metaphor.

With its different floors, the house represents the goals and stages of DBT. Pretreatment takes place just outside the house, the place where patients are oriented to what happens in the house, learn about the agreements and expectations, and are asked to make a commitment to the work that takes place in the house, starting at the basement and working up to the third floor. The therapist uses contracting and commitment strategies at this stage, with the goal to get patients to make as strong a commitment as possible to the treatment. When I taught the House of Treatment at an intensive DBT training in 1999, one imaginative participant (Erik Thompson) added a piece to the metaphor. He drew a picture

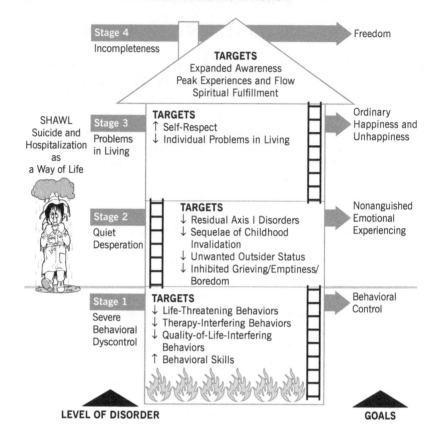

FIGURE 7.1. DBT House of Treatment. Adapted with permission from Marsha M. Linehan.

of a person outside on the ground, outside but next to the house, with a shawl around her neck to protect her from the elements. Torrential rain is pouring down, making the shawl insufficient—a scene that makes the house look more inviting. Using the word *SHAWL* as an acronym, he suggested that some patients considering DBT have been using Suicide and Hospitalization As a Way of Life.

Having gone through pretreatment, most patients proceed to Stage 1, which is depicted as the basement. In the basement the patient experiences intense emotional reactivity and suffering, and regulates the emotions with behaviors that threaten life, ruin treatment, and/or destroy the quality of life. The basement is illustrated with flames coming up from the floor, which represent the experience of burning in hell. Individuals in the basement gain only temporary relief from certain problematic behavioral patterns such as self-cutting or substance use, and some see suicide as the only way out. But there is another way out, represented by a ladder that extends from the floor of the basement to the ceiling, leading up to the first floor. This is the ladder of skills and commitment; I visualize the steps of the ladder as the skills necessary to climb out of the basement, and the two rails that hold the steps in place to be the commitment necessary to stick with it. Each step up the ladder represents the use of adaptive behaviors, step by step replacing the problem behaviors. The overall goal of climbing from the basement to the first floor represents the replacement of severe dysregulation and dyscontrol with behavioral control. Getting to the top of that ladder represents having accomplished the four targets of Stage 1 by (1) decreasing life-threatening behaviors, (2) decreasing therapy-interfering behaviors, (3) decreasing severe quality-of-life-interfering behaviors, and (4) increasing the use of skills.

Getting to the top of the first ladder requires behavioral control but does not eliminate the suffering that prompted the problem behaviors in the first place. For this reason, many patients get to the top of the basement ladder, realize that intense pain remains, and therefore "drop back down into the basement," returning to the recently relinquished problem behaviors. The metaphor captures the clinical dilemma very well, helping patients and therapists to see the necessity of "hanging on" as they get higher up the ladder.

When the patient arrives on the first floor of the house, she has reached Stage 2 of DBT, the goal of which is to become capable of experiencing intense emotions in a nontraumatizing way. Engaging in Stage 2 treatment tasks can be painful (e.g., in some cases, it involves the processing of traumatic memories and affects), and must take place on a solid foundation of skills and commitment built during Stage 1. Otherwise, the work of Stage 2 can catalyze a slip back down to the basement. This need to build skills and maintain behavioral control during Stage 2 can be depicted by "putting a solid cover" over the hole where the ladder ends at the first floor.

Another ladder from the first floor, Stage 2, to the second floor, brings patients to where the work of Stage 3 gets under way. The nature of the ladder in Stage 2 will vary from case to case, depending on the primary sources of suffering. When PTSD plays a primary role, moving up the ladder represents the work of exposure and response prevention. It is best defined to date in the work of Melanie Harned, who has synthesized Edna Foa's prolonged exposure therapy with Linehan's DBT (Harned, Korslund, & Linehan, 2014). In this Stage 2 treatment protocol, Harned and colleagues recommend that the therapist of a patient who "slips down the ladder" into Stage 1 problem behaviors shift back temporarily to the goals and methods of Stage 1 treatment, until the patient reestablishes behavioral control.

(By the way, please note that the House of Treatment metaphor can be slightly confusing in that the first floor corresponds to Stage 2, the second floor corresponds to Stage 3, and so on.)

The patient who accomplishes the work of Stage 2 has reduced the intensity of suffering and has increased his capacity to experience emotions without anguish. Then he can focus on the work of Stage 3, which takes place on the second floor of the house. The goal of Stage 3 is twofold: to establish, or reestablish, self-respect; and to pursue the accomplishment of individual goals in living, whatever they may be. The methods of treatment in Stage 3—getting up the ladder to the next floor—are less well defined, per se, and they depend significantly on the nature of the individual goals. Generally speaking, CBT-based assessment and problem solving will play a central role, augmented by acceptance-oriented approaches and dialectics, as needed. For some patients, the work of DBT ends with the problem solving that takes place in Stage 3.

The patient who progresses to the work of Stage 4, represented on the third (uppermost) floor of the house, pursues increased freedom, meaning, and sustained joy. The methods of Stage 4 are the least defined of all the stages to date, but rely heavily upon mindfulness theory and practice. The achievement of Stage 4 goals will require maintenance of the work that was accomplished all the way from the basement to the top. Whether trying to get out of hell or to get to the top of the house, the three paradigms of DBT—mindfulness, behaviorism, and dialectics—provide an extraordinarily potent vocabulary of options.

Used with patients in treatment, the metaphor can be illuminating and motivating. They can easily see that DBT is a stage-based treatment, and that each floor of the house represents a necessary step on the way to a life worth living. For patients with behavioral dyscontrol who enter DBT wanting to jump immediately to the processing of trauma memories, they can see that trauma processing is central to DBT (in Stage 2), but that the work must begin with laying a foundation of skillful emotional regulation. Seeing parts of the treatment and the whole of the treatment in one diagram helps to orient patients and to elicit a commitment to the treatment as a whole.

Following the old adage "A picture is worth a thousand words," the metaphor can also play a significant role in assessment. On our inpatient DBT program, we introduced the metaphor to each newly admitted patient. We would give a diagram of the house and ask the patient to draw a stick figure to represent his or her location in the house of treatment. This led to some meaningful insights and even transformative dialogues. One of our patients, who had a terrible history of trauma and for whom episodes of dissociation were frequent and debilitating, placed herself on the floor of the basement. She drew a square box in the corner of the basement and put herself inside it. She explained that the basement was "unbearably hot," and that she had found a tolerably cool spot inside the box, something like an area of refrigeration. She related the drawing to her episodes of dissociation, during which she got relief from the constant emotional pain. At the same time, she recognized that the relief was temporary, that when she came out of the box she was still in hell, in the basement, having made no progress. We began to discuss with her the challenge of skillfully tolerating the "heat" and distress without going into the box of refrigeration and dissociation.

Another of our patients had an eating disorder. She was invested in the pursuit of thinness and would use the usual behaviors of anorexia and bulimia in striving toward her goal. An excellent student in college, she managed her intense emotions and almost intolerable sense of imperfection, even while getting good grades, by controlling her eating. Occasionally her eating disorder behaviors would spiral out of control, and she would descend from her status as an excellent and well-managed college student into a world of binging, purging, suicidal ideation, suicide attempts, self-neglect, and impulsivity. She would enter the hospital and twice was sent to our inpatient program. When she was oriented to the House of Treatment and asked to locate herself in it, she added a tall rectangle adjoining the right side of the house. It was narrow, and it extended from the bottom of the basement to the top of the second floor. She explained that the rectangle represented an express elevator, made of glass, running between the basement and the second floor. On the second floor, she was pursuing well-defined goals as a college student, whereas in the basement she experienced emotional dysregulation and behavioral dyscontrol, accompanied by self-hatred. She clearly demonstrated her pattern of moving between the basement and the second floor, between hell and college success. We could all see, as could she, that she never stopped on the first floor, where the treatment of suffering, including self-hatred, takes place through exposure and other methods. This tangible illustration helped her to accept that she needed to do more work establishing stability, tolerating distress, and doing the work of Stage 2.

ARRIVING AT THE TARGET
PRIORITY LIST DIALECTICALLY

Linehan's crystal clarity about the target priority list and how to use it can make it look easy. Some therapists can overlook the fact that establishing a given patient's list of targets cannot effectively be done by simply plugging the patient's problem behaviors into the right spots in the template. This way of proceeding entirely misses the fact that the list must be constructed collaboratively, consistent with the staged approach of DBT, and done with care and attention to what will work for the patient. To impose a list of targets will simply not work. In fact, working with the patient to create a viable list of target priorities is an opportunity (1) to teach an effective way to approach problems, (2) to build the relationship, and (3) to model the essential principles of DBT. Setting up the target list is not "preparation" for treatment; it *is* treatment.

We can conceptualize this process as a search for syntheses of two different dialectics. The first is the overarching dialectic about what is driving the treatment agenda: the pursuit of the patient's goals versus the resolution of the patient's problems. The second is a dialectic that emerges when therapist and patient place the various targets into a specific order. The therapist typically refers to DBT's target priority template to arrive rationally at the order of priorities whereas the patient is likely to advocate for an agenda that prioritizes the rapid reduction of emotional pain. With respect to each of these two dialectics, the therapist works toward a synthesis that includes the validity of both sides.

Regarding the first dialectic, the agenda of treatment needs to be driven by the patient's pursuit of particular life-worth-living goals, but also by the sequential reduction of dysfunctional behaviors. To focus primarily on goals, articulated as hopes, dreams, and practical steps, can contribute to optimism, but also can underemphasize the problems to be solved. To focus primarily on problem behaviors can lead to a concise and detailed work agenda, but may discourage the patient while doing it, as she comes to feel that the point of treatment is to focus on problems rather than to build a satisfying life. The best-made target priority lists are syntheses of the patient's most cherished goals and the problems that stand in the way.

I typically begin treatment by eliciting and exploring the patient's goals, as detailed in the first chapter on the life-worth-living conversation. By taking this perspective, problems can be seen as difficulties that interfere with the accomplishment of goals. I usually capture the dialectic on a piece of paper. I draw a line down the middle, and on the left I list the goals as articulated by the patient. On the right, I list all problems that have been identified in the assessment sessions and in documentation from prior treatment providers. The problem list is usually overly inclusive, including problems identified by others but not relevant to the patient him- or herself. Next, the patient and I look at the two lists together and clarify which goals are most important to him. We look at all the problems and consider which ones will truly interfere with accomplishing those goals. In this way, the synthesis consists of a collaborative process, creating the agenda driven by the patient's goals, but also clothed with the patient's problem behaviors. It is more motivating to reduce the use of alcohol in order to realize one's values, one's concrete hopes and dreams, than to reduce the use of alcohol as an end in itself.

The first dialectic comes about in determining what is on the treatment agenda; the second one involves the specific ordering of targets. On the one hand, the prioritized order should be aligned with the template presented earlier in the chapter. For instance, life-threatening behaviors should be prioritized over therapy-interfering behaviors. On the other hand, priorities should be aligned with the patient's desires to reduce pain and build a life worth living. Both approaches are valid, and yet they sometimes lead to conflicting priorities. For instance, it is not unusual for patients to arrive in therapy wanting to begin by processing the traumatic memories from earlier in life. They may reason that this is the cause of all of their problem behaviors and therefore should be addressed immediately. It is understandable. It is equally understandable that as therapists, we are aware that it can be counterproductive to address trauma too explicitly before patients have acquired some capacity for emotion regulation. Therapists are likely to prioritize the task of gaining better behavioral control and emotion regulation before delving explicitly into traumatic memories. The difference between these two perspectives can become entrenched. However, if we think dialectically, we see the wisdom of each patient's wish to get on with the trauma work, while at the same time recognizing the wisdom of starting to establish stability and safety through skill building. Each case is likely to be different.

Years ago, I began working with a 16-year-old boy, referred by his parents and guidance counselor because of a number of problems: angry outbursts during which he would do damage to his bedroom, self-cutting behaviors, excessive use of alcohol, recent alienation from peers, poor judgment in promiscuous sexual relationships, conflict with family, depression, and deteriorating school performance. It appeared that his alcohol use played a major role in his other problems. He would sneak away from home on weekends, go to dorm parties at the local university, get intoxicated, sometimes with "blackouts," and wake up in strange dorm rooms with no recall of how he got there, or be awakened on the lawn by campus police. He got into fights at the parties and at times suffered significant injuries about which he would lie to his parents. I learned that he had been "fired" from three prior therapies, ostensibly because he refused to give up drinking.

Given how discouraged he had grown, we initially focused on what would make him feel that his life was worth living. For the past 4 years he had found his life to be an endless swirl of excitement, chaos, secrecy, self-destructiveness, and a total loss of the "positive kid" he used to be. In spite of the fact that his "positive self" had been "buried," as he put it, he was able, with encouragement and repeated reinforcement of the notion of himself as a capable individual, to remember and endorse some goals that he had had as a 12-year-old: to succeed in school, to have better friends, to eventually attend college, and ultimately to get a job helping other people. At the same time, he wanted to continue to "have fun": to go to college dorm parties, meet girls, drink alcohol, and have sex.

We constructed the lists of his goals and his problems. We agreed on most items for his target list, and on the order of priority of targets, with one exception. We disagreed profoundly about his use of alcohol. While I was certain that his episodes of drinking hugely contributed to his bad judgment, painful experiences, alienation from peers, depression, and deteriorating school performance, he was not. "I love alcohol, I really love it, and I will not stop." He agreed that he wanted to stop "doing stupid things," as he put it, including "doing stupid things" while intoxicated, but he did not want to target any reduction in his drinking. We arrived at a synthesis that allowed us to move forward with the following target priority list:

TARGET PRIORITY LIST FOR A PATIENT
WITH SELF-CUTTING AND ALCOHOL ABUSE

Pretreatment stage: Increase commitment.
• Strengthen focus on a life worth living
• Strengthen commitment to the treatment plan

Stage 1: Increase behavioral control and stability.
• Decrease self-cutting behaviors.
• Maintain excellent record of attendance at sessions.
• Increase behaviors of collaboration with therapist.
• Maintain excellent record of attendance at skills group sessions.
• Decrease angry outbursts with damage to his bedroom
• **(Decrease use of alcohol.)**
• **Stop doing "stupid things."**
  • **Stop driving while drunk.**
• **Stop making bad choices regarding sex (especially when drunk).**
• Strengthen school attendance and performance.
  • Begin to gather information about colleges.
• Increase quantity and quality of friendships.

Stage 2: Increase capability of adaptively experiencing emotions.
• To be defined as we learn more.

As our initial "working target priority list," it synthesized goals and problems, and it synthesized his "agenda" and mine. The contentious areas of the list are in **bold** font. We agreed to include "decrease use of alcohol" on the list, but putting it in parentheses indicates that it is a target that I proposed but that with which he disagreed. We included "stop doing stupid things" on the list, as he wanted to end this behavior, but without any reduction in drinking. In practice, we agreed not to formally target his alcohol use, but to keep it under assessment. We would monitor the impact of alcohol use upon other targets. It was a synthesis.

Needless to say, it was a challenge to arrive at a treatment plan to "stop doing stupid things" without directly targeting his excessive use of alcohol. But that is exactly what we did. I kidded him, saying that if we developed a therapy that could help people stop doing stupid things when they drank, which allowed them to keep drinking, we could market it and make millions. We proceeded to develop a set of guidelines, something of a "mini-manual," for ways to stop doing stupid things when he went to parties and drank. We subdivided his drinking episodes into three parts and came up with strategies and skills for each part: what he could do prior to the party, during the party, and afterward. I told him I would work with him on this plan under two conditions: (1) He would not drive if he had been drinking; and (2) if there was no change in "doing stupid things" after 3 months, I would discontinue treatment.

He agreed to both conditions and appeared eager to get started. He completely stopped cutting himself almost immediately, faithfully attended individual and group sessions, and his schoolwork improved. He continued to do "stupid things," showed no change in his use of alcohol, and after 3 months there was little change in the pattern. He was saddened when I told him that, per our agreement, I had to stop treating him. About 3 months later, having not seen him since we'd stopped, he called me: "Charlie, I think I'm an alcoholic. Can I come see you?" We commenced work on his alcoholism. Within months he had stopped drinking, was attending Alcoholics Anonymous meetings, was doing well in school, was beginning to look at colleges, and in psychotherapy was addressing the ways in which he responded to an invalidating familial–social context by adopting a secretive, renegade, substance-abusing lifestyle.

In retrospect, I believe we laid the foundation for success of this treatment in our difficult but honest handling of the pretreatment stage, including the life-worth-living conversation, which rekindled his memories of previously buried hopes and dreams, and the careful, dialectical process of setting up the target priority list. Our differences regarding what to target, and in what order, were transparent; the target list upon which we settled represented a synthesis such that we could both "own it," and the treatment agenda was clear as we got under way. We agreed to disagree about the drinking, giving it special status by monitoring it but not directly targeting it. Having set up the conditions with a time limit, he was eventually convinced, through experience if not conversation, that his alcohol use had to be targeted. Had we avoided the acknowledgment of differences and not searched for a synthesis in a prioritized target list, those differences could easily have led to a standoff, resulting in a premature ending as had happened to him before.

USING THE TARGET PRIORITY LIST
TO ESTABLISH THE SESSION AGENDA

Insofar as DBT with each patient involves a long-term "mission statement"—the image of a life worth living, broken down into a "strategic plan" comprised of the prioritized list of treatment targets pursued in stages—it can be seen to resemble a business enterprise. The work on the specific behavioral targets is monitored and executed in a weekly (therapy) meeting, the agenda for which is driven by the highest-priority targets of the moment. The therapist collaborates with the patient in setting the agenda at the beginning of each session, in a process of targeting.

After the initial greeting and brief but important check-in period, which might take anywhere from 30 seconds to several minutes, the therapist asks for the diary card. The card is a record, to be completed daily, of the occurrence of the patient's targets, including the use of skills. It's the "report card" of the week. There are more and less effective ways to review the diary card. It presents opportunities not only to set the stage for the session, but also to do "diary card therapy": that is, to engage the patient in a meaningful practice by modeling the treatment principles and strengthening the therapy relationship. Consistent with behavioral principles, the review should be disciplined, target-focused, and practical—a laboratory for the practice of executive functioning: keeping larger goals in mind, accurately remembering, consistently self-monitoring, and reliably reinforcing on-task behaviors. Consistent with the principles of acceptance, it is a perfect opportunity to encourage mindful attentiveness to treatment goals, to validate the pain that results in target behaviors, to validate the difficulty of staying on track, and to cheerlead the patient's capabilities in completing the diary card. If the therapist can balance the change and acceptance principles, and use dialectical interventions as needed, the diary card review can result in a stronger relationship. All of this requires actively engaging the patient throughout the review, rather than the rather common process in which a therapist quietly reviews the card and then proposes a session agenda. Over time, the process of completing the diary card every day and reviewing it every week creates an infrastructure for consistency and problem solving. It is the aspect of DBT that resembles the often onerous tasks of home life, school life, and work life that are so challenging for those with severe emotional dysregulation. If the patient fails to complete the card effectively or at all, it is an opportunity for the therapist, on the spot, to assess and treat whatever problem behaviors contribute to the noncompletion.

Having reviewed the diary card, the therapist moves on to set the agenda for the session, which is a way of answering the question, "Which target(s) will we work on today?" I might, for instance, begin that brief discussion by saying, "Given that we are still trying to get the self-cutting behaviors under control, let's assess and work on the factors that led to the cutting episode on Wednesday, OK?" And then I am likely to add, "Is there anything else that you want to talk about today?" Between the two of us we will come up with an agenda driven by a variety of factors: behaviors reported on the diary card; information that may have come to me from my consultation team meeting where I heard about other modes of treatment that week; and by the patient's additional wishes. We will create an agenda of two or three items, rarely more, including what we need to discuss and what the patient would like to discuss, using the prioritized list of treatment targets to establish the order of priority. Once the agenda is firmed up, we move on to the work on the first target of the session, which is likely to begin with a behavioral chain analysis. During the course of the session, of course, more information could come to light that will add another item to the target list of the day or change the order of priority of targets on the agenda.

As therapy proceeds through the months, the target list requires care and attention. From time to time it needs to be revised as some targets are accomplished, new targets are added to the list, and the order of priority may change as more information comes to light. For instance, whereas excessive use of substances may have been targeted at the beginning of therapy as a quality-of-life-interfering behavior, it might ascend the target list to the category of therapy-interfering behaviors if the therapist learns that the patient has been arriving intoxicated to sessions. It might possibly move up the list to a life-threatening behavior if it comes to light that the patient's suicidal or homicidal behaviors are routinely associated with substance use. The structural aspects of DBT—including the use of the diary card, adherence to the agreements, and formal targeting at the end of the diary card review—can undergo drift during treatment. Structures that could be maintained with rigor at the beginning, when the relationship was new, can be challenging to maintain as familiarity between patient and therapist grows. Both parties can easily let the structures fade as they each come to feel that they "know" what needs to be done session by session. Maintaining the structures of the treatment requires a kind of discipline that sometimes grates on both parties. In my experience, the discipline pays off more often than not, and does not have to interfere with the development of a potent attachment, which is also critical in DBT.

I once treated a young woman who, while living in another country, had married into a violent gang, where she had been mistreated by gang members and physically abused, even tortured, by her husband. She escaped from her husband and the gang, which put her in great jeopardy. She moved to the area where I was working, and that's when she entered treatment with me. She presented with PTSD, as indicated by intrusive memories, nightmares, sleep disruption, hypervigilance (although this seemed realistic), and an intense fear of leaving her apartment. She cut herself on her arms every day. She used substances, especially marijuana and occasionally cocaine, to regulate her emotions. Naturally she tended to mistrust people, and that included me. At the end of the assessment, when we considered her life goals and her problematic behaviors, we established the following prioritized list of treatment targets:

TARGET PRIORITY LIST FOR A PATIENT WITH PTSD,
SELF-CUTTING, AND SUBSTANCE ABUSE

Pretreatment targets
• Increase commitment to treatment plan.

Decrease life-threatening behaviors.
• Decrease self-cutting.

Decrease therapy-interfering behaviors.
• Increase willingness to share information with therapist.

Decrease quality-of-life-interfering behaviors.
• Decrease use of cocaine.
• Decrease use of marijuana.
• Decrease avoidance of community life.
• Increase safe social relationships.
• Increase efforts to get a job.

Increase skills
• Increase distress tolerance, emotion regulation, interpersonal effectiveness, and core mindfulness skills.
• Increase self-management skills.

Decrease posttraumatic stress.
• Decrease intense fear response to safe cues.
• Decrease avoidance of and escape from cues.
• Increase capacity to detect likelihood of unsafe behaviors in others.
• Increase capacity to recognize trauma cues.

Within a short time the patient was sufficiently committed to move into Stage 1, which started with the targeting of self-cutting behaviors. She was especially motivated by the prospect of treating the PTSD. She did not agree at first that we needed to address the Stage 1 targets before treating the PTSD, but after orienting her with the House of Treatment metaphor, she understood and seemed to accept the stage-by-stage treatment plan. I emphasized that we would already be addressing aspects of her PTSD as they emerged in Stage 1, and all work in Stage 1 on trauma-related behaviors would add to her readiness for the exposure treatment that would be the centerpiece of Stage 2. After about 6 weeks of treatment, during which we assessed the controlling variables of her self-cutting behaviors with behavioral chain analyses, she reported that she was no longer cutting herself. I had the impression that once she understood that the prerequisite for addressing the trauma memories, and discussing other things in detail, was to stop cutting herself, her capacity to do so was reinforced. When therapists are disciplined in holding to the target priorities, these kinds of changes are not unusual.

As it appears in retrospect, our next target (to "increase her willingness to share information with the therapist") became both the most stubborn and most important one to solve. In spite of her positive statements about me, and her seeming willingness to engage, her mistrust of me proved to be deep and strong. She was withholding information that was central to her treatment: She was actually continuing to cut but was lying about it on the diary card; she continued to use substances when she claimed to have stopped; and she exaggerated her accounts of constructive involvement in her community. The discrepancy between her presentation to me and her actual behaviors during the week was substantial. She was not changing the behaviors we were targeting. The momentum of the entire treatment stalled around the target of increasing collaboration with me.

This stalemate stretched over several months, and it wore us both down. She wanted to move on to the treatment of her PTSD in Stage 2, but by withholding behavior about Stage 1 targets, we could not get there. I began to wonder if we should bypass this impasse and attempt to do the work of Stage 2. I wondered if we perhaps should move on to the processing of trauma responses, trying to build trust and make progress in that area, which might then result in more honesty about her Stage 1 targets. My consultation team listened to my thoughts and validated the frustration that I was feeling, but they pointed out that practicing DBT included adherence to the target priorities. I knew that, of course, but their compassionate reminder helped me to stay the course. I intensified our focus on the target behavior of her mistrust of me, as evidenced by withholding information from me. As we analyzed the antecedents and consequences of keeping the truth hidden in the sessions, the sources of her mistrust of me emerged more clearly. Most importantly for this discussion is the fact that when she realized I would not move on until we solved the noncollaborative behavior target, she revealed a crucial piece of information that she had kept to herself. Her father, with whom she was living, had been lying to her for months, telling her that he routinely spoke with me on the phone. He told her what my "true" opinion was about how she "should behave," and he was using it against her. Because her fear of her father prevented her from challenging him, and because she feared that if she were to challenge me, she would learn that her father was correct, she never told me what her father said about me. Once it was out in the open and I was able to clarify matters with her, trust came rather rapidly. Our work in this area also helped her to see her father more accurately.

In sum, this case evidences the need for the target priority list to be an enduring structure. Despite the fact that this structure is a product of dialectical tensions, that it undergoes change during treatment, and that it can be used with some flexibility, it is a reliable and stable format for setting the agenda and monitoring progress. The DBT therapist holds on to it, much as one takes a road map or a GPS into unknown territory, but like the hiker who needs to change course due to unanticipated impediments, the clinician retains flexibility when alternative paths reveal themselves. It is an important tool to be used on the journey that should serve the therapy relationship, but not control it. Finding that balance is a clinical art.

USING TARGET PRIORITIES
TO STRUCTURE OTHER MODES OF DBT

To provide comprehensive DBT, inclusive of all five functions of treatment, is to provide several modes of treatment. One of those is individual therapy, the primary function of which is to improve the patient's motivation. The target priority list discussed so far in this chapter is used to structure individual therapy. When the individual therapist is the "quarterback" of the overall treatment, as is the case in standard outpatient

DBT, his target list can also be considered to be the main target list structuring the whole treatment. With the support of the consultation team behind him, the individual therapist is the guardian of the treatment as a whole and of the list of primary treatment targets.

However, other functions of the treatment are carried out in other treatment modes. For example, the function of enhancing the patient's capabilities is addressed in the skills training group. The function of helping the patient to generalize skills to the natural environment is enacted through the mode of telephone coaching calls. The function of enhancing therapists' capabilities and motivation is centered in the mode of consultation team. Each of these modes has a more specific agenda than the broad agenda of the individual therapist, and a much briefer and focused target priority list. Each mode is structured around its own unique target list, separate from but related to the target priority list of the individual therapist. Sticking to the mode-specific target priority list helps to keep the work of that mode on track, centered on the intended function.

As an illustration of some principles in the structuring of mode-specific target lists and how to use them, I examine the target priority list of the skills training group next. In order of priority, the three targets for the therapist leading the skills group are:

1. Decrease behaviors likely to destroy therapy (i.e., the skills group).
2. Increase skill acquisition and strengthening.
3. Decrease therapy-interfering behaviors.

First, notice that the second target, "increase skills acquisition and strengthening," is the primary function of this mode. If the group leader had her preference, she would spend 100% of the group's time on this activity. In a group that is going well, it is almost always possible to do that. The only target higher than that is the first one, "decrease behaviors likely to destroy therapy," and it is the highest priority because it must be. If a patient in the group behaves in any manner destructive to the group skills training process, thereby ruining the possibility of helping everyone to acquire and strengthen DBT skills, those behaviors have to be addressed until they are eliminated. I once had a patient with a bipolar disorder who was presenting with manic behaviors in the skills group. He was excited about every teaching topic and about every individual in the group and enthusiastic about the possibility that the group might change his life. He could barely stop talking even when asked to stop. Naturally, this behavior destroyed the possibility that other patients could learn from me or each other, and even my ability to think straight. Eliminating or reducing his excessive talkativeness in the group became the highest-priority target. Despite several warnings and requests, the patient kept up his continuous chatter, so we found a dialectical intervention that would, on the one hand, honor his desire to learn the skills, and on the other hand, protect the group's need to learn the skills. We placed a chair outside the circle and made an agreement with him that if I asked him, he would move to the chair against the wall, which we called the "silent chair." When sitting in the silent chair, he was to say nothing, but when he thought he was ready to better restrain his speech, he could move back into the group circle. This plan worked well, and I was able to return to helping all group members acquire and strengthen their DBT skills.

To lead skills groups with emotionally dysregulated individuals can be challenging. The leader encounters passivity, social anxiety, and emotional reactivity, which can lead to disruptions, inertia, tension, and conflict. Since these groups are led in a classroom format, there is little room for the verbal processing of in-group problem behaviors. Therefore the group therapist has to be alert to maintaining structure and momentum. What we covered above will help guide the group therapist toward quickly and firmly intervening to reduce or eliminate destructive group behavior. But notice that the third target, lower in priority than skills acquisition and strengthening, is to reduce therapy-interfering behaviors. In other words, there is a category of problematic behaviors that interferes with therapy that is distinct from the category of behaviors that destroys the group, and that is the lowest priority of the three.

In one of my first skills groups, there was a young woman who wore sunglasses in a dully-lit room and turned her chair to face away from me and from the group. Even when directly addressed, she remained silent. I had to decide whether her behavior was therapy-destroying or therapy-interfering. Was her behavior destroying my capacity to teach and the capacity of other patients to learn? If so, I had to insist on immediate behavioral change. In this case, it was not therapy-destroying. It might have been interfering with her own learning process (though, in fact, she was learning throughout the time she was silent and facing away from the group). This is a critical decision and it comes up regularly. The vast majority of problem behaviors in the group are therapy-interfering, not therapy-destroying. In the case of most therapy-interfering behaviors, the group leader ignores them, putting them on an extinction schedule. The most typical therapy-interfering behaviors are eye rolling, doodling, remaining silent, failing to complete the practice assignment, refusing to enter into a role play, seeming to not pay attention, and voicing criticism of DBT or the group leaders but not in a demoralizing way for other group members.

Whether the group leader regards a given behavior as therapy-destroying or therapy-interfering can be a personal matter. For instance, if a given behavioral pattern crosses the personal limits of the group leader, distracting him to the degree that he cannot teach effectively, it is therapy-destroying. The same behavior pattern might be less difficult for another group therapist. As I have grown more familiar with what I consider to be group-destroying behaviors and more comfortable in intervening in such patterns quickly and decisively, while ignoring therapy-interfering behaviors, my groups have run more smoothly. Keep in mind that even if one ignores therapy-interfering behaviors in the moment, the persistent ones can be addressed by asking the patient to address the related issues in individual therapy. In general, bear in mind that therapy-interfering behaviors taking place persistently in the group may be the lowest-priority target in the group format, but are rather high on the target priority list of the individual therapist.

The target priorities used to structure the brief telephone skills coaching calls play a similar role as those used to structure the group. The three targets for the individual therapist in setting and maintaining the agenda for phone calls initiated by patients are as follows:

1. Decrease suicide crisis behaviors.
2. Increase generalization of skills.
3. Decrease sense of conflict, alienation, and distance with the therapist.

Just as in using the target priorities for the skills training group, the second target is the central work of this mode. The "perfect" phone call would be focused entirely on how to generalize skills in the context of the ongoing crisis. But if the patient is experiencing an episode of suicide crisis behaviors, with potentially high lethality, the targeting of generalizing skills takes a temporary back seat to a suicide risk assessment or the implementation of a suicide crisis protocol. As soon as the crisis has been sufficiently addressed, the therapist can revert immediately to coaching skills used in the face of high risk. Notice that the third target focuses both patient and therapist on current problems in the therapy relationship, wherein the patient is feeling conflict, alienation, and distance from the therapist. According to Linehan (1993a, pp. 189, 501) if the call is not a suicidal crisis or a request for help in generalizing skills, but instead consists of a contact to discuss problems in the relationship, the response should be a brief phone chat, much as might take place between two friends who are suffering an episode of alienation. If it can't be resolved in the phone call, the therapist can bring it to the next therapy session.

When I developed our inpatient DBT unit, the lessons I learned from studying the mode-specific targets were remarkably helpful in structuring my staff's work. In an inpatient program, there are a number of modes not present in the standard outpatient DBT treatment covered by the manual. When nursing staff members met for check-ins with patients for 5, 10, or 15 minutes, we conceptualized it as the "check-in mode." When I led the entire community on the unit in a "community meeting," I conceptualized it as the "community meeting mode." Even in my job as "unit chief," I considered it to be the "unit chief mode." And in each case, we started with the primary work of that mode, and from that vantage point, identified other targets of that mode and where they fit in the list of priorities. We saw check-ins on the inpatient as functionally akin to phone calls in outpatient DBT. Generalization of skills was the central work of the mode. We specified three targets, the second one being the main work of that mode: increasing the generalization of skills to the milieu environment. The highest target, akin to the situation in telephone coaching, had to be behaviors that presented immediate danger: suicidal, homicidal, or unit-destroying behaviors. We lumped them into one category, which we called "egregious behaviors." The third target for check-ins almost exactly paralleled the third target for phone calls: efforts to reduce the sense of alienation, conflict, or distance from the staff member or the program as a whole. By having a clear set of three targets in order of priority, which were often the focus of staff training exercises, staff members found a sharply defined role on the unit, rather than what I have seen in so many inpatient programs, where these extremely important and frequent check-in meetings lack a guiding focus or structure.

DBT has been implemented in a huge range of settings and with a number of patient populations. As a result, DBT programs have developed a myriad of modes, serving typical DBT functions. This multiplicity helps to account for DBT's flexibility in implementation. We can extrapolate from the above discussion to designating some guidelines for the use and development of mode-specific target priorities. Clarifying the function of each mode will link that mode to the larger goals of the treatment program (e.g., generalization of patients' skills during the nursing check-in mode is part of the larger program goal of enhancing and generalizing capabilities). Clarifying the target priority list of the mode will provide shape and structure to it, and help the treatment provider stay on track. Generally, the central work of the mode will be embodied in the *second* target priority on the list. And, in general, the first target priority of the mode will target those behaviors that prohibit the central work of the mode. If the patient attacks the individual therapist, eliminating the attack is a higher priority than the desirable work on improving motivation. When a skills group member is overly critical of another group member, in that moment reducing finger-pointing will be a higher priority target than teaching skills. If a patient on an inpatient unit tries to harm herself during a check-in with a staff member, reducing the self-harming behavior is a higher priority in that moment than the work on generalizing skills to the environment. The third target provides for other matters that can be addressed if the top two targets have been accomplished. The individual therapist might hand over the agenda to the patient; the skills trainer might address therapy-interfering behaviors that do not prohibit the teaching of skills in the group but that do interfere with an individual's learning. And during a telephone coaching call, the therapist might focus attention on repairing a rift in the therapist–patient relationship if there is not a higher-priority target that needs attention. It is not always feasible to fit this formula exactly, since in some cases a mode will have a larger list of target priorities, but still the principles can be applied.

USING THE TARGET PRIORITY LIST TO STRUCTURE AND MAINTAIN A VIABLE, COMPREHENSIVE DBT PROGRAM

We have discussed the nature of the target priority list in DBT and have seen how it serves to structure the work of the individual therapist, the agenda of each session, and the work of each mode of DBT treatment. Were it not for this kind of target-driven structuring, therapy would inevitably be driven by emotional dysregulation, overwhelmed by the number and magnitude of problematic behaviors, and paralyzed by passivity or persistent conflict. Similarly, the implementation and maintenance of a comprehensive DBT program takes place amidst pressures that can collide with treatment philosophy or evidence-based decision making. Program leaders contend with pervasive institutional agendas to avoid crises, prevent friction among administrators and their departments, minimize utilization of resources, reduce high-level complaints by families and patients, and accommodate to certain staff personalities. Akin to the use of goals, stages, and target priorities to keep order and direction in therapy, program leaders do the same thing in a wider context in DBT implementation. To remain clear and vigilant about overarching program goals and stages, and about prioritized targets for patients in each treatment mode provides a backbone for programmatic decision making that keeps things on track. We cannot simply maintain a program philosophy in the abstract by knowing the principles; instead, we rely on structures consistent with those principles.

When I first implemented DBT in an inpatient setting, the determination of our goals, stages, and targets guided us, from that point forward, in decisions about treatment, staff training agendas, and communication with families, administration, and other "third parties." As a result, over time, the goals, stages, and targets became embedded as a "deep structure" within the program. Even as seismic changes took place in our fiscal and institutional environment, this deep structure helped us to make decisions that maintained the essence of the program.

For instance, we determined that one of our overarching programmatic goals was to increase our patients' capabilities to acquire, strengthen, and generalize the skills they needed to pursue their life-worth-living goals outside the hospital. As a result, we kept our focus on targets related to those tasks, choosing to ignore work on some other possible targets, or to defer that work to outpatient treatment. We realized that it would be unrealistic to target the elimination of suicidal behaviors and ideation in our inpatients; instead we targeted an increase in the patients' capacities to do that work in outpatient treatment without repeated hospitalizations. We did not target the large number of serious quality-of-life-interfering behaviors that would have been on the target list of an outpatient DBT therapist; instead we focused on those quality-of-life-interfering behaviors that prompted or prolonged hospitalization. The length of stay was too short for us to target the wider range of behaviors, and in DBT our preference is to address problem behaviors in the natural life context. These targeting decisions carried implications for how we oriented new patients to the unit. We let them know that our job was not to solve all of their problems but to help them get through a crisis and to build the capabilities to solve their problems outside the hospital. This clarity helped us stay on track with patients who were disappointed in the limited agenda. Many patients enter the inpatient setting with high hopes of solving everything.

After doing this work for a couple of years, we came to define our program as solving three main sequential goals, in three stages. Stage 1 was "getting in." This encompassed steps of assessment, orientation, developing a treatment plan, and getting a commitment to the treatment plan. It also included an emphasis on establishing enough behavioral control to take part in the various aspects of the program. Stage 2 was defined as "getting in control." This was the middle stage of treatment and focused on assessing and treating those behaviors that prompted and prolonged hospitalization, with an eye to teaching patients skillful ways to avert them in outpatient life in the future. Stage 3 was defined as "getting out." This was the stage of transition from inpatient to outpatient life, and revolved around setting up viable outpatient structures and acquiring and strengthening skills to work on important targets without having to return to the hospital. Once we were clear about our three stages, the targets on which we would focus, the targets that we would defer until outpatient life, and the interventions that would accomplish these goals, we arrived at a new and realistic level of organization that strengthened our program. This is just one example of how a DBT program is organized around specific goals, stages, and targets; how that specificity delimits the tasks of the program; and how it keeps all the various modes, interventions, and protocols aligned with one another in the service of the program's target priorities.

THE ROLE OF THE TARGET PRIORITY LIST IN ADAPTING DBT TO ALTERNATIVE TREATMENT SETTINGS AND POPULATIONS

In this chapter, we've seen that the list of target priorities plays a central role in organizing and staging the overall treatment, establishing the agenda for each session of individual therapy and of all other treatment modes, and even structuring a treatment program as a whole. When I adapted DBT to inpatient care, I realized that I had to get the target priorities right. I had to design a template for the whole program, prioritizing the categories of behavioral targets that could then also be tailored to each case. This was an example of using the goals, stages, and targets to structure DBT treatment in a context for which it was not originally designed. Similarly, the specification of goals, stages, and targets is key to adapting DBT to any patient population for which DBT was not originally designed. I discussed an example of this in the previous chapter regarding the DBT Tree, where I identified and discussed the list of treatment targets for individuals with substance use disorders. I needed to locate where in the larger standard DBT target categories I would insert the substance use targets, and then I had to specify the "subtargets" for the treatment of substance use problems. In order to consolidate this growing understanding of how to apply the goals, stages, and targets to different disorders and problem behaviors, I conclude this chapter by discussing the adaptation of DBT to an individual with both borderline personality disorder and a binge-eating disorder.

First, where in the overall standard DBT target list will we target the eating disorder behaviors? After all, the patient might present on a given week with self-cutting behaviors, suicidal ideation, nonattendance at the skills training group, binge-eating and purging behaviors, dysfunctional interpersonal patterns, and poor compliance in medication management.

Just like our considerations in the treatment of substance use disorders, we first determine whether the eating disorder behaviors present as commitment challenges (pretreatment target), life-threatening behaviors (target category 1), therapy-interfering behaviors (target category 2), or severe quality-of-life-interfering behaviors (target category 3). Any of these options is possible. The patient might present with ambivalence about targeting eating disorder behaviors, which will require attention to commitment during pretreatment. She might present with a low body weight that nearly poses a threat to life, or with a disrupted esophagus secondary to violent purging episodes that could also pose a threat to life. In either case, the eating disorder behaviors will be targeted along with other life-threatening behaviors. She might lie about her eating-related practices, or might be thin to the degree that she disturbs or distracts the psychotherapist. In either case, these will be targeted along with therapy-interfering behaviors (in one case, as a noncollaborative behavior; in the other case, as a behavior that violates the personal limits of the therapist).

But in most "ordinary cases" of binge-eating disorder, the eating disorder behaviors will be targeted as part of the set of severe quality-of-life-interfering behaviors. If the DBT program specializes in the treatment of eating disorders, these behaviors will probably be targeted as the highest priority among the quality-of-life-interfering behaviors, unless one of the others in that category is causing an immediate crisis. If you recall, these considerations are exactly parallel to the determinations of where to target substance use behaviors in the treatment of such disorders.

Having located the place for eating disorder targets within the larger target hierarchy, it remains for us to specify the sequence of subtarget behaviors leading to the successful treatment of the binge-eating disorder. The same kind of strategy used for the substance abuse subtarget sequence is used here. To do so, however, requires considerable familiarity with the disorder, and how it is successfully resolved in step-by-step fashion. For binge-eating disorder a typical pathway—often called the "path to mindful eating"—follows:

1. Stop binge-eating and purging.
2. Eliminate mindless eating.
3. Decrease cravings, urges, and preoccupations with food.
4. Decrease capitulating—close off options to binge-eat and purge.
5. Decrease apparently irrelevant behaviors (e.g., buying binge foods "for company").
6. Increase skillful emotion regulation behaviors by learning and practicing skills from three modules: Mindfulness, Emotion Regulation, and Distress Tolerance.

With this level of clarity and specificity, the DBT therapist is appropriately prepared to take on the challenge of treating binge-eating disorder within the overall DBT treatment approach.

CONCLUDING COMMENTS

We have reviewed the central importance of DBT's goals, stages, and targets in individual psychotherapy, other modes of treatment, implementation and maintenance of DBT programs, and the adaptation of DBT to other settings and populations. Without this crucial structure at the core of DBT, therapy and implementation tend to drift, driven by priorities other than those based on treating the patient with effectiveness and compassion. It is useful to have a framework that specifies not only what to treat, but also what not to treat or what to defer until later.

CHAPTER 8

Dialectical Dilemmas and Secondary Targets

Doing DBT is like climbing a mountain. The therapist and patient need to chart their course together, stock up on all necessary equipment in advance, work as a team, and handle a wide range of predictable and unpredictable challenges along the way. The ultimate goal in climbing is to reach the summit, which in DBT is for the patient to experience a life worth living. This will usually require scaling several smaller summits along the way. Similarly, the DBT therapist works with the patient to scale several "smaller summits," sequentially, to achieve a strong commitment to the journey; bring an end to life-threatening behaviors; overcome significant therapy-interfering behaviors; resolve a number of quality-of-life-interfering behaviors; acquire a repertoire of skills; and proceed onward to scale the summits of Stages 2, 3, and 4. Having successfully negotiated the sequence of primary targets, the patient arrives at a life worth living.

The climber can often see the next summit or locate it on a topographical map. It is discrete, definable, there for the taking. Its presence provides direction and motivation. But the truth is, to ascend the summit may require forging raging streams, scaling steep rock faces, enduring sudden storms, slogging through swamps, losing and finding the trail several times, and pushing through discouragement and fatigue. In other words, the real work of getting to the next summit in view is the work of traversing these challenges. The identifiable summits in DBT, the primary targets, can be described rather succinctly as well: to increase commitment, decrease self-cutting, increase attendance at therapy, decrease substance use, and so on. To accomplish any one of these primary targets requires slogging through the resolution of complex behavioral patterns—the DBT equivalent of swollen streams, steep rock faces, sudden storms, scary swamps, fatigue, and discouragement. The swamps in DBT—the complex and problematic behavioral patterns encountered daily in therapy—present as obstacles standing in the way of the resolution of the primary target behaviors. In so doing, they tend to maintain the primary target behaviors.

In contrast to the discrete and definable primary targets, these patterns are anything but clear-cut. They involve constellations of emotion, thought, and action; they can be extensive, with unclear boundaries around them. In fact, the therapist might not recognize them as patterns at all, and could end up unwittingly colluding with them. I once treated a patient with a debilitating combination of self-hatred, self-harm, substance abuse, and violence toward inanimate objects. Her behaviors occurred in episodes of emotional and behavioral dyscontrol, culminating in dramatic self-harming behaviors. Two months into therapy, our most consistent primary target, session after session, had become the reduction of self-injurious behavior. For several consecutive weeks, we assessed episodes of self-harm with behavioral chain analyses. A pattern gradually emerged: The self-harming behaviors were functioning to terminate painful episodes of emotional dysregulation and behavioral dyscontrol; these behaviors provided a kind of punctuation point, quickly reducing emotional pain while creating psychological distractions such as trips to the emergency room and crisis assessments. These episodes resulted in enhanced behavioral control and a sense of relief.

Once we identified the nature of the pattern leading up to the self-harm, I recognized that I was inadvertently perpetuating the pattern. I was compassionate and validating when assessing the episodes, with the intention of reducing the intensity of her shame. But I learned that she experienced my compassion as a form of "forgiveness," which actually reinforced the episodes. In other words, I was participating in a dysfunctional cycle: (1) Her emotional dysregulation, accompanied by behavioral dyscontrol, was "solved" through an episode of self-cutting; (2) as she reviewed the episode with me in sessions, accompanied by intense shame, I responded with compassion and validation; (3) she interpreted my interventions as akin to "forgiveness," similar to her experience of confessing her sins to her Catholic priest as a child; (4) it felt to her as if our interchange "cleaned the slate"; and (5) this "confession" would set the stage for another episode. Until I could understand the whole sequence, I didn't perceive my own role in reinforcing the episodes. Had I been able to recognize the behavioral pattern more promptly and objectively, I could have treated it more efficiently and effectively.

In Linehan's early years of developing DBT, while assessing and treating primary treatment targets, she encountered a multitude of similar problematic behavioral patterns. She categorized those patterns. As different as they were in each case, there were common themes. She noticed that they presented in pairs, such that one problematic pattern could be seen as existing at one end of a certain dimension, with another at the opposite end. The paired patterns often seemed to be polar opposites, and seemed in some respects to be interdependent with one another. She named six such patterns, existing in three pairs.

1. Along one dimension related to the theme of emotion modulation, a dysfunctional pattern that she named "emotional vulnerability" lay at one end, opposite to a dysfunctional pattern called "self-invalidation."
2. Along a second dimension related to the theme of asking for help, a dysfunctional help-seeking pattern of "active passivity" lay at one end and an equally dysfunctional help-seeking pattern of "apparent competence" lay at the other.
3. Along a third dimension related to the theme of processing loss and trauma, dysfunctional patterns of "unrelenting crisis" and "inhibited grieving" lay at opposite ends of the continuum.

Because these dialectically related pairs of behavioral patterns stood in the way of successfully treating primary treatment targets, Linehan (1993a) called them, collectively, the "dialectical dilemmas." They can be seen in relationship to one another in Figure 8.1.

Notice that the three dimensions intersect at a midpoint. Linehan (1993a) posited that the patterns above that point were influenced more by biological factors, and that the patterns below that point were more heavily influenced by responses coming from the social environment. For instance, at one end of a dimension, represented by the vertical line, the pattern of emotional vulnerability is hypothesized to be the result of biological factors; the pattern of self-invalidation is hypothesized to be the cumulative result of environmental responses to the individual's emotional vulnerabilities. The three patterns that are thought to be influenced more by biology are interrelated in a meaningful way to each other, and sometimes present in overlapping fashion in therapy. They all represent extremes of underregulation, or dyscontrol, of action, thought, and/or emotion. The three patterns thought to be influenced more by environment also tend to cluster together to one degree or another, and they seem to represent extremes of overregulation, or overcontrol, of actions, cognitions, and/or emotions. Of interest, the three dialectical dilemmas

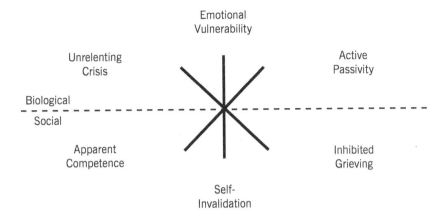

FIGURE 8.1. Dialectical dilemmas.

proposed by Rathus and Miller (2015) to understand the relationship patterns between adolescents and their families also revolve around the opposition of patterns of undercontrol (e.g., excessive leniency) and those of overcontrol (e.g., authoritarian control).

In spite of the fact that the dialectical dilemmas occupy a central role in DBT case conceptualization and in clinical practice, they are sometimes understated in training and literature. Recognizing, labeling, and treating these patterns in real time during therapy is invaluable. Here I spotlight the nature, functions, and clinical utility of the dialectical dilemmas. In addition, an understanding of the principles underlying the construct allows a therapist to tailor the dialectical dilemmas flexibly to each case, and to derive dialectical dilemmas other than the six proposed by Linehan. In this chapter, we consider (1) the crucial theoretical relationship between DBT's biosocial theory and the dialectical dilemmas; (2) the nature of the three dialectical dilemmas in clinical context; (3) how we derive the secondary targets in DBT (those behavioral patterns that cause and maintain the primary target behaviors) from the dialectical dilemmas, and how we use them; and (4) how we can identify additional dialectical dilemmas and secondary targets.

BIOSOCIAL THEORY
AND DIALECTICAL DILEMMAS

Beginning with Linehan's manual for comprehensive DBT (1993a), DBT's biosocial theory has been described in detail in multiple contexts.

Although we are not interested here in comprehensively restating or reconsidering this fruitful theory, a brief review of its essential ingredients will set the stage for understanding the relationship between the biosocial theory and the dialectical dilemmas. Currently being subjected to empirical study, the theory is a set of hypotheses offered to explain the causation and maintenance of problem behaviors treated in DBT. The overarching proposition is that chronic and severe emotional dysregulation results from an enduring transaction between an individual's biologically based emotional vulnerabilities and the pervasive environmentally based invalidation of these vulnerabilities. This proposition is represented in Figure 8.2.

Linehan (1993a) proposes that the term *emotional vulnerabilities* encompasses three biologically based features: (1) higher than average emotional sensitivity to environmental cues, (2) higher than average emotional reactivity (amplitude), and (3) slower than average return to baseline. The biological influences could come from genetics, the intrauterine environment, radical postnatal influences of neglect and abuse, and/or significant psychological trauma during development. Presumably, anyone who inherits or acquires these biologically based vulnerabilities will be more sensitive and more reactive than the average person to emotionally salient stimuli throughout development. In learning to experience, recognize, and manage these vulnerabilities, the individual will be heavily influenced by the responses of the relevant environment(s), such as parents, caretakers, teachers, coaches, peers, and society in general.

Linehan (1993a) further proposes that the emotionally vulnerable individual raised in predominantly validating environments will learn effective means for living with, and making the most of, emotional sensitivity and reactivity. Key environmental figures will show a measure of tolerance, compassion, and understanding for the vulnerabilities, and will address them with a combination of effective buffering, modeling, and coaching. This type of thoughtful and constructive response, when consistent, is unlikely to result in the behavioral patterns of borderline personality disorder. But the same emotionally vulnerable individuals raised in a relatively *invalidating* environment, where the predominant responses to the their emotions as children are undermining, are placed at high risk for developing the problematic behavioral patterns of borderline personality disorder. Linehan (1993a) proposed three characteristics of invalidating environments to be the tendency to (1) judge, disregard, dismiss, pathologize, or otherwise punish the individual's valid emotional responses; (2) intermittently reinforce the escalation of emotional responses; and (3) oversimplify the ease of solving emotional problems. As a result, the individual who is already contending with a biologically

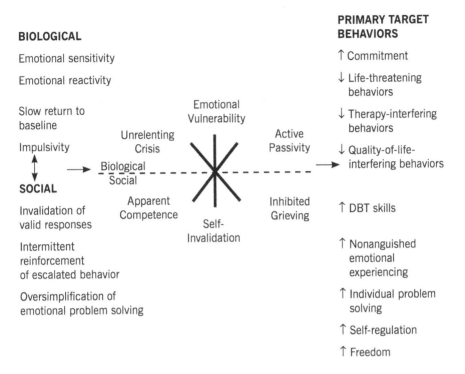

FIGURE 8.2. Biosocial theory, dialectical dilemmas, and primary treatment targets.

based excess of poorly regulated emotional responses, fails to acquire the capacity to accurately discern and label her emotional responses, to understand her emotions in a compassionate manner, or to use strategies to regulate those responses.

Linehan (1993a) further highlights four capabilities that emerged in research on the development of emotion modulation in children (Gottman & Katz, 1989). These capabilities are crucial for the individual with high emotional vulnerability: the ability (1) to inhibit inappropriate behavior related to strong negative or positive affect; (2) to self-regulate physiological arousal associated with affect; (3) to refocus attention in the presence of strong affect; and (4) to organize oneself for ongoing action in the service of an external, non-mood-dependent goal. These relative capacities, which could heavily determine a person's "emotional intelligence" and success in life, seem to occupy an intermediate location between the biologically based and environmentally based factors. At times Linehan has suggested when teaching workshops that there may be some evidence for genetic input into these capabilities, but it is also easy to see that their presence could be reinforced or inhibited by environmental factors. I have often found them useful as an inventory of emotion modulation capabilities, which I apply to my patients in assessment and treatment.

The theory is a transactional one. Prolonged exposure to the invalidating environment actually worsens the individual's problems of emotional vulnerability; the individual's worsening problems of emotional vulnerability further challenge the environment, which can then become more invalidating. The spiraling transaction eventually results in the problem hypothesized in DBT to be at the core of borderline personality disorder: chronic and severe emotional dysregulation. Once the core problem has taken root in the individual, in whatever form, it can be rekindled again and again by encounters with relatively invalidating responses in new environments. These include encounters in psychotherapy, where the therapist's push for behavioral change almost ensures that the patient will feel invalidated and will become emotionally dysregulated. As uncomfortable as this dysregulation is for both parties, it offers repeated opportunities for the *in vivo* treatment of the core problems in real time.

The three primary concepts in the biosocial theory—*biologically based emotional vulnerability, invalidating environment,* and *chronic and severe emotional dysregulation*—are seen from the perspective of the outside scientific observer. Each concept is defined objectively, in ways that can then be subjected to research. The outcome of the biosocial transaction takes shape in the form of certain complex behavioral patterns in the individual patient, and these are the dialectical dilemmas. But although the biosocial theory and the dialectical dilemmas are intimately related to each other, with the former giving rise to the latter, they represent very different perspectives. Rather than the objective, scientific perspective of the biosocial theory, the dialectical dilemmas represent the subjective perspective of the individual. For instance, *emotional vulnerability* is a scientifically defined construct, seen from the "outside-in," when we are considering the biosocial theory; but the same term, when used to name one of the dialectical dilemmas, refers to the "inside-out" perspective of one who is suffering from uncontrollable, agonizing emotional responses. Similarly, in biosocial theory the term *invalidating* refers to an objective construct with several defined features, whereas the term *self-invalidation,* as one of the dialectical dilemmas, refers to the painful subjective experience of self-criticism or self-hatred. We move from the language of theory to the language of personal experience.

The six extreme patterns that comprise the dialectical dilemmas represent six "faces" of severe and chronic emotion dysregulation as experienced by the patient and, in treatment, seen by the therapist. When optimally understood, the dialectical dilemmas serve as a window into the various painful results of the transactional developmental process, and as a bridge of understanding between therapist and patient that can foster collaboration on transforming the patterns. Not every pattern or dilemma will be present in every DBT patient; it is always up to the therapist to assess for the presence and the role of the patterns in causing or maintaining primary target behaviors. Once the particular dialectical dilemmas and patterns are identified, and a language to describe them that fosters collaboration is developed, the therapist and patient can work persistently on fading out the extreme patterns and replacing them with skillful ones that are conceptually located in the middle path between the two extremes.

THE NATURE OF THE THREE DIALECTICAL DILEMMAS IN CLINICAL CONTEXT

Having reviewed the biosocial theory and considered the general nature of the dialectical dilemmas, we can examine the nature of each of the dilemmas and how each is generated by the transactional influence of the two poles proposed in biosocial theory. Regarding the dilemma of *emotional vulnerability versus self-invalidation*, these two extreme, dialectically opposed patterns result when the child, already emotionally vulnerable within a pervasively invalidating environment, is learning the basics of how to modulate emotions. As to the dilemma of *active passivity versus apparent competence*, these two patterns arise as the emotionally vulnerable individual in a pervasively invalidating environment learns the basics about feeling distress, communicating distress, and asking for help as needed. Finally, the emotionally vulnerable individual learning the basics of managing and processing losses and trauma in a pervasively invalidating environment arrives at the dialectically opposed patterns of *unrelenting crisis versus inhibited grieving*. Next, I consider the three dilemmas one at a time.

Emotional Vulnerability versus Self-Invalidation

Let's start with the process of learning to modulate emotions. When the emotionally vulnerable child expresses emotional responses, often imbued with intensity and often aversive to those who receive them, he places demands on the environment. If the environment is ill equipped to handle those demands in a constructive way, the emotional expressions will be met with low tolerance, harsh judgment, and pejorative labeling. The figures in the environment have no room and show little compassion for the kind of responding that might allow the individual to experiment with, to "play" with, emotional expressiveness. Little effort is made to help the individual label and tolerate painful emotions. And there is likely to be almost no step-by-step coaching or modeling for the child in the crucial tasks of structuring his environment to reduce the frequency or intensity of emotional stimuli; experiencing, tolerating, and managing the onset of an emotional response; naming an emotion once it is activated; regulating himself effectively in the face of strong emotions; and interrupting the momentum and perpetuation of a painful emotional process.

The emotionally vulnerable individual is therefore lost at sea in wave after wave of intensified emotions that are felt to be painfully spreading, bleeding into other painful emotional responses. Linehan (1993a, pp. 67–71) has written that the patient has "no emotional skin"; the slightest winds can set off bouts of emotional agony. The patient may sense that the emotions will never stop; life is experienced through the windows of these emotions. The sense of time and perspective gives way to totalistic experiences of intense fear, shame, guilt, sorrow, anger, or other painful emotions. Without having the capabilities to regulate the process, the individual eventually finds behaviors that temporarily alleviate the otherwise relentless pain. These behaviors are reinforced because they work, and the individual comes to rely on them. Typical examples are suicidal attempts, self-harming actions, homicidal assaults, the use of substances, episodes of dissociation, dropping out of treatment, or engaging in extreme interpersonal behaviors. These behaviors become the destructive but reliable answer to unstoppable emotional vulnerability. It is easy to see how unchecked emotional vulnerability could drive an individual to suicide accidentally or intentionally. In DBT, these behaviors become the primary treatment targets for elimination.

Emotional vulnerability is an experiential manifestation—a magnification—of the biologically based emotional vulnerability noted in biosocial theory. At the other extreme, self-invalidation is a magnified experiential inheritance of the harsh perspective of the invalidating environment. Imitating the invalidating figures of the environment, the individual harshly judges and labels her own emotional responses, ignores and suppresses them to whatever degree possible, occasionally erupts emotionally in a way that brings some measure of attention and support, and arrives at unrealistic and simplistic goals for regulating emotions. In some patients, it appears as if self-invalidation is the verbal equivalent of vicious self-cutting. One patient spoke of putting her hand through a meat grinder because it was the only thing she could imagine that would capture her aggressive self-hatred; not surprisingly, she had been the target of denigrating attacks throughout her childhood. To direct critical attacks toward the self can transform the pain of undercontrol—the consuming, spiraling, emotional agony without boundaries of emotional vulnerability—to the pain of overcontrol—the focused, disciplined, self-denigration of self-invalidation. Emotional agony is replaced with harsh self-judgment, self-control, aggressive self-discipline, and self-hatred, as the patient's attitude toward self becomes, in essence, "You are an idiot! You are weak! What's the matter with you?" There is even a measure of hope implicit in the self-judgments—"If only you were not so stupid, weak, and incompetent, then you could manage your life better." At the extreme edge of self-invalidation, it is easy to see that the individual's intolerable degree of self-hatred could lead to suicide.

Although some patients may remain in one of these opposing patterns more enduringly than the other, in many cases patients alternate between the two. When you grasp the subjective flavor of the two different dysfunctional ways of coping with the task of emotion modulation, it is possible to feel the flow back and forth between them. While emotional agony continues, the sense of self-judgment and self-hatred for being so emotional can grow until that person flips to self-invalidation as a predominant experience. While immersed in the throes of self-invalidation, the individual may experience a growing sense of emotional dyscontrol until the switch back to emotional vulnerability takes place. By flipping back and forth between these two "channels," there is no new learning of a middle path, which might include self-awareness, self-compassion, self-validation, and/or skillful means for modulating emotions. There can be a sense of stagnation and growing despair.

I was once asked to do a thorough retrospective review of the case of a teenage girl who committed suicide months after being raped and subsequently humiliated by the online distribution of photographs depicting the rape. As I pieced the story together, I learned that in those final months she had failed to notify her parents, law enforcement, or school authorities about the rape or the photographs, that she felt herself to be the laughing stock of the school, and that she vacillated wildly between unstoppable sadness, fear, and hatred of her perpetrators, and terrible bouts of shame, hating herself for "letting it happen." During one of those shame episodes she viciously attacked her legs with scissors, resulting in multiple sutures and a hospitalization. When the details of her traumatic experience came to light during her hospitalization, her parents suggested that she keep those details mostly to herself so that her social standing in the school would not be further jeopardized. They suggested that she might have been exaggerating the degree to which she was victimized. By all accounts, her biology and her environment did fit the profile of the biosocial theory, as she showed high emotional sensitivity and reactivity, and her home environment emphasized emotional suppression and social appropriateness above all. She was caught between the two poles of emotional vulnerability and self-invalidation, the disclosure of the facts brought even more invalidation, both patterns of this dialectical dilemma moved to more extreme forms, and she saw no way out. She killed herself and left a suicide note in which she emphasized her self-hatred, omitting any mention of the invalidating experiences with her perpetrators or her parents.

Active Passivity versus Apparent Competence

The second pair of dialectical dilemmas grows out of the fact that every child needs help with painful experiences. The child with high emotional vulnerability in the context of a pervasively invalidating environment is not likely to learn an effective way to communicate painful experience and ask for help. Envisioning how this is likely to work, it begins as the child experiences distress of some kind. Not having yet developed capacities to manage and resolve it, he communicates his distress, in one way or another, to those in his environment, seeking support. In a relatively validating environment, those around the child might notice his expressions of distress, receive them with concern and interest, and help him to name the emotions. They might then help the child solve the problem causing the distress, coach him in how to regulate the troubling emotions, assist him in tolerating the distress temporarily and safely, and reinforce him for coping adaptively. If the environment is pervasively invalidating, the child's indications of distress and implied requests for support are met with some flavor of dismay, disapproval, judgment, and/or rejection. As the caregivers are often dysregulated themselves, or incapable of knowing how to parent the distressed child, his emotions are seen as undesirable, exaggerated, invalid, and even manipulative. The consistent invalidation pushes the child toward emotional suppression.

The child's efforts to hide his emotions, and to extinguish them if possible, grow into one of the two extreme patterns in this dialectical dilemma: apparent competence or active passivity. *Apparent competence* refers to the masking of emotional distress in the context of those who could conceivably provide assistance. The individual with this syndrome does not learn to experience or express emotions accurately, and may develop considerable confusion about whether he is in need of help or not. If asked how he is doing, this person may answer, "Fine,"

"OK," or "I'm good," and deflect attention by focusing on the one who is asking. Such individuals in psychotherapy not uncommonly begin the session by asking the therapist how *she* is doing, or respond to the therapist's inquiries with "Don't worry, I'll be fine." The suppression of emotional distress and the failure to communicate it to those in the environment result in a situation in which no one around the patient actually appreciates his degree of distress. Consequently, people treat him as if he is "OK." Still, he may think that people should be able to "read" his distress and respond to it. The fact that they don't do so worsens his sense of isolation, of being "unknown" and invisible. This very isolating pattern can lead to considerable loneliness, resentment, and despair, and it is easy to see that taken to an extreme, it could eventuate in suicide as a means of extinguishing intolerable pain or punishing a callous environment.

In the increasingly pressurized situation that takes place behind the mask of apparent competence, it is likely that the individual desperately needs interpersonal support. Prior efforts to get help have been extinguished and punished. At a certain point he flips over to the dialectically opposite pattern of active passivity. *Passivity*, in the term *active passivity*, refers to the passive approach to procuring needed support. Yet the individual is "active" in recruiting help, usually through a loss of behavioral control—a crisis behavior of some kind that elicits support from those around. The passivity is active, so to speak, and functions to elicit support. To be very clear, this is not a conscious choice. Active passivity is a pattern of behavior that evolves in the context of invalidation, that secures much-needed attention and support, and that has been intermittently reinforced multiple times in development. It is not unusual for the mental health system to reinforce the pattern of active passivity by offering attention and support only when the patient evidences a more serious loss of control. Given the behavioral dyscontrol that is part of the pattern of active passivity, and the intensity of internal distress that drives it, it is easy to understand that suicide could result from this pattern either accidentally or intentionally.

As was discussed regarding the dialectical dilemma of emotional vulnerability and self-invalidation, it may be that an individual evidences primarily one of these two patterns, in which case the therapist assesses it in detail and works to reduce it and replace it with more skillful means for communicating distress and asking for help. But not uncommonly, the emotionally vulnerable individual who experiences distress and requires help in a pervasively invalidating environment flips back and forth between the two opposing patterns, never learning adaptive ways to solve the problem in the "middle path" between the two.

At one point I was working in a DBT intensive outpatient program. It was the end of the day and nearly everyone had left. One patient remained, as did her therapist. The patient was experiencing intense distress and did not want to go home to her apartment where she would be alone. She appeared at the door of her therapist's office. When asked how she was doing, she responded: "Great! I'm fine. I just happened to still be here so I thought I'd say hello. But I should leave now, I can see you've got work to do." The therapist: "Really, if you want to hang around, you can stay until I lock up." Patient: "No, I think I'll head out. I'll see you tomorrow." Therapist: "OK, good night." Twenty minutes later, when the therapist locked up, left the building, and went to the parking lot, the patient was lying on the ground in front of the right front tire of the therapist's car. The therapist spoke to the patient, who remained mute. She would not move when addressed. The therapist called the emergency services team, which evaluated and hospitalized her. This an example of how an individual in need of distress but lacking the skills to ask for it, can flip between apparent competence and active passivity in the search for rescue. The likely outcome of this scenario, in which the distressed patient received the attention and support of the emergency room and hospital, is that the "actively passive" behaviors were reinforced.

After years of teaching DBT, it is clear to me that active passivity is the most poorly understood of the six behavioral patterns. The term is sometimes used as shorthand for almost any kind of loss of behavioral control. Sometimes therapists use the term with a judgmental tone: "There she goes with her active passivity again." For me it is reminiscent of the way in which inpatient staff members in psychodynamically oriented programs loosely use the term *acting out* to refer to almost any undesirable behavior, without specific reference to the more disciplined meaning of the term in psychodynamic theory. In the case of active passivity, it is important that we have an accurate understanding, and one that helps us approach it with empathy.

Toward this end, I recall a metaphor that Marsha Linehan used when teaching an intensive workshop (1993, New York Hospital–Cornell Medical Center, Westchester Division, White Plains, New York) to convey the meaning and function of active passivity. Imagine that a shipwreck occurs near an island in the middle of the ocean. The sole survivor swims to the island. Over several years she learns how to survive: creating an effective shelter, protecting herself from predators and the elements, and learning how to eat off the land and from the sea. No ships come near the island and only rarely does a plane fly overhead. She is assumed to have died with the others from the ship, so no one is looking for her. Although she has learned to survive, she is desperately lonely (compare the internal experience of the individual with apparent competence). She remains on the lookout for the rare event of a low-flying plane. The question for us in this context is this: In the event that a small plane should pass overhead, low enough to see her and her surroundings, how should she behave when it comes by? If the pilot looks down and sees the situation, with a well-maintained shelter and a waving woman, he may totally fail to recognize that the individual needs help. He might even think, "How quaint, romantic, and courageous; I really should do something like that myself," in which case he might simply smile, wave, and fly away. If the sole survivor wants to maximize the possibility that the pilot will land the plane and rescue her, she needs to appear frantic and desperate. A wiser approach might be to set her shelter on fire and to flail and roll around on the ground, making it obvious that things are not right. Using our term, she would employ *active passivity* as the only means to elicit desperately needed support. Understood correctly, active passivity is a perfectly sensible strategy for individuals who cannot effectively communicate distress and ask for help. Of course the most effective path would be, if possible, to learn to recognize internal distress, express those feelings, and ask for help. That would constitute the middle path between the two extremes.

Unrelenting Crisis versus Inhibited Grieving

Whereas the first dialectical dilemma revolves around the effective modulation of emotions, and the second revolves around the communication of distress and the effective request for help, the third one revolves around the processing of significant losses and traumatic events. Of course, losses and traumatic events, defined broadly, are common early in life, but for the individual with borderline personality disorder, typically the number of such events is way beyond average; grief overload and PTSD are common. Within a validating environment, the individual beset with loss or trauma is met in a supportive way that helps him recognize and process the loss or trauma, helps him develop a realistic narrative that gradually allows him to put it in the past and move on in life.

But the invalidating parental environment, for a range of reasons, is ill equipped to help the individual manage and process losses and traumatic events. Not only do the caregivers show disinterest in the individual's negative life events; they are likely to communicate that those events didn't really happen or were not that serious. We might recall the example earlier in this chapter, in which the parents of the teenage girl who was raped and then committed suicide minimized the traumatizing events of their daughter. By invalidating the nature or the extent of the painful experience, parents in these situations implicitly or explicitly insist that the young person bury his grief and traumas, and "stop complaining." This pervasive message activates the two previously discussed dialectical dilemmas (emotional vulnerability vs. self-invalidation, and active passivity vs. inhibited grieving), and furthermore contributes to the third dialectical dilemma, inhibited grieving versus unrelenting crisis. Unable to process or tolerate the globally disruptive impact of negative life events, and unable to get effective help from the environment to do so, the highly sensitive, reactive individual reacts with affective dysregulation, distractibility, rigid and unrealistic thinking, faulty anticipation of consequences, and confusion. In this state, he acts impulsively and makes errors in judgment, resulting in the pattern of "unrelenting crisis." It can be difficult even for a therapist to recognize that the pattern of impulsivity and poor judgment, fostering chaos, is related to an incapacity to tolerate and process responses to loss and trauma. Having an awareness of this pattern during careful listening and a systematic study of antecedents may help the therapist formulate the "underlying" problem: the failure to process life events in a safe and effective manner. Obviously, unrelenting crisis, driven as it is by unrealistic thinking and poor decision making, can lead to chaos, despair, and in the extreme case, suicide.

Whereas unrelenting crisis is the pattern in this dilemma that is characterized by global dyscontrol (i.e., cognitions, emotions, and actions), its dialectical partner, inhibited grieving, heavily influenced by the invalidating environment, is characterized by overcontrol. The patient automatically avoids cues related to grief or trauma, and when exposed to them, attempts to escape from them and from his initial response to them as quickly as possible. The individual is engaged in a constant effort to block awareness and extinguish memory of negative events. As a result, he loses access to memories of those events and they continue to haunt him, living in the shadows of daily life, ready to return and hijack somatic and behavioral processes in a moment's notice. Inhibited grieving can result in temporary shutdowns of emotional experiencing altogether, which then set the stage for sudden eruptions of suppressed experience resulting in unrelenting crisis or the other two biologically driven patterns of active passivity and emotional vulnerability. Inhibited grieving, taken to the extreme, can result in a level of suppression and detachment that lends itself to extreme loneliness, despair, and suicide.

To summarize, the biosocial theory posits a transaction that takes place between a biologically based emotional vulnerability and an invalidating environment. Burdened with this transaction, the individual undertakes the processes of learning to relate to the world and to her own responses to that world. Three of these processes are to modulate emotions, to ask for help, and to process painful life events. Rather than developing relatively balanced and effective solutions to each of these challenges, as might occur under more optimal conditions, the individual develops two dialectically opposed types of extreme behavioral patterns. Because each pattern is inherently unstable and temporary, the individual alternates from one of these patterns to another, a bit like switching from one bad channel to another, leading to a growing sense of hopelessness and helplessness. The DBT therapist tries to help the patient to develop, in the case of each of the three dilemmas, a "middle path" channel whereby she can effectively modulate emotions, ask for help, and process loss and trauma.

DERIVING DBT'S SECONDARY TARGETS FROM THE DIALECTICAL DILEMMAS

As DBT therapists, we make our way through behavioral chain analyses in the assessment of primary target behaviors and thereby identify behaviors and behavioral patterns that promote or maintain the primary target behavior. For instance, we may find that for a given patient, her self-cutting behaviors often take place in the context of an explosion of shame. Self-cutting is linked with shame for that patient, and the treatment of self-cutting will require the treatment of shame. Improving the management of shame becomes a "secondary target," or "instrumental target," in that it is secondary, and instrumental to, the treatment of the primary target.

Having characterized the three dialectical dilemmas, which can result in six problematic behavioral patterns, we can see that each of the patterns could function to promote or maintain a given primary target behavior. Therefore, the resolution of each pattern might become a secondary target: the treatment of self-cutting for a given patient might require the treatment of self-invalidation, or the treatment of problematic substance use might require the treatment of unrelenting crisis in another patient. Furthermore, the presence of any one of the six patterns can give rise to two secondary treatment targets. On the one hand, we can work to decrease the problematic pattern: for instance, to decrease self-invalidation. On the other hand, we can work to increase the acquisition, strengthening, and generalization of the skill set that can replace the dysfunctional pattern: for instance, to increase self-validation.

Beginning with the first dialectical dilemma discussed above, we can derive four potential types of secondary targets, two for each pattern. With respect to the pattern of emotional vulnerability, we work to

(1) *decrease emotional reactivity* and (2) *increase* its "antidote," *emotional modulation*. With respect to the pattern of self-invalidation, we work to (3) *decrease self-invalidation* and (4) *increase* its "antidote," *self-validation*. Each of these four secondary targets refers not to simple and singular behaviors but rather to a complex pattern of emotion, cognition, and action, with a different profile in each case. In other words, the effort to increase or decrease a given pattern serving as a secondary target will require an understanding of the ingredients of that pattern. For instance, one patient's "apparent competence" will involve different specifics than another patient's "apparent competence." Treatment of the secondary targets that are derived from the dialectical dilemmas must be individualized and spelled out in each case.

Although they sound almost like the same thing, *decreasing self-invalidation* and *increasing self-validation* are two distinctly different processes. For example, let's say that I hate myself, convinced that I am stupid, fat, and ugly. This self-denigration is based in the pervasive attitude of my original invalidating environment, but I perpetuate the attitudes in my own self-hatred. Almost any reference to appearances or attractiveness by someone around me sets off a litany of self-invalidating statements, self-hatred, shame, and eventually I cut myself, which "gives me what I deserve" and at the same time provides temporary relief. In this scenario, the reduction of self-cutting behaviors is the primary target; one of the secondary targets is to decrease self-invalidation. My DBT therapist will have me monitor my self-invalidating episodes, communicate the details to him, and he will work with me strategically to reduce my self-invalidation. Another secondary target would be to increase self-validation. In contrast to the effort to reduce self-invalidation, this target would involve working with me strategically to increase my capacity to validate my own thoughts, emotions, and actions; that is, to see that my beliefs that I am fat, ugly, and stupid are understandable, given my history. It would involve turning an understanding and compassionate tone toward my own suffering, my own shame, and the chain of events that led me to this point. And it may involve validating some of my capabilities with cheerleading statements that create an alternative point of view toward myself.

I was assessing the primary target behaviors of bingeing and purging in a woman who communicated disgust about the shape of her body. She was forever wanting to be thinner. All of her efforts to extinguish her rather normal appetite were unsuccessful, and she alternated between restricting and bingeing. The battle with her body and her appetite was distressing, but it seemed to define an area, something of a battleground, in which she felt a measure of control and hope—hope that if she could reduce her intake, she might become thinner and feel more worthwhile. When she wasn't battling her weight, life seemed meaningless to her, empty, and she experienced waves of sadness and hopelessness. It became painfully clear that when she was not focused on controlling her weight, the memory of certain terrible losses in her life came back to mind, bringing grief and sorrow.

The eating disorder behaviors of restricting, bingeing, and purging were the primary target behaviors. Maintaining the target behaviors were several dialectical dilemmas: emotional vulnerability versus self-invalidation, active passivity versus apparent competence, and the pattern of inhibited grieving. Identifying the dialectical dilemmas active in this patient pointed toward several secondary targets: decreasing emotional reactivity, increasing emotion modulation, decreasing self-invalidation, increasing self-validation, decreasing active passivity, increasing active problem solving, decreasing apparent competence, increasing accurate expression, decreasing inhibited grieving, and increasing the processing of cues related to loss and trauma. The battle to end the eating disorder would be fought within the territory defined by several patterns of dialectical dilemmas. To the degree that the therapist has specified the problematic behaviors within a particular patient's dialectical dilemmas, she can be quite specific about how to target them within the treatment plan.

Whereas the "first draft" of a treatment plan might include the targets of reducing active passivity and reducing apparent competence, the more specific plan breaks these generic targets down further. With respect to the pattern of active passivity, the therapist may be working toward (5) *decreasing behaviors that solve problems by eliciting rescue from others* and (6) *increasing active problem solving*. With respect to the pattern of apparent competence, the therapist may be working toward (7) *decreasing mood dependency* of behaviors and (8) *increasing accurate communication of emotions*. Once the secondary targets are fleshed out in sufficient details, the therapist can employ DBT strategies to accomplish them. For instance, *increasing active problem solving* may require improved emotion regulation skills that help to reduce avoidance, better interpersonal effectiveness skills to sharpen the capacity to self-assert and to say "no," or more enhanced self-management skills to strengthen executive functioning.

Increasing accurate communication employs several skills: exercising mindful and nonjudgmental awareness of one's negative emotions, expressing emotions accurately through verbal and nonverbal channels, checking to see if the intended communication has been received, and being specific in asking for help. With regard to the secondary target of *decreasing mood dependency*, Linehan (1993a, pp. 163–164) emphasizes that the patient must learn to separate his current mood from his current actions such that actions are aligned with goals rather than moods. The process of active passivity, with its loss of behavioral control, is fueled by the deep belief that one must act in accordance with one's mood. If I am depressed, I act depressed; if angry, I must demonstrate my anger; and so on. If I am in need of help and no one is offering it, I must act in a manner that brings me the support I need, even if it requires "falling apart." To decrease mood dependency and to decrease active passivity will require acting in a manner consistent with my long-term goals rather than my immediate mood. Radical acceptance of reality, along with a range of problem-solving skills, will be crucial in achieving this secondary target.

When primary target behaviors are functionally related to patterns in the third dialectical dilemma, unrelenting crisis versus inhibited grieving, four more secondary targets are potentially at work. With respect to unrelenting crisis, the therapist is helping to (9) *decrease crisis-generating behaviors* and (10) *increase realistic decision making and judgment*. With respect to inhibited grieving, he is helping to (11) *decrease inhibited grieving* and (12) *increase emotional experiencing*. Once again, note that these are *types* of secondary targets, not secondary targets themselves. The particulars need to be assessed case by case.

Decreasing crisis-generating behaviors will require different approaches for each individual, but the above-discussed problem of mood dependency is usually important here. If a patient "feels a crisis coming on," he needs to learn ways to act against that "feeling." The therapist needs to challenge the patient's sense that crisis after crisis is inevitable and work on ways to structure the environment, manage emotions, and make behavioral choices that reduce the likelihood of generating a crisis. Increasing realistic decision making and judgment is the "positive" skill set required here. Often individuals with borderline personality disorder have become accustomed to being the recipients, often the victims, of the decision making of others, and have not acquired the attitude and skill of determining their own course, generating possible action plans, evaluating those plans with respect to possible outcomes, and coming to their own choices.

Decreasing inhibited grieving must take place in a therapeutic relationship when trust has developed. Within such a safe context the therapist helps the patient to understand that she has suffered crucial losses and traumas, that these are real and have exerted real impacts, that the process of inhibiting such memories and experiences has negative consequences, and that, with assistance, these negative life events can be approached safely and thoughtfully without losing control. The therapist will work with the patient to increase emotional experiencing in general, rather than relying on inhibition as a primary approach, and emotional experiencing in particular with respect to losses and trauma after more trust has developed, more skills have been acquired, and the patient wants to do it. To stop inhibiting grieving and to increase the capacity to experience emotions will require skills from the modules of core mindfulness, emotion regulation, and distress tolerance.

Having the menu of six dialectical dilemmas and the twelve associated secondary targets helps to conceptualize the case and treat the patient. I once treated a 19-year-old woman who lived in a prominent family in which all members appeared to be quite successful. They were all attractive, had a beautiful house, and in their community they were admired or respected. It took about eight sessions before the 19-year-old revealed to me that she was hurting herself. In fact, she was using a hammer to smash her wrists. She had broken bones twice, in each case claiming that she was having skateboarding accidents. When I assessed the primary target behavior of hitting and breaking her own bones, I used the dialectical dilemmas as a menu of possible controlling variables, as a sort of scanning procedure. First, considering emotional vulnerability and self-invalidation, I found her to be harshly judgmental toward herself, considering herself to be "an idiot, a failure, and a huge disappointment." She was emotionally vulnerable with respect to shame in particular; when she hit her own bones it was almost always in the context of subjecting herself to harsh verbal attacks. Second, considering active passivity and apparent competence, it was the latter that stood out. She almost always presented as appealing, engaging, capable, and "fine," matching the family presentation style. Behind that mask she wanted to die, was intensely humiliated, and lived with the fear of being "unmasked." Her apparent competence had prevented her distress from being recognized, and it was only due to a savvy college advisor that she was referred for treatment. After a short while in treatment, she was crying out for help. I never saw real evidence of active passivity that elicited rescue from others. Third, considering unrelenting crisis and inhibited grieving, once again this patient showed little evidence of the biologically based pattern (unrelenting crisis) but prominent evidence of the environmentally based one (inhibited grieving). In her case, it did not seem that there were any notable losses (other than the terrible loss of a safe and connected childhood!) or any point traumata; it was more that she had felt pervasively invalidated within her family, with its focus on appearances, for years. So, in her treatment plan, I prioritized the focus upon self-invalidation, emotional vulnerability to shame in particular, apparent competence, and inhibited grieving. Accordingly, these four patterns suggested eight secondary targets. I aimed to:

1. Decrease the harsh judgments, criticisms, and punishments that she directed toward herself.
2. Increase her validation of her own feelings, thoughts, actions, and strengths.
3. Decrease her passivity and helplessness with respect to her emotions.
4. Increase her capabilities in modulating her emotions, including shame, which required increased recognition of her emotions first.
5. Decrease her "mask-like" presentation, which first involved helping her to become aware of this automatic feature.
6. Increase her direct communications of emotional distress and her willingness to ask me for help.
7. Decrease suppression regarding her memories and reactions to invalidation.
8. Increase processing of the memories of significant invalidation.

It isn't that I constantly scanned for these eight secondary targets and treated them in every session; it's that I had them in mind as a series of possible foci as time went by in treatment, and each of them became a project at different points in time. Each took shape around particular events and trends. While I kept my eye on the primary targets, beginning with self-hitting, I watched for the ways in which these eight secondary targets aligned themselves with the primary target at hand. As I mentioned, treatment time and effort are spent on the secondary targets; it is the "grunt work" of DBT.

SOME SUGGESTIONS FOR WORKING WITH PATIENTS AROUND DIALECTICAL DILEMMAS

1. Having discovered the presence of a particular extreme behavioral pattern, consider whether there is evidence for the presence of the dialectical partner of that pattern. For instance, if you identify apparent competence as a pattern, be on the lookout for elements of active passivity. Sometimes you can notice that while an individual is engaged in the process known as apparent competence, thereby masking her distress from others, there may be evidence of growing distress and tension without any adaptive outlet, setting the stage for an episode of active passivity. It can be helpful to see the two of these patterns in tandem.

2. In orienting the patient to the presence of a certain pattern, trying to cultivate collaborative work on that pattern, see if you can come up with a language for it that works for the individual. This may involve a metaphor or a story, even a drawing. It is very difficult to target these patterns without the patient's willingness, and the willingness is often influenced by the nature of the orientation and the language used, in particular. A therapist might choose the term *masking emotions* rather than using the term *apparent competence*, which sounds rather impersonal and can be confusing. She might use a metaphor such as *reduce episodes of drowning* rather than the clinical term *decrease emotional reactivity* for a given patient, if that works best. On one of the early inpatient DBT programs for adolescents, the program evolved the term *turtling* for social withdrawal and nonexpressiveness. Temporary *turtling*, in the service of then coming out of the shell to face reality, was adaptive. Extremes of *turtling*, such as staying in the shell forever to avoid life, were problematic.

3. Help the patient see how the behaviors associated with this pattern are linked to, indeed are even perpetuating, the primary target behavior and elicit the patient's collaboration with you on the secondary target. For instance, if you have oriented the patient to the presence of apparent competence when his distress grows, have helped him to name it and to see the outcome (a growing internal sense of distress, accompanied by a growing sense of isolation and not being recognized), highlight how it is that this pattern of growing internal pressure and no interpersonal outlet is likely to lead to emotional eruptions that could keep ruining his life. If you can get the patient to "co-own" the pattern and to see what skills it will require to "take the middle path," you stand a better chance of reducing the pattern and strengthening the "antidote" skill set.

4. Once the process has been clarified and seen several times, it can be useful to put the secondary targets, using whatever user-friendly language has evolved, on the diary card alongside the primary targets, so that the patient can monitor their occurrence and outcomes. For instance, the patient may benefit from monitoring the number of occurrences per day of "masking," "self-invalidation," or crisis episodes.

5. Once you identify an extreme behavioral pattern and associated secondary targets that are functionally related to a primary target, try to generate a concrete idea, an image, of how this patient can move toward a middle path of effective behaviors that could replace the problem pattern. It is my experience that the more clearly I can conjure up this image of my patients as functional individuals in their particularly troublesome domains of functioning, and the more I can specifically identify skill sets that will serve them toward actualizing that functional

image, the more likely I am to make constructive skills-oriented interventions in sessions.

FROM DIALECTICAL DILEMMAS TO SECONDARY TARGETS TO TREATMENT PLANNING: A CASE EXAMPLE

A psychiatrist referred a 22-year-old man to me for DBT. The young man saw the psychiatrist at the insistence of his mother after he was arrested for shoplifting three times in 3 months. The psychiatrist learned that he also had a history of self-cutting for relief of social anxiety and showed impulsive judgment in relationships. He was taking a year off college after episodes of self-cutting came to light, along with taking hallucinogenic drugs and skipping classes. He met criteria for borderline personality disorder due to emotional lability, relationship chaos, suicidal and other self-harming behaviors, a chronic sense of emptiness, and identity disturbance. He agreed to enter DBT.

I learned during the assessment that his home life had been peculiar and troubling: His mother drank alcohol almost constantly, his father spent most of his time in the basement, his sister had a serious autoimmune disorder that required whatever attention the parents could muster, and it sounded as if my patient had raised himself. No one in the family had seen him as having problems or needing emotional support even though he was erratic in his functioning. In his peer relationships, others often relied on him for support and he resented that they rarely reciprocated when he was in need. He did not ask for support, but he thought it should be obvious that he needed it. On weekends he took hallucinogenic drugs with peers; he felt that it was the one time that he opened his mind to what was going on inside. He wanted to finish college, get a degree in studio art (he was a talented sculptor), and travel to Europe where he thought he might want to live.

He was obviously intelligent and engaging, and was quirky.

In sessions, and sometimes via lengthy text messages, he would relay things that had happened to him, sometimes troubling events resulting from shortsighted decision making, such as the time his car was stolen after he loaned it to someone he barely knew. Whenever I showed interest and inquired further into experiences that struck me as painful or problematic, he would tell me that he was fine, the event was over, he had "learned my lesson," and he wanted to move on. In a certain respect he was cooperative with me in therapy and showed great interest in the skills, but he usually claimed to have "already resolved" every problem before he came to sessions.

In the initial weeks of treatment, his primary treatment targets were to (1) stop shoplifting, (2) maintain good attendance at therapy (since in prior therapies he had shown poor attendance and eventually dropped out), and (3) "find a friend who is like me, changing all the time." Several months had gone by since the last episode of self-cutting. He would not agree with me that taking hallucinogenic drugs was a problem behavior; he felt that he was safe in using these drugs and that it constituted another "form of therapy." He did, however, agree that shoplifting was a problem, and he wanted to stop it. During our first 6 weeks he was caught shoplifting twice. It was always in "big box" stores, involved sneaking relatively minor items under his shirt or coat, and experiencing great suspense about whether he would be apprehended.

We did several behavioral chain analyses of the shoplifting behavior. It was clear from the start that the most potent reinforcing consequence of shoplifting for him, whether apprehended or not, was the sense of excitement and suspense. Whatever his emotional state was prior to stealing, his immersion in the "game" of shoplifting removed him from that state and made him feel better. Consequently, the treatment plan targeted the reduction of shoplifting behaviors and the search for legal activities that would help him reduce negative moods and create positive excitement.

Through the behavioral chain analysis of several shoplifting episodes, past and present, we identified the following. First, his unrealistic thinking, terrible judgment, and repeated negative events fit the profile for *unrelenting crisis*. Second, his insistence that he was "fine," that he was "moving on," and that any genuine distress seemed to be yesterday's news fit the profile of *apparent competence*. He was masking his distress, repelling invitations to express his painful feelings. This pattern seemed to be in keeping with his experience that he was the "OK" one in the family, that he was the more emotionally capable one in friendships, and that he was upset that others could not reciprocate his support for them even though he did not ask for it. The suspense and drama surrounding each shoplifting event, serving as it did to "rescue" him from unsolvable negative emotional states, could be seen as a variant of *active passivity*, the dialectical partner of *apparent competence*.

Early in the therapy I oriented him to the profiles of unrelenting crisis and apparent competence, and we began to work on developing his capacity for more realistic judgment to reduce his crisis-generating behaviors and on his capacity to observe and describe his feelings in sessions to reduce apparent competence and increase accurate emotional expression. Identifying two (and to some degree, three) dialectical dilemma behavior patterns that appeared to be associated with shoplifting, formulating the corresponding secondary targets, and intervening to change them provided a sense of direction and a rich set of therapeutic opportunities.

But what really turned the corner in our work together, taking it to a deeper and more potent level, began with my observation that although the pattern of *unrelenting crisis* was obviously present, I could see no clear evidence for the presence of its dialectical partner, the pattern of *inhibited grieving*. It was the case, however, that he seemed to object to processing negative events after the fact, and that he minimized the invalidating nature of his childhood. I was far more upset about his descriptions of what happened at home than he was. I became convinced that he did, in fact, fit the profile for *inhibited grieving*, and I pushed more forcefully to learn from him about losses in his life, the negative impact of his previous and current invalidating environments, and about his emotional reactions to some of my less on-target interventions.

As I probed, I was soon rewarded with references to "bad things" that happened in the basement sometimes when he would go down to see his father. Reluctant at first to reveal anything, he began to tell story after story about how his father, under the influence of alcohol and drugs, would plead with my patient to stimulate him sexually. On two occasions he described being beaten by his father for refusing to participate. He was afraid to go to the basement, and afraid not to, and he had never told anyone. Although the precise links between these terrible experiences and his shoplifting behaviors never became crystal clear, it was noticeable that as he revealed these memories and processed his emotional responses in sessions, the shoplifting behaviors lost their urgency and faded from his behavioral repertoire. Later he couldn't remember why the "shoplifting games" had been so compelling.

In sum, what begins with the attempt to solve a primary target leads to the recognition of dialectical dilemmas that interfere with the solution. Once dialectical dilemmas are recognized and fleshed out, they result in the specification of secondary targets. Once there is sufficient clarity about the secondary targets, the therapist can employ strategies and skills to solve them, and through that process ultimately solve the primary target.

WHY JUST THREE DIALECTICAL DILEMMAS?

Although I have no empirical evidence for what I am about to explain, I have found it a productive way to think about dialectical dilemmas. It has occurred to me that each of the three dialectical dilemmas represents a dysfunctional outcome of a normative developmental process. Emotional vulnerability versus self-invalidation represents a miscarriage of the process of *learning to modulate emotions*, which every child needs to do. The child with heightened, biologically based emotional vulnerability, who undertakes this developmental task in the pervasively invalidating context, experiences two dysfunctional patterns with respect to emotion modulation, one more biologically driven (emotional vulnerability) and the other more socially driven (self-invalidation). The presence of a strong emotion is processed in one of these two problematic ways, and the functional skill set for modulating emotions does not develop.

Similarly, when the developmental task of *learning to accurately identify, tolerate, and express distress, and seek support* takes place in this biosocial crucible, two dysfunctional patterns come into being rather than the functional skill set of accurately expressing emotions and asking for help. Active passivity is the one more driven by the biological factor, including a measure of dyscontrol as it does, and apparent competence is the one driven more by the social factor. And when the important developmental task of *managing and processing loss and traumas* takes place in the biosocial transactional force field, the dialectical dilemma of unrelenting crisis versus inhibited grieving is the outcome, the former more driven by the biological factor and the latter by the invalidating environment. The miscarriage of these three developmental tasks results in the six behavioral patterns, each of which could eventually function in a way that maintains primary target behaviors, including suicide attempts.

So if we understand the model in this manner, there is no a priori reason why there should be only *three* dialectical dilemmas. If we consider other developmental tasks that could be negatively impacted by the factors noted in biosocial theory, we might discover other dialectical dilemmas. For instance, consider the task by which the growing child differentiates herself from others in relationships, with distinct and clear boundaries between "self" and "other." One might predict two dysfunctional outcomes, one in which the child is chaotically overengaged with a caregiver and the other in which she is disengaged to a problematic degree. The child with the neurobiology of attention-deficit/hyperactivity disorder (ADHD), who faces the developmental task of learning to accept those features and to function effectively in the world, may end up instead with a dialectical dilemma, extreme ADHD vulnerability versus self-criticism of deficits. The child who experiences auditory hallucinations early in life, or other unusual perceptual experiences, and who needs to develop a compassionate, accepting point of view along with a set of skills for coping in the face of those perceptions, may instead evolve a dialectical dilemma of "hallucinatory vulnerability" versus self-criticism. In other words, rather than thinking of the three dialectical dilemmas as the only possible ones, and looking to fit every case conceptualization into them, we can think of them as three excellent and typical examples of a formula by which the *miscarriage of a developmental task results in two dysfunctional patterns related to that task*. This use of the construct underlying dialectical dilemmas frees us to (1) assess our patients' problem behaviors with an open mind, (2) look for the extreme behavioral patterns that maintain those behaviors, (3) look for the dialectical relationship between those patterns, (4) link the patterns to the task that the individual was trying to accomplish within the biosocial crucible, and (5) try to move the patient from the extreme behavioral patterns to the particular middle path with its skillful behaviors.

CHAPTER 9

Case Conceptualization in DBT

Standing precisely between theory and practice is case conceptualization. Theory finds its way into treatment through a case conceptualization, which then drives treatment planning and interventions. Practice, which includes ongoing assessment and treatment interventions, gives rise to in-the-moment "outcome" data, which inform the case conceptualization, sometimes confirming it and sometimes leading to revisions. Much as a contractor periodically consults the blueprints while building, the therapist refers back to the case conceptualization. Because a case conceptualization is that crucial link between theory and practice, we can expect it to be the clearest, most concise, and most practical illustration of the particular therapy model.

For instance, the case conceptualization in Kernberg's (1975) transference-focused psychotherapy (TFP) revolves around the activation of intrapsychic object relations units, with self and object representations and linking affective states. The therapist identifies intrapsychic splitting of self and object representations as they emerge in the transference relationship, and intervenes to illuminate and resolve the activity and the products of splitting. The case conceptualization in mentalization-based therapy (MBT) revolves around the activation and deactivation of the patient's mentalizing capacities and modes. MBT guides the therapist toward interventions that strengthen the patient's capacity to mentalize and to restore and maintain that capacity in the face of increased emotionality and the pressures of an attachment relationship (Bateman & Fonagy, 2004).

In this chapter, we examine the nature and role of case conceptualization in DBT. Unlike some models, DBT therapists do not actually "conceptualize the case," they conceptualize the variables that maintain a given target behavior. The conceptualization of an individual's self-harm behaviors might differ significantly from the conceptualization of the same individual's substance use behaviors. Even within the range of self-harm behaviors, the case conceptualization of a given individual's self-cutting behaviors might differ distinctly from the case conceptualization of his self-burning behaviors.

Case conceptualization begins with, first, identifying the target behavior of interest, typically the highest-priority target behavior at that moment of the treatment. Although it is the case that the DBT therapist assesses and conceptualizes one given high-priority target behavior, in fact the patterns and controlling variables discovered in that enterprise are likely to provide a "head start" in conceptualizing other target behaviors of the same patient. Second, the therapist identifies the stage of treatment. It matters. To target a self-harming behavior during the pretreatment stage, when the goal of treatment is to get a commitment from the patient, is different from targeting the same self-harming behavior during Stage 1, when the goal of treatment is to increase behavioral stability and control. That same behavior, if it reemerges during Stage 2, when the goal of treatment is to increase the patient's capacity to engage in nonanguished emotional experiencing, will be conceptualized in a different way.

COGNITIVE-BEHAVIORAL PRINCIPLES AND VOCABULARY IN CASE CONCEPTUALIZATION

The template for a DBT case conceptualization is the behavioral chain. Indeed, the behavioral chain serves as the organizing structure and platform for the assessment and treatment of a given high-priority target behavior. Antecedents will be found to the left of the behavior and consequences to the right. During the first occasion of a behavioral chain analysis for a particular behavior, in collaboration with the patient to define the links preceding and following the behavior, the therapist cannot tell which of those links, and which patterns among those links, will prove to be key in determining the controlling variables of the behavior. The therapist often quickly concludes that a certain link—or pattern of links—was instrumental in perpetuating that problem behavior, only to learn later that it was a red herring, hardly central to the maintenance of the behavior. In one treatment of a patient who was traumatically

raped by a friend and who subsequently presented with PTSD and suicidal behaviors, I was initially convinced that the experience of being
penetrated against her will was the most important determining variable.
Only later did I discover that the more profound "link in the chain" came
an hour prior to that one, when she had noticed but dismissed the significance of a relatively minor action by her good friend and perpetrator-to-
be when he had brushed the back of her neck almost incidentally as they
entered a room.

The therapist must proceed with careful attention, hypothesizing as
she goes, with the humble appreciation that her initial hunches are very
likely to be wrong. Better to proceed with an attitude of curiosity and
openness. The second and third and fourth times she spells out the links
of a chain of that problem behavior, the therapist and the patient begin to
discern the nature of the links and patterns that are associated, again and
again, with that behavior. Furthermore, the evolving "generic" chain for
that behavior begins to take on more shape and more detail. After a number of chains have been constructed, the therapist grows more confident
that she has found associated patterns, and even if they may not cause
the behavior, they are at least correlated. They invite further attention.
As they collaborate in defining the controlling links and patterns, patient
and therapist can work on solutions to those patterns and thereby impact
the targeted behavior.

Let me give you an example. I began work with a woman who had a
long history of suicide attempts and self-harming behaviors. She also had
episodes of dissociation, chronic and refractory major depression, PTSD
based on sexual abuse as a child, and alcoholic binge drinking. For some
time, her highest-priority target behaviors were her suicide attempts. In
particular, we were undertaking the assessment of her suicide attempts by
overdose. Having engaged in several chain analyses, the following patterns began to become evident:

1. She seemed more likely to harm herself on days when she had not
   slept at all during the prior night.
2. It seemed that attempts were more likely to follow when she had
   been with a group of people, rather than having been alone or
   with a friend or two.
3. She noted a severe degree of self-hatred most of the times when
   she was with a group.
4. It appeared that in those chains that included a suicide attempt,
   there was some kind of antecedent reference to her body: for
   example, "I went swimming with friends today"; "I noticed I'm
   gaining some weight"; "I'm afraid I'm getting a sunburn." Upon

further inquiry, she noted that any reference to her body set off
visceral disgust toward herself.
5. Suicide attempts by overdose resulted in lengthy episodes of
sleep, and when she awoke, her desire to kill herself had gone.

Every time we could characterize and further define a pattern in
these chains, we had another potential point of entry, and therefore
another possible solution. As we slowly but surely arrived at a "typical" or "generic" chain for her problem behavior, we carefully built and
tested a treatment plan, or rather a series of "mini" treatment plans for
each pattern. By trial and error we were discovering which variables
were associated with suicide attempts, which variables lent themselves to
change-oriented interventions, and which variables had to change before
others could be approached. One of the challenges of being a DBT therapist, conceptualizing the controlling variables as the therapy proceeds,
is the practice of keeping in mind a range of hypotheses regarding different "locations" on the chain, making trial-and-error interventions to
further clarify their roles, and holding back from arriving prematurely at
conclusions about where to intervene. The process of conceptualizing,
reconceptualizing, and refining those conceptualizations over time, probing and assessing, intervening and observing, can be a helpful way for the
therapist to stay engaged in a process of inquiry and intervention without
submitting to the temptation of "knowing" what is the critical variable
before the data are sufficient. In and of itself, this process of collaborative
inquiry is an important therapeutic activity.

To become clearer and more prosaic, a case conceptualization in
DBT requires the determination of the links and patterns of the generic
chain, and treatment planning is based on that determination. It takes
place collaboratively, involves a logical (deductive) approach along with
trial-and-error (inductive) interventions, and evolves through insight
about patterns that might be discovered by the patient and/or therapist.
Consistent with the central theses of this book, a case conceptualization of DBT is shaped, at its core, along the lines of a rational, logical,
cognitive-behavioral framework, and then modified and augmented by
bringing in principles associated with mindfulness and dialectics. I now
launch into the rational, CBT-based framework and then consider how
this framework is modified with principles of mindfulness and dialectics.

Consider the "vocabulary" of a DBT chain. It is a chronological,
horizontal representation of an ongoing stream of behavior, comprised
of links and patterns. Every link is either a behavior of the patient—an
emotion, a physiological event, a cognition, or an action—or a behavior
or feature of the environmental context with which the patient interacts.

Based on DBT theory and guided by the principles of cognitive-behavioral science at its core, as DBT therapists we are especially interested in certain kinds of links. First, there are those links that reflect the patient's biologically based emotional sensitivity, reactivity, and slow return to baseline. Second are the links that reflect invalidation of the patient by the environment. The more we know about the patient, the more sensitively we can identify emotional vulnerability in the chain, and the more accurately we can identify those contextual events that are invalidating for her. In the patient mentioned above, it was not easy at first to recognize signs of emotional vulnerability because she had masked them in the invalidating contexts that characterized her early life. But as the subtle signs of sensitivity became more apparent, and as she grew to recognize and communicate them in therapy, our identification of these moments grew more accurate and more frequent. For each individual, an "invalidating environment" has a unique signature. In her case, she experienced invalidation every time she thought someone should know she was upset. Even though her masking was effective in disguising her upset, she still thought it should be obvious to others. As we characterized this kind of "invisible" invalidation, it became more evident that it was happening nearly all the time, including in the therapy. Our "instruments for detection" grew more sensitive and valid, and as they did we were able to deepen and broaden our understanding of the most relevant causal patterns. More importantly, we began to find more ways to help her get what she needed to modulate her emotions and communicate her distress.

If the first two relevant categories of links in the DBT chain are instances of emotional vulnerability and environmental invalidation with direct reference to biosocial theory, the next six are links, or sequences of links, that represent any or all of the six behavioral patterns described as polar opposites of the three dialectical dilemmas, discussed in Chapter 8. To review, three of them represent the patient's subjective experience of the biologically based emotional vulnerability: active passivity, emotional vulnerability, and unrelenting crisis. The other three seem to manifest the influence of the invalidating environment: apparent competence, self-invalidation, and inhibited grieving. Anytime we notice the presence of links that seem to be part of one of these six patterns, we consider the possibility that these links are important in determining and maintaining the problem behavior. In the above-mentioned patient, her "masking" was part of a syndrome of apparent competence, which, once identified, was seen by both of us to play a huge role in her escalating spirals of hidden distress, and ultimately in her suicide attempts. Deprived of the opportunity to constructively find help, while hidden behind her mask of apparent competence, her suicide attempts served a function of a "cry for help," which was a form of active passivity. Her instances of self-hatred and disgust toward her body were links in a pattern of self-invalidation, a crucial pattern to understand and treat. While she conveyed a sense of reserve and control, "behind the scenes" she was very frequently—several times per day—experiencing episodes of emotional vulnerability: the feeling that she had no control, that her emotions were overwhelming her, that she could die simply from having unregulated emotions. It took longer for us to discern that a deep and persistent pattern perpetuating her suicide attempts involved her inhibited grieving: She was persistently suppressing and guarding against the emergence of any thoughts or feelings related to her traumatic past. And in doing so, any cue that set off those memories and feelings would trigger crisis episodes of many kinds—that is, unrelenting crisis as a pattern.

In this particular case, all six patterns belonging to the three dialectical dilemmas came into play very actively and frequently. In other cases, one finds the predominance of one or more, but not all six. There are some patients with borderline personality disorder and anorexia nervosa, for instance, in whom the most prominent patterns are those of overcontrol derived from an environment that was perceived to be overcontrolling—primarily characterized by apparent competence ("I'm fine!"), self-invalidation ("I'm never good enough, never skinny enough"), and inhibited grieving. In any case, the determination of the six categories of patterns mentioned up to this point, all consistent with DBT's biosocial theory, contributes to a growing understanding of the functions—the driving forces and the purposes—of the problem behavior. Armed with this kind of pattern-based understanding, the therapist can further monitor the patterns and propose procedures to change them.

Then there are four more categories of potential controlling variables for which therapist and patient should be scanning while doing behavioral chain analyses. Each category is based on one of DBT's CBT-based change procedures. Associated with the procedures for contingency management, there are the problematic contingencies that reinforce the continued practice of the problem behavior. In the above-mentioned patient, who rarely got enough sleep and for whom exhaustion seemed to play a role in her growing distress, the suicide attempts by overdose could bring her distress to a (temporary) end and reliably provide her with several hours of restorative sleep. These were contingencies that revealed some of the functions of her suicide attempts, which could be taken into account in problem solving.

A second CBT-based category of relevant variables pertains to powerful emotions that are set off, automatically and instantaneously, by emotionally salient cues in the environment. Once we discover the unique and potent role of such cue-based emotional responses, which have been classically conditioned to traumatic and disturbing stimuli, we can organize interventions around the recognition, modification, management, and ultimately the therapeutically effective exposure to those cues.

In addition to the important roles that problematic contingencies and problematic emotions can play in a chain leading up to dysfunctional behaviors, there are two other categories: problematic cognitions and skills deficits. We "scan" for dysfunctional cognitions such as "I'm incompetent"; "No one will ever like me"; There is no way I can succeed"; "I'm just a bad seed and I deserve all the punishment I get"; and so on. Locating these kinds of cognitions, working with the patient to understand their role and to appreciate the fact that they are thoughts, not facts, provides another avenue along which to change the chain. Finally, the behavioral chains of most individuals with borderline personality disorder, when the chains include severely damaging behaviors, are punctuated with multiple skills deficits in tolerating distress, regulating emotions, maintaining balance, and interacting effectively with others. As is obvious in DBT, the therapist routinely targets such multiple skills deficits.

Having identified eight categories of links and patterns derived from DBT's biosocial theory and dialectical dilemmas, and four more derived from cognitive-behavioral science, it may be useful to list them here before adding a few others.

1. Emotional vulnerability, objectively identified in biosocial theory as heightened sensitivity, reactivity, and slow return to baseline
2. Invalidating episodes, in which the patient is invalidated by the environment
3. Emotional vulnerability, subjectively experienced as agonizing by the patient
4. Self-invalidation
5. Active passivity
6. Apparent competence
7. Unrelenting crisis
8. Inhibited grieving
9. Problematic contingencies
10. Problematic emotions
11. Problematic cognitions
12. Skills deficits

As a psychiatrist who also is trying to determine whether the patient suffers from a psychiatric disorder that may be responsive to psychotropic medications, I consider a 13th category: the presence of a psychiatric condition. Although it is true that almost any condition will manifest in ways already represented in the 12 categories just listed, I find it clinically useful to identify any such biologically based condition that may indicate the use of psychotropic medications. If I determine that my patient shows convincing evidence of a major depressive disorder of a moderate to severe nature, I can target that disorder with medications (among other behavioral interventions). If my patient has evidence of a prominent bipolar disorder or a panic disorder, I can consider medication options to treat one of these potent controlling variables.

All 13 variables identified to this point are focused on the patient's behavioral presentation and behavioral chain. But there are still other variables in the patient's environment that may be driving the target behavior: namely, contextual variables. The first set of relevant contextual variables can be found in the patient's familial–social context. A case conceptualization is often incomplete without identifying problematic interactions with family members or individuals that are part of the patient's social network. DBT's usual interventions involve consulting with the patient to deal with these kinds of environmental contexts, but in some instances the therapist directly intervenes with contextual factors—with the individuals or circumstance in the environment. This is most obviously the case in the treatment of an adolescent patient in DBT, where the family is involved in the treatment, but can be true with adult patients as well.

The other set of important contextual variables are those in the DBT treatment context. If the individual therapist and the group skills trainers are not "in synch," or the consultation team is not providing sufficient support to the individual therapist, these non-patient-related factors can play a quiet and facilitating role, culminating in a suicide attempt. They too should be assessed and attended to as part of the case conceptualization and, if indicated, part of the treatment.

The "vocabulary of controlling variables" enumerated to this point are those factors that might contribute to the cause or maintenance of problem behaviors that we want to decrease. Equally important is the attention paid to variables that are suppressing functional, skillful behaviors that we want to increase. The building of skills and of constructive living patterns should parallel the reduction of problematic patterns, but sometimes this process suffers while we focus on pathology. The therapist needs to scan for functional links and patterns: supportive contextual variables, resilient and favorable behavioral patterns in general, and, in particular, use of skillful, adaptive behavioral patterns. In the case of the above-mentioned patient with numerous suicide attempts, her favorable factors were hidden behind the chaos and dysfunction of her daily life, barely noticeable after years of living on the edge of death, going in and out of hospitals. Little did we recognize, until we deliberately cultivated them, that her intellectual abilities were substantial, had been important in her adolescent years, and would prove to be instrumental in her ultimate success in treatment. Whereas reading, and thinking, had been "reasons for living" and the cornerstones of an imagined life years ago, they had been buried for many years. When she acknowledged, upon inquiry, that she had not read a book in years, and that she just could not settle her mind enough to focus on a written story, she agreed to an "off-label" use of stimulant medication to enhance her ability to focus on reading. Within 2 weeks she was reading again, which proved a huge solace and a constructive focus for her. This discovery of a long-unused resource turned out to be one of the building blocks in her progress. Just as important as recognizing and activating underutilized resilient behavioral factors in the patient, we must include recognition of the relationship of the environment to those adaptive features. If the environment is not reinforcing them, or worse, is even punishing and suppressing them, this becomes part of the case conceptualization and might be addressed in treatment.

Adding the contextual factors and the resiliency-building factors to our assessment vocabulary, we have a menu of 17 types of links or patterns comprising a DBT case conceptualization.

1. Emotional vulnerability, objectively identified as heightened sensitivity, reactivity, and slow return to baseline
2. Invalidating episodes, in which the patient is invalidated by the environment
3. Emotional vulnerability, subjectively experienced as agonizing by the patient
4. Self-invalidation
5. Active passivity
6. Apparent competence
7. Unrelenting crisis
8. Inhibited grieving
9. Problematic contingencies
10. Problematic emotions
11. Problematic cognitions
12. Skills deficits
13. Manifestations of a biologically based psychiatric disorder
14. Contextual factors reinforcing problem behaviors: family, social network, professional (non-DBT) network

15. Contextual factors reinforcing problem behaviors: DBT treatment program
16. Resilient and adaptive behavioral factors
17. Contextual factors strengthening resilient and adaptive factors

MINDFULNESS PRINCIPLES
IN CASE CONCEPTUALIZATION

If the menu of relevant controlling variables, derived from CBT and DBT, represents the rational, blueprint-like template for case conceptualization, the template is used in a manner additionally informed by principles of mindfulness and dialectics. Among the principles underlying mindfulness is the one of non-attachment to one's own thoughts, judgments, and perceptions. As much as the therapist applies the template above in a scientific manner, and invests in it with diligence and discipline, he also realizes that it is a formulation, a set of thoughts, a set of hypotheses. Having a logical template to apply to such a chaotic and often confusing set of problems can be tempting and satisfying. But to believe in it in a manner that filters perceptions and interventions, that preselects data supporting it, can blind the therapist to the reality of the next moment, the next session, the information contradictory to the propositions up to that point. So, as much as the therapist embraces the blueprint as a road map to change, he does not become attached to a particular equation to explain the outcome of the chain. And as much as he is convinced that he has fashioned a degree of predictability and order, organized around a view of the future of the treatment and of the patient, he lets himself, session by session, reside within that one current moment, given that the only reality is the one in this very moment. The case conceptualization, logically derived, is in the past, and it may or may not predict the future. In the present moment of treatment is the reality of the patient and the therapist, and everything that transpires in them and between them at any given moment. If the therapist can apply the case conceptualization as a set of hypotheses that inform the present moment *but do not replace it*—if he proceeds with "beginner's mind" as defined in Buddhist thought—he remains open to new data all the time.

Another mindfulness principle involves the recognition that everything in reality is impermanent. This includes all aspects of a case conceptualization, no matter how convincing. If the therapist views the case conceptualization as a representation of reality *and* recognizes that reality is changing every moment, then she will also realize that the written case conceptualization is perpetually one step behind. If the therapist maintains this principle, she is more likely to make judicious use of the hard-won case conceptualization, allowing it to guide and inform her in assessment and treatment, without letting it control her.

Finally, as discussed in Chapter 3 on the acceptance paradigm, the other mindfulness-based principle holds that "reality is perfect as it is." In the course of the ongoing, ever-evolving case conceptualization, the therapist keeps in mind that every link, every pattern, and the entire presentation are "exactly as they should be." In other words, the therapist assumes the "wisdom of the data" even if he cannot understand it yet. Staying in the current moment, building *and* letting go of the case conceptualization over and over again, bowing to the impermanent and constantly changing nature of reality, including the constantly changing nature of the case conceptualization, and assuming the wisdom and "perfection" of everything as it is in this moment, the therapist is then prepared to make the most effective use of the scientifically derived approach to case conceptualization in the context of accepting reality in the moment. The reality of the present moment, the reality of the individual sitting in front of the therapist, trumps the "road map" provided by the case conceptualization, every time.

When we fully understand that the actual, real-time case conceptualization is changing moment by moment, it is possible to make maximal use of the conceptualization without getting trapped by it. In a sense, whatever is the explicit case conceptualization is not only partial, but is also temporally behind the progression of reality. I once worked with a man in his mid-20s who presented with desperate suicide attempts alternating with deliberate aggressive actions toward others. The aggressive actions were designed to frighten others, even making them fear for their lives in spite of the fact that he did not actually hurt them. He was willing to commit to a full course of DBT, to attend a DBT skills group, and to target both his suicidal and aggressive behaviors. Not surprisingly, the behavioral chains associated with his suicidal behaviors were quite different in nature than the chains associated with his aggressive behaviors. Behavioral chain analyses of the latter revealed several patterns linked to a DBT framework. In masking any distress or need for help, he showed apparent competence. The syndrome of inhibited grieving was suggested by his careful avoidance of any topics related to prior losses, which had been profound. When he was engaged in frightening other people, he seemed to be in a damaging spiral with considerable momentum, a form of unrelenting crisis. He showed problematic cognitions ("People are idiots; they deserve to be scared"), problematic emotional responses (showing a "hair-trigger" aggressive reaction to any comment that could even vaguely be interpreted as an insult), and skills deficits in anticipating and managing troubling triggers, in approaching others effectively to ask for things, and in experiencing and regulating intense negative emotions without retaliatory action. We worked from several behavioral chains of his aggressive behavior and worked on a number of solutions to the problematic links in the chains.

Although his presentation was complicated, I began to think I had a handle on his typical behavioral chains, to a point of some predictability. One day this patient arrived at the session with a mask covering his face. I asked him to remove it, which revealed substantial bruises on both cheeks. It looked as if he had been beaten. I asked him about it, and he said he had gotten into a fight in a bar, which was unusual behavior for him. He seemed to be almost smiling, in an eerie and uncomfortable way, as if he were proud but in an altered state. I experienced fear, wondering if he had any harmful intent toward me. I asked him. He said no, but that he had had thoughts about driving around my house. I made it crystal clear that any such action would be a violation of my personal limits and I asked him to respect those limits. When he smiled in response, I was further worried and inquired again into his thoughts, feelings, and motivations toward me. By the end of the session, I was feeling more reassured that he would respect my limits and that our usual fairly good working relationship had been reestablished. At the same time, I realized as the session ended that we had spent little time on the assessment of the incident that had damaged his face.

By that point in the treatment, I had conceptualized his aggressive actions in frightening others as behaviors driven by several controlling variables: a history of invalidation that included physical beatings by his father and teasing by other children; a smoldering resentment toward anyone who seemed, in even the slightest way, to insult or demean him; skills deficits in emotional regulation and interpersonal effectiveness; blanket suppression of any thoughts or feelings of loss or trauma; general lack of progress in his life toward any goals; and potent reinforcement of the aggressive behaviors in that they enhanced his feelings of control and incited fear in others.

Late that night I was unable to fall asleep. I got out of bed and sat in the kitchen drinking tea. I found myself thinking about him, wondering what had happened to his face. I realized that the bruises were symmetrically placed on both cheeks, mirroring each other, not likely to have been the outcome of a physical fight. I wondered if he had self-inflicted the bruises, though there had been no other evidence in his presentation or history of any kind of nonsuicidal deliberate self-harm. I was puzzled. I found myself letting go of my conceptualization of the case, as if I were "looking underneath" that conceptualization. I saw something else, all

at once, in my mind's eye. I saw someone who was much more vulnerable, frightened, prone to being teased and hurt. Even his smiling in the
session that day looked less like a smirk of satisfaction and more like an
uncontrollable smile of discomfort. I still could not fathom what he had
done to his face, but I entered the next session as if starting over, knowing
nothing. I asked what had happened to his face, which still had significant bruises. He said he was not about to tell me. It suddenly occurred to
me that he had had surgery. I remembered that prior to the session when
he entered with the mask, he had missed two consecutive sessions.

I asked him, "Why did you have surgery?" He looked surprised, not
unpleasantly so, as if he was pleased to be found out. He told me he had
had his face altered because it had always been so ugly. This was the first
presentation of a quite full-fledged and serious case of body dysmorphic
disorder. As I carefully, and compassionately, inquired into his thoughts
and feelings about his face, which extended back into his childhood as
far as he could remember, his presentation softened and he began to seem
rather depressed. Over time it was rather easy to see how his aggressive
behaviors were part of a secondary emotional response, an escape from
the primary emotional responses of self-hatred, self-disgust, and the fear
of others' insulting behaviors toward him. This radical shift in perspective led in promising directions.

In that case, and in a number of others, I have noticed that the
arrival at a case conceptualization with considerable data can serve as a
straitjacket. Sometimes, in fact perhaps many times, it is wise to shed the
case conceptualization up to that moment, much as a snake sheds its skin
and begins to grow a new one. Case conceptualizations are extremely
helpful in providing guidance, but they can also be seriously constricting
and narrowing. It might be useful to think that the case conceptualization does not represent reality, but that it provides a scaffolding based on
the observations up to that point, and by standing on that scaffolding,
perhaps the therapist has a chance to see reality and to intervene.

DIALECTICAL PRINCIPLES
IN CASE CONCEPTUALIZATION

When we add the principles of dialectics to the process of case conceptualization, we acquire a richer, more flexible, more fluid, and more creative
process. This happens in several ways. There is the dialectic between the
explicit case conceptualization and the implicit one. The explicit one is
the one that we write down, that incorporates many of the behaviorally
based elements described above, and that helps us to predict behavior

and design targeted interventions. But in fact, all of us, in every case, whether we explicitly conceptualize it or not, have an implicit case conceptualization, an unarticulated working model sitting just outside of full awareness. Although we create a sharp and explicit conceptualization, guiding us thoughtfully as we do treatment, we also operate with freedom, openness, and spontaneity. In the latter respect we intervene more, in the moment, from the implicit formulation. We "know" what to look for based on our educated and explicit understanding, and in another sense we "know" what to do guided by intuition and our implicit understanding. When we try on the explicit model in sessions, and find that it fits the situation, it may become implicit over time and become part of our automatic way of understanding and intervening. Sometimes, as in the case I just described, the explicit model, although intelligent and perhaps on target in some ways, may constrict our understanding, block our awareness of our intuitive and implicit interpretations of the data, and only shift when we "wake up" for one reason or another. In the process of case conceptualization, as an ongoing activity assumed to have both explicit and implicit forms, we are wise to continue to "wake up" by letting in data that do not fit.

Dialectics is practiced with movement, speed, and flow. As such, it also helps to think of case conceptualization as a moving, experimental, trial-and-error process. We come up with an idea, recognizing a pattern or considering a solution, and we bring it up with the patient. We talk about it, consider it together, expand upon it, and may decide to intervene to change it. In discussion, or with trial interventions with the patient, we may learn salient truths about the behavioral chain under discussion. This is much in the way that a good surgeon works. She has a "case conceptualization" based on history, physical exam, laboratory findings, and radiological findings on x-rays and a variety of scanning techniques. She decides to operate and has a pretty good idea of where to find the pathology and a plan for resolving it. Then she operates. And as she does so, she finds surprises, anomalies, unexpected twist and turns, more or less pathology than expected. She might find out that she was almost perfectly correct in her explicit model, that she was partially correct, or even that she was amazingly wrong. She adjusts as she goes; because she uses trial and error, intuition and discovery, the outcome is likely to be better. It is much the same when driving with a global positioning system (GPS). The GPS provides an explicit conceptualization of how to get from here to there, but in the process of driving, of looking out the window and seeing reality as it is at this moment, adjustments are constantly being made. It is useful to bring the same dialectical process to psychotherapy.

Central to the concept of dialectics is that any current situation is the product of a transaction that led to it. The person who makes repeated suicide attempts may be dying to live, but without having figured out how to make life worth living. Instead, he engages in an unsuccessful attempt to die. The individual who comes to therapy sessions but then barely speaks, may be longing for contact and terrified of it at the same time. When we encounter a persistent behavioral pattern that won't move forward or backward, as one might characterize these, we can scan for the presence of an unresolved dilemma, a temporarily impossible conflict, a chronic collision between X and anti-X. And if we can think of it in this way, we may tease out the opposing elements, identify them intuitively or explicitly, and look to bring about some kind of synthesis that allows things to move forward. Assuming that reality, in its essential nature, is filled with opposites, can prompt us to search for the opposing sides, to find the validity in both sides, and to facilitate movement toward synthesis.

I once worked with a 16-year-old girl who presented with self-cutting behaviors, episodic alcoholic binges with blackouts, a sense of hopelessness about ever being successful in school or in life, and a chronic sense of being an "outsider" with respect to various circles of friendships at her school. In sessions she could be thoughtful, insightful, curious about herself, and open to considering a range of influences on her sometimes troubling, even dangerous, choices. But between sessions, especially during weekend nights, she resorted to partying, drinking heavily, and acting in dramatic bold gestures that brought her significant attention as someone willing to "go to the edge." On one occasion she went to a concert in her hometown, with other girls from her school, and became so intoxicated that she passed out on the sidewalk. The other girls, not wanting to expose my patient's outrageous behavior (and their own), took her to an abandoned building rather than the emergency room. She woke up hours later, being looked over by several girls.

In my case conceptualization of this girl's extreme use of alcohol, I included several factors typical to a DBT formulation. She was rendered vulnerable by her social isolation, her "outsider-ness," her estrangement from her family (who knew nothing of these episodes), her downward spiral in school, her lack of confidence about her worth to others, and by the fact that she had found a temporary "solution" to her discomfort by heavy drinking with other teens. Her vulnerabilities were activated when she faced weekend evenings, knowing that other girls were out socializing together, and when she was feeling particularly estranged and alone. Once her painful emotions of sadness, loneliness, and humiliation were activated, she was relatively incapable of effective modulation: that is, of recognizing them, experiencing them as transient emotions, communicating them to people who might understand, and using skillful means to cope with the painful feelings. The tried and true path of getting drunk, getting wild, getting involved with others, being a dramatic individual rather than a retiring one was far too compelling to pass up for a more "boring" evening. Her problematic behavior with alcohol "worked" in the short run, each time, and it brought her increasingly close to a position in which others would attend to her and try to protect her. Meanwhile, it did nothing to provide a longer-term constructive solution to the problems.

There was nothing wrong with my conceptualization as far as I could tell. It was comprised of sensible ingredients all consistent with a DBT model, leading to some suggestions about recognizing her vulnerabilities, increasing her use of emotion regulation skills and strategies, and finding means to enhance her self-respect and to build more meaningful relationships. But as is often the case, although this conceptualization pointed to a number of reasonable ingredients in a treatment plan, it was missing something more experience-near: more in the moment, improvisational, real and heartfelt in the therapy—an ingredient that would bring things into focus in a way that could provide a "tipping point." I am tempted to call this the "human element" in the case conceptualization, but that would unwisely suggest that the other, more explicit elements were less than human. I found myself thinking, "Why is this girl, who has a caring and involved family, for whom she has a great deal of affection, living out the life of a lost teenager?" Focusing away from any one behavioral pattern, but just taking in the larger picture, I wondered what was not working in her life. How could her parents be unaware of such profound trouble? How could it be so easy for her to fool them? In other words, I widened my purview of the case to include the "big picture," the larger pattern she was enacting, and the surprising disengagement of her reasonably well-functioning family. And while considering this big picture, I realized that in some way my own responses to her, although appropriate and thoughtful, were also lacking some measure of intensity. Similarly, I realized that my own sense of outrage and disappointment— the kind that could arrive because being a therapist to a 16-year-old can evoke parental feelings—seemed surprisingly minimal. I felt that she had somehow managed to drift, in relation to her parents and to me as her therapist, into something of a vacuum, as if she were an orphan, trying to find her way in the jungle of peer relationships, as if she had already left home. If I were to state the polarization within her now, in retrospect, she was torn between the girl who wanted to be part of her family, developing more constructively, and the girl who also desperately wanted to belong to someone. She wanted to matter to someone, to block out her painful feelings, and she found all of that in her friends and her drinking.

In the next session I jumped in with both feet, increasing my intensity and spontaneity. "What has happened to you? What has happened to you as your parents' daughter, someone with a valued place and a hopeful set of life dreams? How is it that, right in front of me, you have slipped into a kind of disenfranchised place that leaves you feeling so alone that you have to drink yourself into unconsciousness in order to find your way into being cared about? What has happened to you and me that you are doing that and that I am somehow accepting it, when I know you are capable of building your life in more constructive directions? Really, what is going on with you? Where did you get lost? Where did I lose you? Where did your parents lose you? Where did you lose your parents?" She looked stunned. She could feel the strength of my concern, and the directness. She teared up, began sobbing, and over the next 50 minutes she unfolded a story of having "lost my parents" as they spiraled into marital conflict over their older child, who had run away from home and who was doing rather poorly. Literally, she described herself as an orphan, finding her way on the streets. She knew that her parents were so preoccupied that they were blind to her own paralysis and waywardness. That session proved to be a turning point, returning her to herself, her more hopeful and skillful self, and we moved on to address the sources of her orphan-like directions, eventually involving her parents in sessions.

As I think back on this episode in this treatment, I am curious about how I arrived at this intervention and how I carried it out in a meaningful and effective way. It did not follow directly from the case conceptualization I was building up to that point. And yet it was not incompatible with that conceptualization either. It's just that the explicit conceptualization, rational and multifaceted as it was, was just missing a big-picture ingredient, a heartfelt ingredient that could "reach" her and potentiate her insight and her efforts. I don't find this to be an unusual occurrence. As a therapist, I work along well-formulated lines, in keeping with treatment protocols, strategies, and skills, and I build a framework of understanding. I find it essential to do so even if it does not provide that tipping point. From that framework I intervene. And still something can be missing. I might overlook a "hidden link" in the behavioral chain, a contextual factor in the patient's interpersonal or vocational environment, or a sense of disengagement in myself, the patient, and/or the family. *Dialectical assessment* is listed as a DBT dialectical strategy, which involves always looking for what is left out of the current picture, the current formulation. And often I find that what is left out is the ingredient that moves everything else forward. And often that missing ingredient is not to be found by a logical review of the case, but more implicitly, intuitively. This is part of the dialectics of case conceptualization. It involves movement, flow, engagement, and improvisation, finding what is left out, looking beyond the obvious. Perhaps it would be fairest for me to say that a standard behaviorally based case conceptualization is necessary but not sufficient in DBT to meet the greatest challenges.

Remembering that the worldview of dialectics is systemic, understanding every element of reality to be part of a system and part of a transaction, we can expand the field of inquiry to the context around the patient. Perhaps the ongoing problem behavior is being maintained by an unrecognized polarization between patient and therapist, therapist and team members, patient and family members, patient and doctor, patient and society, and so on. Thinking dialectically while conceptualizing a case brings more elements of time and space into the equation. Although this may seem daunting, threatening the therapist with "possibility overload," it need not be experienced in that way if the therapist sees the work as an ongoing process of inquiry, unfolding moment by moment, subject to forces in and around the patient.

I once assessed a 17-year-old boy who presented with perfectionistic academically based anxiety, rigid social interactions, and as I quickly learned, extreme lack of confidence bordering on self-hatred. What was surprising is that he was an honor-roll student at his school and was a fine athlete who was publically recognized for his accomplishments. I met with him and his parents during the evaluation and as far as I could tell, they were supportive of him and his accomplishments. While we began to work on his perfectionism, social rigidity, sense of isolation, and lack of confidence, I had a sense that I was missing something that would help me conceptualize the depth of his troubles. Simultaneously I was treating the parent of a different child in the same high school class. Coincidentally, that parent began talking in therapy about the family of the boy who was lacking self-confidence. She was friends with his parents, but was troubled about how they treated their two children. While both children were highly competent and performing well in school and sports, they spoke of their 14-year-old daughter as if she was a superstar, and about the boy, my patient, as if he was lacking. While I could not share that information with the boy I was treating, or his parents, my case conceptualization shifted to include this possible systemic variable. Almost immediately, even without explicitly asking my patient about his sister, he began to talk about his sense of inferiority in relation to her. Armed with the information I heard from my other patient, I was able to provide a convincingly validating response to his comments and to ask about differences in how he and his sister were perceived by the parents. We never know in advance where the key elements of the case conceptualization reside: in the patient, in the family, in the therapist, in the team, or in someone or something else. We proceed with an open mind, alert to fresh observations and surprises; they are more the rule than the exception.

PRACTICAL SUGGESTIONS FOR CONSTRUCTING AND USING CASE CONCEPTUALIZATION

1. Even after carrying out just one behavioral chain analysis on a particular target behavior, construct your first case conceptualization. It is only a beginning, but it leads to careful thinking and hypothesizing, which in turn leads to thoughtful interventions in the early sessions. After a second and third behavioral chain analysis of the same behavior, the new data will require revisions in the initial case conceptualization, but your therapy will already have the quality of figuring out the controlling variables in an organized way.

2. Steep yourself in your case conceptualization, so that it is on the tip of your tongue during sessions, but at the same time totally "let it go," forget about it, and conduct sessions from the heart as well as the head. This dialectical movement between explicit and implicit, head and heart, comprehensive explanation and in-the-moment reactions will serve you and the patient well.

3. Of course you need not confine yourself to information derived from behavioral chain analyses in developing and revising your case conceptualization. You will make use of everything you learn about the patient and his behavioral patterns, including things that you learn from the history, from others, and from the in-the-moment "behavioral chain" that is happening as you conduct the session.

4. There is a distinction between behavioral chain analysis and "missing link analysis," but they are similar in nature and they both contribute to the case conceptualization. A behavioral chain analysis is a technique to identify the controlling variables of problematic or ineffective behaviors; a missing link analysis is a parallel technique to identify the controlling variables explaining the *absence* of an effective behavior in the chain.

5. Work hard on specifying the case conceptualization. At the same time realize that it does not exist in reality; it is simply a way of ordering data in a format that is superimposed by our minds.

6. Certain data are more relevant than other data, and certain hypotheses are considered over other hypotheses, because some kinds of data and some kinds of hypotheses are consistent with a DBT-based con-

ceptualization. We look for evidence of emotional vulnerability, invalidating environments, dysregulated emotions in the chain, skills deficits, contingencies reinforcing problematic behaviors and suppressing effective behaviors, and problematic cognitions. We are always asking, as we review a link in the chain, is this a dysfunctional or a functional link, and if dysfunctional, can we imagine and elicit a functional alternative to get to the same valid goal?

7. Similarly, our hypotheses should be consistent not only with the tenets of biosocial theory, but also consistent with DBT's assumptions (i.e., the "practical philosophy" of DBT).

8. At the same time, while considering hypotheses explaining the dysfunctional sequence of links, try to envision a functional sequence of links that might work for this patient in lieu of the problematic sequence.

9. Even if the case conceptualization, subject to revisions as time passes, is "wrong," it can still function constructively for the therapist. It gets the therapist thinking conceptually and strategically, and it can organize confusing or disparate experiences and information for the therapist in a manner that promotes his own cognitive regulation, emotional regulation, and motivation. It "clears the field" and allows him to think.

10. A case conceptualization need not be complex, especially early on in the treatment. It might consist of a few links that repeat frequently in the chain, such as the same dysfunctional cognitions again and again, or the same primary or secondary emotions, or the same type of prompting event. On the other hand, it might be quite complex, involving many steps and sequences, even putting together data from different individuals (e.g., a systemic or familial case conceptualization). A DBT therapist needs to be free in determining the complexity and nature of case conceptualization to fit the data.

11. Think of case conceptualization as something that not only goes on in the head of the therapist; think of it as a lively, collaborative construction to be shared with the patient, tried out in interventions, and then altered as a result of collaboration and trial-and-error processes.

12. To highlight one point that was made in this chapter: When there is considerable data from the patient, or a complex field of interaction between the patient and others, you might deliberately consider a metaphor to grasp the big picture. If done in a creative and playful spirit, this may allow you to locate connections between different elements that are not so obvious and that can lead to parsimonious explanations and interventions.

CHAPTER 10

Commitment and Commitment Strategies

THE NATURE OF THE COMMITMENT PROBLEM

The argument for using enhanced commitment strategies in DBT begins with the obvious: Solving any difficult life problem requires a sufficient level of commitment. Take an easy and common example in modern life, and yet surprisingly challenging to solve. Imagine that for health-related reasons, you want to change your sedentary habits and begin exercising on a treadmill for 30 minutes each day. You acquire a serviceable treadmill and locate it in the most ideal setting in your household. You certainly already have the skill of walking, even running, on the treadmill. You have already indicated a significant intention by creating the conditions, and you have made a commitment in your mind. Still, though, you find it a boring and onerous task, you always have something more pressing to attend to, and you avoid the exercise with a multitude of excuses. You may have the skill for walking and running on a treadmill, but the skill for *getting yourself to walk and run on a treadmill* is not so strong or enduring. Even the individual who is healthy, well intended, well supported, and well equipped can lack the requisite degree of commitment to change a stubborn behavioral pattern.

    Commitment does not refer to any one step in the process of changing behavioral patterns. We don't simply commit, and then do. There is no invisible "on–off" commitment switch located somewhere in the body or mind. In spite of that, we can hear others—parents, teachers, trainers, therapists, even ourselves—make definitive statements about patients, out of frustration: "He lacks commitment," "She really doesn't want to get better," "She just isn't ready for this program," or "He obviously has no interest in improvement." When not at our best, we talk as if commitment were a *thing*, something tangible that belongs to an individual and that is either present or absent.

Linehan (1993a) wisely placed the need to elicit a commitment up front in DBT. The pretreatment stage, accompanied by the life-worth-living conversation (Chapter 1), focuses solely on eliciting a commitment that is sufficiently strong, durable, and meaningful to carry the patient through the challenges of behavioral change. But it does not mean going from no commitment to full commitment, or getting it once and for all. From a DBT perspective, commitment is comprised of a collection of behaviors—including thoughts, emotions, and actions—and a set of contextual conditions—including time, space, materials, monitoring, and supportive relationships—needed to establish it, build on it, and attend to it throughout the treatment process. And there is no absolute definition of what constitutes commitment; it can be defined as what is required in a given case, for a given task, to get oneself to do what is needed to meet a goal. Getting oneself to run daily on a treadmill requires an alignment of hopeful and realistic cognitive content, emotional readiness, facilitative action patterns, a strategy for holding oneself accountable, and contextual factors that permit and reinforce the behavior. As Linehan wrote in her manual, "Commitment itself is viewed as a behavior, which can be learned, elicited, and reinforced" (1993a, p. 285).

Getting a commitment to making a behavioral change from someone without psychopathology is challenging enough. If you add to that the additional burdens imposed by the presence of emotional sensitivity and reactivity; a baseline of depression or high anxiety; a tendency toward avoidance, withdrawal, and fatigue; and a syndrome of mood-dependent behavior, you magnify the problem of commitment multiple times over. If self-injurious behaviors have evolved as the most and only reliable strategy for bringing emotional relief, and the therapist is asking the patient to give them up and use more adaptive behaviors that don't work as well in the short run, the challenge is understandably enormous. Now consider further that the patient with whom you are trying to elicit a stronger commitment has been profoundly shaped by negative experiences of making such efforts in prior, pervasively invalidating environments. The mere thought of pushing oneself forward to realize life-worth-living goals and constructive intentions can elicit memories of being dismissed, criticized, demeaned, and blamed. For example: "What makes you think you can do this? What makes you think you are better than all the rest of us? Just give up!" A backlog of life and treatment failures infiltrates the woodwork of memory. For example: "I can't do this no matter how hard I try and they can't help me with this! I have never been able to stick with anything or succeed." Now we are considering the monumental challenge of getting someone with borderline personality disorder to commit wholeheartedly to a defined challenge, whether it be to enter DBT treatment, to sign on to the agreements in DBT, to target destructive behavioral patterns that have been reinforced a thousand times, or to try new skills. DBT has within it a huge range of strategies, skills, and protocols that facilitate behavioral change, but none of them will work without the requisite level of commitment, and the set of behaviors associated with commitment require attention throughout the treatment process. If you have a great set of tools and materials for building a house, and you have the skills to do it and the blueprints in front of you, you still will not build the house if you cannot generate and maintain the necessary commitment to exert the required effort. This basic reality was the discovery that launched the development and widespread application of motivational interviewing in the world of substance abuse treatment (Miller & Rollnick, 2012).

Because the concept of getting a commitment goes well beyond getting someone to think about commitment, speak about commitment, or even to evidence commitment in any one behavioral pattern, the process of getting a commitment is conceptualized as: (1) eliciting commitment-related behavioral patterns of all sorts and (2) structuring a reinforcing context. Sometimes it is difficult to know whether a failure to make a desired behavioral change is due to a problem of commitment. It might not be obvious. For instance, an individual whose commitment is rather strong might be unable to accomplish a certain behavioral change because dysregulated emotions or problematic cognitions override the best intentions, or because needed environmental supports or reinforcements are not in place. If the therapist in such a case can locate the factors interfering with progress and focus the work on those instrumental targets, the patient's level of commitment to those tasks often strengthens.

For instance, a 19-year-old female patient with borderline personality disorder and ADHD suffered from a series of disappointing relationships in college, which left her isolated, lonely, depressed, and less productive at school. She had shown evidence of a strong commitment early in therapy, and had successfully addressed problems with suicidal behavior and an addiction to pain medications. But the relationship problems were more stubborn, and sometimes it felt to me as if she were simply not as committed to do what was necessary to have more reliable, reciprocal relationships. But as it turned out, it was not a commitment problem. She simply could not see, nor could I in the early stage of treatment, exactly how her subtle interpersonal behaviors consistently alienated potential friends. Her tendency to relate everything to her own life situations, as a way to understand others and connect with them, was done in such a way as to lead others to think she was "self-centered." This particular social skills deficit was not sufficiently addressed in DBT's module on inter-personal skills, but once we accurately assessed the problem, through a careful study of her encounters with potential friends, she brought her commitment-related set of behaviors to bear on altering her usual com-munication patterns. She deliberately experimented with only listening to others and validating them, noticing her urges to relate everything to her experience without acting on it, and she saw sudden successes in relationships. What appeared to be a problem of commitment was in fact a stubborn social skills deficit to which she was blind, and to which I was blind, until we objectively assessed and treated it.

In other cases where an individual appears to be committed, thera-pists may discover, upon closer inspection and assessment, that the level of commitment is not what it appears to be. I once agreed to teach skills one-on-one to a 19-year-old woman with anorexia nervosa, whose weight was dangerously low. Her psychotherapist, who was not practicing DBT, wanted the patient to learn behavioral skills to help her in regulating her emotions, improving her self-esteem, and asserting herself more effec-tively in relationships. The patient's relentless pursuit of thinness seemed to be a multipurpose solution to these problem areas, and several months of supportive, insight-oriented psychotherapy had resulted in little to no change. The rationale made sense to me, the patient agreed to the justifi-cation and the requirements of skills training, and I began to meet weekly with her to teach her the DBT skills. At the end of each session I gave her a homework assignment to practice the skills.

Within 3 to 4 weeks, it was noticeable that in spite of her apparent cooperativeness with me during sessions, she was strikingly unengaged in practicing skills between sessions. By bringing this to her attention and asking a series of questions, I attempted to assess whether her lack of skills generalization was due to problematic emotions, cognitions, actions, or environmental contingencies, or to a deficit in commitment. I wondered whether her attachment to me was sufficient to provide me with therapeutic leverage, whether I validated her accurately and effec-tively, or whether I was pushing for change with sufficient intensity. In fact, she acted as if she were attached to me, and my assessment questions did not illuminate the situation.

Finally I asked her, directly, "I have to know: Do you really, really, *really* want to use these skills to change your eating-related behavioral patterns, because it doesn't seem like it?" Without guilt or shame, she admitted that the only change she wanted in her eating-related behaviors was to increase her capacity to tolerate and overcome hunger, to stop eating entirely, to get rid of any remaining (even "invisible") fat, and to be as skinny as possible without dying. She knew she was risking death, but she claimed that if death were a side effect of her quest, it would be OK; it was worth it. It was shocking to hear. I tried to paint a verbal picture of what she would look like and be like if she succeeded, to further assess and challenge her shocking belief. With little hesitance, and with a bit of embarrassment, she told me she had always admired, even envied, the Holocaust survivors whom she had seen in photographs in the process of leaving the concentration camps. Once identified, it appeared that her lack of commitment to the goals of treatment was profound and unshakeable, in that her immense capacity for commitment was devoted entirely to goals that were opposite the stated treatment goals. When I asked her why she had gone to such lengths to give the impression that she wanted to learn skills to change her behaviors, she admitted that she didn't want to disappoint her therapist or her parents; she didn't want them to know how profoundly she was committed to thinness even if death was the side effect. I worked toward a dialectical solution. Given that she had an immense capacity for commitment, but the goals of treatment were opposite to her current goals, I suggested that we reframe the treatment goals, such that she was working toward an increased capacity to speak the truth and to say "no" more effectively. She seemed interested at first, but her lack of interest and commitment to this more assertive interpersonal style quickly became apparent. Within a few days her weight dropped below a "medically acceptable weight" and she was put in a hospital against her will.

So the problem of commitment in DBT is extremely important, often formidable, sometimes difficult to assess, and requires attention throughout treatment because it waxes and wanes over time and in relation to different goals and tasks. As conceptualized by Linehan (1993a, p. 284), there are several levels of commitment. First is the commitment to the treatment as a whole. This includes the agreement to target life-threatening behaviors, to work to maintain and strengthen the therapeutic relationship, to attend skills training, and to comply with the other expectations of DBT defined in the initial contracting process. Second is the commitment to the typical problem-solving procedures in DBT: skills training, cognitive modification, and exposure procedures. And third is the commitment to specific agreements and assignments made within the individual therapy relationship. Linehan described seven commitment strategies to be used again and again, woven into therapy as needed to strengthen the initial commitment and then to bolster or rekindle a flagging commitment during the therapeutic process. Over the years of teaching and supervising DBT, I have seen many good therapists who rely on the seven commitment strategies in an overly mechanical way. Even if they accurately identify a problem with commitment, they assume that the next step is to use one or more of the commitment strategies. Experiences such as the one I had with the patient with anorexia have strengthened my belief that DBT therapists need a more thorough understanding and application of the principles underlying the strategies. Such an understanding leads to a more fluid, flexible, and tailored use of those strategies. In the remainder of this chapter, I first explore the broader topic of the "spirit" of commitment; then consider the role of the principles belonging to the behavioral, acceptance, and dialectical paradigms as they inform the process of getting commitment; and lastly discuss the use of the formal commitment strategies in that principle-based context.

"TRY" VERSUS "DO": THE SPIRIT OF COMMITMENT IN DBT

By highlighting the *spirit* of commitment, I am referring to something broader than any specific set of strategies or interventions; indeed I think of it as something that surrounds those strategies. Let's begin with understanding the difference between deciding to *try* to accomplish a goal versus deciding to accomplish the goal. "I'll try to do it" is a markedly different statement than "I'll do it." For example, if a high school teacher gives a difficult assignment to the class, some students might say, "I'll do my best, I'll try," and others might say, "OK, I'll do it." For good reasons, the teacher likes hearing the latter. If I were standing at the bottom of a mountain that was more challenging than any mountain I had climbed before, unable to know for sure whether I could successfully get to the peak, I might say to myself, "OK, this might be hard, but I will try." Alternatively, I might say, "I know it's going to be hard, but I am going to do it!" Of course there is no way to guarantee success; even a solid commitment, good climbing technique, and personal stamina could run aground in the face of impossible terrain, a powerful storm, or an unexpected injury. But my claim here is that, all other things being equal, the self-statement of the person most likely to succeed is the "I will do it" statement. It's a bold attitude; it is an in-your-face stance toward the "Gods of Difficulty and Interference," and psychologically it brings the accomplishment of the goal closer. More importantly, the bolder claim tends to recruit other behavioral patterns and contextual resources that will be required to succeed. This is what I mean by the *spirit* of commitment. The therapist who pushes the patient toward the bold "I will do it" statement, and who is reluctant to accept "trying" as the goal, is likely to create more momentum and purpose. Given that our patients often come with a biologically based sensitivity and reactivity, and pervasive environmentally based invalidation, getting this kind of commitment can be incredibly challenging, and at the same time it becomes critically important. My expectation that my patient can and will commit to the task with the "I-will-do-it" attitude communicates my belief in her capabilities. Obviously, the therapist has to have a rough idea of whether the patient is capable of what is being asked, and has to have a good idea of how high to set the bar. Generally I would prefer to elicit a 100% commitment to a lesser goal than a "I'll-give-it-a-try," 75–90%, commitment to a higher goal.

I worked with a 30-year-old woman with borderline personality disorder, a history of sexual trauma in childhood, and a series of high-lethality suicide attempts that had resulted in a "revolving door" pattern of hospitalizations for many years. Among other problem behaviors, she relied on self-cutting incidents every day to regulate her emotions. In about the third session, after she had shown an interest in working with me in DBT, I told her that I would want her to commit to not injuring herself for at least 1 year. She was taken aback, reminding me that she tended to cut herself every day and that she thought it had helped her to stay alive. She also told me that she didn't want to make a promise that she couldn't keep by telling me she could succeed in stopping her self-cutting behaviors all at once. I told her that I could understand that, and that I respected her commitment to honesty, but that it had become clear to me that she needed to make the all-out commitment to stop cutting if she was to have a better chance at succeeding. She took me seriously and told me that she could try. I told her that I respected her for her willingness to try, but that I was more interested in her doing it rather than trying. I was setting the bar higher. She had been in a large number of psychotherapy treatments of different kinds, and she told me that no one had ever asked her to definitively give it up. She said she had to think about it, because it was a frightening idea. She returned to the hospital where she was residing at the time, and she proceeded to tell all of the staff and many of the patients that I had asked her to totally give up cutting. From what was reported to me, she was not only frightened by the prospect, but also evidenced some pride and hope. In fact, our therapy got off to a good start as she committed to not cutting herself, which led to significant behavioral changes rather quickly. As mentioned in the first chapter, integral to the successful strengthening of commitment is the capacity to visualize the desired outcome, to visualize the picture of a life worth living.

As this example demonstrates, the seeds of commitment and the spirit of commitment must begin in the therapist, and the DBT consultation team must help each therapist strengthen his or her level of commitment to DBT, to the goals of each patient, and to the treatment tasks undertaken by each patient. This kind of commitment by the therapist is not to be taken for granted. I was once supervising a young and talented psychodynamically oriented therapist who was in the early stages of learning to practice DBT. Week after week she reported on her efforts to prompt her patient to fully comply with completion of the diary card—not an easy task in many DBT treatments. Week after week her patient handed in a diary card that was only partially completed, and the therapist assessed the factors interfering with full compliance. As far as I could tell, the therapist was seriously engaged in working on this therapy-interfering behavior target, but compliance hardly improved. I asked her to videotape the upcoming sessions so that I could see how she was intervening. Within minutes of beginning to watch a therapy session, it was obvious that the therapist's heart was not fully into making her case. She was willing to accept it when the patient said, "OK, I'll try harder next week," when in fact she had said that several times before. This therapist was not insisting on the kind of 100% spirit of commitment that would be represented by the statement, "OK, I will do it fully next week." It was my assumption that her prior training, which did not include the use of self-monitoring procedures such as diary cards, had left her somewhat reluctant to make such activities mandatory in treatment. This clarity about the problem led to our role playing in supervision, in which I played the role of the therapist asking her for the diary card. She immediately understood that the therapist needs to embrace the completion of the diary card as mandatory. She was immediately able to change her approach, and it quickly translated into a stronger and more complete commitment from the patient.

It would be understandable to question my insistence on the 100% commitment to "do it." After all, what is the likelihood that a patient who cuts herself every day will be able to guarantee she would stop cutting herself altogether for the coming year? It's not likely. But what we are focusing on here in gaining the strongest possible commitment is not a discussion of the odds of succeeding in reality; we are talking about a committed frame of mind, in this moment. We want to cultivate and support the patient in arriving at a committed frame of mind that leads to the recruitment of as many commitment-related behaviors as possible. If the patient says, "But what if I don't keep my commitment—will I be kicked out of treatment?," I say something like this: "No, you won't be kicked out. If you make the maximum commitment you can make right now, and get your mind around it, and do everything you can to honor that commitment, and then something overrides your commitment or your commitment decreases, we will figure out what's going on and reestablish the commitment. This has nothing to do with punishment, criticism, or kicking you out. We just do it this way because you are more likely to succeed at your goals."

The 100% commitment approach can be considered *abstinence* if it involves ending an addictive behavior such as substance use or self-cutting, and the approach to ending the relapse and reestablishing the commitment can be called the *harm reduction* approach (also borrowed from substance abuse treatment). The combination of the two, emphasizing abstinence up to the point of relapse and then shifting over to harm reduction upon relapse, has been called *dialectical commitment* in DBT. Although it began in the context of applying DBT to the treatment of substance use disorders, the concept has been incorporated into standard DBT in relation to self-harm behaviors. The challenge for each therapist is to bring the strongest commitment to the therapy and to insist on the strongest commitment from the patient. In my experience as a therapist and supervisor, there are some patients who seem to automatically elicit this commitment in their therapist, and other patients toward whom the therapist does not so readily and strongly commit. When the spirit of commitment is present, it is a valuable resource, leading the therapist to set the highest standard and push for the most change, which then helps the patient respond in kind. It is probably a quality associated with a heightened therapeutic attachment that comes easily in some cases and not others. DBT therapists have to be alert in those treatments where this kind of therapeutic attachment is not so strong. With the help of their consultation teams, therapists should work to generate the attachment, strengthen their own commitment, and thereby increase the likelihood of eliciting a strong commitment in their patients.

CONTRIBUTIONS FROM THE BEHAVIORAL PARADIGM

A number of typical steps in eliciting and strengthening a commitment in the patient are part and parcel of standard CBT. We try to be clear and direct in arriving collaboratively at specific treatment targets. We establish a means to monitor progress on those targets, particularly the diary card in DBT. Having oriented to the targets and the specific strategies to accomplish them, we orient the patient to the problem of commitment. We reinforce evidence of progress on the targets and progress on commitment. When the patient cannot meet these expectations, we use shaping procedures, reinforcing successive approximations of behaviors "on the way" to the desired behaviors. If we find that the strength of commitment is inhibited by dysfunctional thoughts and beliefs, we highlight those cognitions and work toward revising them. We maintain a focus on skills training in the insufficiently committed patient, as commitment will sometimes increase as the patient acquires needed skills. Sometimes the blockade in commitment is a result of avoidance of certain emotionally evocative cues that elicit painful emotions, in which case we might use exposure procedures to desensitize the patient to the practice of fully committing to change. Throughout the application of these change procedures, we use didactic interventions to teach the patient about his functioning, about treatment and pathology. Sometimes this kind of psychoeducational intervention can increase understanding of what is needed and can generate hope. In other words, typical CBT approaches that we use to address anxiety, depression, and dysfunctional behavioral patterns can effectively be brought to bear on enhancing commitment-related behaviors.

It may surprise some DBT therapists to realize that if getting a commitment is particularly difficult, therapy might focus on this task for months. I was once teaching the first 5 days of a 10-day DBT intensive workshop, and, in that context, I showed the participants a videotape of a session in which Marsha Linehan was trying to elicit and strengthen a commitment from her patient to stop abusing the drugs to which she was addicted. She was validating the patient, using standard commitment strategies, and reinforcing any evidence of commitment-related behaviors. In spite of what appeared to be effective application of commitment strategies, the patient moved no closer to a commitment to stop using drugs. Even though she seemed to agree with much of what Linehan said, she would not state her willingness to stop using drugs. Six months later, I was teaching Part 2 of the same workshop, in which participants came for another 5 days. Someone asked if I knew whether Linehan had managed to elicit a commitment from that patient. I didn't know, so I called Marsha that night, and she sent a videotape of their latest session in overnight mail. (In those days, the regulations governing the distribution and viewing of treatment videotape were not so stringent.) We watched it the next day. All of us were surprised to see that the entire focus of the session was the attempt to elicit a commitment to stop using drugs, much the same as 6 months prior. We got on the phone with Marsha and asked her about the continued focus on commitment extending so far into treatment. She explained that in spite of our desire to get a commitment within four sessions, sometimes it is a more stubborn problem. She had settled into working on commitment to stop using drugs. She had broken down the concept of commitment into a number of commitment-related behaviors, had oriented the patient to working on this target, and was using all of CBT in addressing the factors interfering with commitment. The patient appeared to be a semi-willing partner in the effort to stop using drugs. In other words, the fact that this most competent DBT therapist had not elicited the needed commitment, even after 6 months, was not a reason to end her treatment; it was reason to use all the principles, strategies, and skills to strengthen commitment. As it turned out, there was something missing in the formulation, which involved an unacknowledged role of a close relative of the patient in supplying her with drugs and reinforcing her for using them. Once this was out in the open, Linehan was able to elicit the kind of commitment she had been seeking.

So we have seen that in the face of stubborn problems in getting a commitment, the DBT therapist can access the entire behavioral paradigm to succeed. He uses targeting, behavioral monitoring, orientation, didactic interventions, behavioral chain analysis, case conceptualization, and all four change procedures: contingency procedures, cognitive modification procedures, exposure procedures, and skills training. In concept it is the same as using the entire behavioral paradigm to treat another primary target behavior such as self-cutting or substance abuse. Beyond these specific uses of CBT strategies and procedures, the DBT therapist brings a behaviorally oriented stance, consistent with principles inherent in CBT, to the problem of commitment.

Consistent with a behavioral approach, the therapist uses an irreverent style to get a commitment: forthright, matter of fact, transparent, bold, optimistic, objective, and disciplined. This stance, itself, can sometimes elicit a stronger commitment. Sometimes therapists are unnecessarily tentative in asking for change, softening the clear and direct approach, as if the direct push for change would be too much for the patients. Even if a patient objects to the direct push for a defined behavioral change, the fact that the therapist presents it sets a tone, communicates direction and hope, and establishes a "can-do" atmosphere for the patient's consideration. Sometimes establishing a direction and pushing for it, even if the patient appears to object to it or dislike it, can plant the seeds for forward movement. From a skills training perspective, the therapist models the interpersonal skill set for getting one's objective. We teach patients to ask very specifically and clearly for their objectives, and when there is opposition or evasion, to continue to ask for them like a "broken record." In asking for commitment, the therapist might appear to be a broken record too.

CONTRIBUTIONS FROM
THE ACCEPTANCE PARADIGM

The principles inherent in the paradigm of acceptance in DBT also inform therapists who are working on increasing commitment in their patients (and themselves). As suggested in the above section on the spirit of commitment, the therapist asks for a commitment *in the present moment*. Naturally, he wants the commitment in this moment to increase commitment throughout the treatment, but the focus is entirely on this one moment. The patient's memories of past failures and disappointments might interfere, as might her anxieties about whether she can accomplish the task under consideration. The therapist wants the patient to set aside judgments and recrimination about the past or pessimism about future success, and to just be in the present, conjuring up an attitude of commitment in this moment. This is a subtle but very important application of mindfulness practice. It involves being mindful of making a commitment, mindful of the various elements that go into making a commitment, and mindful of the tendency to judge the past and to project into the future. When a patient anxiously asks, "But what if X happens, or what if Y happens, and I can't keep the commitment?," the therapist points out that these are frightening thoughts, but they are only thoughts, and encourages the patient to bring her attention back to the focus on making a 100% commitment (or as much as possible) in this one moment.

Inherent in this is another Buddhist principle, *nonattachment*. It's challenging but helpful, since the concept of commitment immediately pulls one's attention to the future, to notice one's attachment to how things should be and should have been. As soon as we think of committing to some behavioral pattern in the future, we tend to become attached to it, to ruminate about it, to assess whether we can do it, to go back over times when we failed to honor a commitment. We multiply our anxiety and our suffering by getting attached to what should happen instead of just staying focused, in this moment, on noticing and strengthening our commitment. We tend (and our patients tend) to get attached to whether we can do what we are saying we will do, and the associated anxiety results in diminishing the strength of our commitment. I am suggesting that we reach for a commitment that is centered *only in this one moment*, even though it is a statement about future behavior. Recently I asked a patient, whose depression and fear were resulting in a pattern of avoidance, to "just commit, right here, right now, to me, that you will get up tomorrow morning, and that whatever is your state of mind, you will get dressed, eat something, and go to school."

She responded with distress, "But what if I can't make it? I can never predict how I will feel the next day or whether I can do something."

I said, "No one can. That includes you. That is simply a fact, and it is not your fault. You cannot predict how you will feel. All you can do is to take care of this, and only this, one moment. And I am asking you, right here, right now, to decide that you are going to get up and go to school tomorrow. And I want you to picture it, to believe it." "But how can I?" she asked, "I just don't know what will happen."

"None of us knows what will happen, none of us. But if we didn't commit to anything, because we can't predict the future, we would never do anything. Just bring yourself into this one moment, create an image of getting up and going to school, a vivid image, and just notice yourself committing to it."

Here the DBT therapist draws from the rich research literature supporting visualization of a positive outcome, something that is also taught to patients during the module of Distress Tolerance Skills.

Another principle associated with Buddhism and woven throughout DBT is the realization that "self" is a construct. As discussed in Chapter 3 on the acceptance paradigm in DBT, what we call self is actually made up entirely of nonself ingredients. While we use the concept of self to differentiate ourselves from others, implying that there is some unique ingredient that establishes the self of each of us, this perspective suggests that there really is no such thing. We can apply the same reasoning to the concept of commitment. We can realize that *there is no such thing as commitment, as there is no such thing as self, and commitment is made up entirely of noncommitment elements.* What we are conveniently calling *commitment* is simply a collection of behaviors that increases one's chances of making desired behavioral change; it is not a real "thing" in itself. There is no real entity of self and no real entity of commitment. We are simply working to increase the collection of elements, energies, or behaviors that will help move things in the direction of the desired goal. This is consistent with the Buddhist principle of emptiness To let go of considering commitment as a solid and unique thing in itself, as a thing belonging to the individual, is to embrace the broader concept that commitment comprises a huge range of interdependent influences without boundaries.

If we abandon the concept of self and of commitment as a real thing, we are less likely to fall into the trap of deciding whether a patient has commitment or not, and whether we can strengthen commitment or not. We just focus on moving things in the desired direction. This can help us think more freely and creatively about how to increase commitment in a given individual toward a given goal or task. For instance, at times the most effective approach will be to stop trying to increase commitment.

Years ago I was at a social gathering that included one of my wife's cousins, a man who had been a dentist into his 50s, but then left dentistry to pursue his real passion, coaching tennis. He was the tennis coach for a college women's tennis team, and on his team was a phenomenally good player. He was talking with me about this player, explaining that she was a champion in her league and in her region, and that if she were to develop a stronger serve, he was convinced that she had a chance to be a national champion. He had tried to arrange for a serving coach to work with this player one-on-one, but the player was not interested. He couldn't understand it. He described his conversation with her:

> COACH: If you improved your serve, you could be a contender at the national level.
>
> PLAYER: But coach, I win all of my matches and I feel like I'm really good.
>
> COACH: I know, but when you play against the very top players, your only weakness is your serve; if you focused in on it with some specialized coaching, I think you could perform at the next level.
>
> PLAYER: It's not worth it to me. I just love to play and I don't care about playing at the next level.

My relative was clearly frustrated with her, and he wondered whether I had any ideas of how to get her to increase her commitment to make it to the next level. I suggested to him that he appeared to be more attached to that goal than she was, and that he was overlooking, and invalidating, her own goals, whatever they might be. He ran the risk of souring their relationship when she sounded quite happy with her tennis. He got the point, and as I learned later, he went back to her and said something like, "I want to apologize for pushing you so hard to improve your serve. I am aware that it seems more like my goal than yours. You are a wonderful player, and you love tennis, and I think you should just do exactly what makes sense to you, and I won't push it any more. I don't want this to interfere with what has been a great experience coaching you." She was appreciative; she thanked him. A week later, she asked him if he could arrange for her to meet with the serving coach: "I might be more interested in it than I thought."

So we have highlighted the value of invoking acceptance principles such as "present moment," "non-attachment,' and the concept of "inter-being" which refers to non-self and the profound interdependency of all phemonena. In addition, we sometimes adopt the acceptance-based perspective of "impermenance" or "transience."

Commitment Is Transient in Its Nature

Like everything else in nature, commitment is not permanent. Made up, as it is, of so many interdependent elements, in a world where everything today is different than it was yesterday, we can expect every commitment to fluctuate in strength and nature. A strong commitment today to stop self-cutting behavior can weaken tomorrow, in the face of a changed mood, a stressful encounter, a shift in a relationship, a renewed level of interest. A weak commitment today could strengthen tomorrow, because of renewed physical energy or mental clarity, an inspiring comment by a valued friend, or sudden recognition of the potential importance of the destination under consideration. Naturally, we are wise to continue to monitor the level and nature of commitment in each patient, and to remain aware that patients may require commitment-oriented interventions again and again as treatment ensues. Rather than thinking that someone "should" remain committed at the highest level, we can expect that high levels of commitment will naturally fade, low levels of commitment will often increase, and by truly grasping this fact of life we can relax, assess, and intervene as needed, without getting caught in the trap of "what should be."

It can be helpful for us as therapists to realize that we cannot "make" someone else commit to something. Commitment is not under our control. We can identify commitment-related behaviors, help patients consider the consequences of various courses of action, work toward establishing conditions that might increase commitment, and push for it—all the while letting go of it at the same time. We don't cause commitment; we intervene in ways that increase the chances that it will happen. And the level of commitment we are looking for is "good-enough commitment"— enough commitment to get the job done—and we sometimes need to notice our own urge to push for a perfect commitment that is more than necessary. And when we find that in spite of all of our efforts, and those of the patient, there is little evidence that commitment is strengthening, especially in the early days, weeks, and months of therapy, we may find that it is our role to "hold" the commitment for a relatively uncommitted patient as it waxes and wanes. I am not arguing here for an interminable pretreatment period aimed at commitment; I am simply defining a stance, a state of mind, in the therapist, that in my opinion is more likely to result in the patient's commitment.

Commitment Is Perfect Just as It Is

The work of increasing a patient's level of commitment to the treatment or a particular task involves persistent and intelligent devotion, and sometimes the fruits are slow to ripen. The cost of that kind of therapeutic devotion might be the experience of therapeutic frustration. No difficult task is ever accomplished without some frustration. Tempering that frustration, which often includes an element of judgment ("This patient is not working half as hard as I am!"), is the Buddhist-based insight that the world is perfect exactly as it is in this moment, the level of commitment is perfect just as it is, in that given the history and evolution of all of the commitment-related elements that bear on the current level, how could it be otherwise? It is as it is; it is as it "should" be. If we truly let go of our attachment to how we think things should be, we can then endorse the viewpoint that it has to be as it is. We might not know exactly why, but we can assume it. Once brought back into balance by this recognition and acceptance of reality as it is, the more relaxed therapist might then be able to push for an increase in commitment from a more balanced and accepting stance.

Once we adopt the perspective that everything is perfect as it is, including the current level and nature of commitment in our patients, it by no means suggests a fatalistic or resigned position. On the contrary, there is nothing predetermined about whether commitment increases, decreases, or stays the same; that is, *everything matters*. Every intervention related to strength of commitment might make a difference. It's just so complicated to know what will strengthen commitment, since everything matters. Will it help to adopt a challenging tone, or a reciprocal and accepting one? Will it help more to say that the commitment is weak, or to proceed without mentioning it? Would the therapist's self-disclosure of a personal experience that required a heightened commitment be useful to share or not? When to push and when to let go? It is so complicated; the choices are complex, and there is much to be said for maintaining an observing, reflective posture with regard to oneself, to the patient, and to the transaction, trying interventions and noticing what seems to work.

In my experience, in situations with patients in whom commitment is difficult to generate, greater successes have arisen from an attitude of trial and error, back and forth, push and pull, and observing what works, than the times when I applied commitment strategies and met success in a straightforward way. Perhaps the most important advice embedded in this perspective is that the therapist remains cognizant of the level of commitment, and remains committed to increasing it if necessary. The therapist keeps the target in view and tries anything, everything that might work, and observes the in-the-moment outcome. Facilitating the development of commitment requires different interventions with different patients, and the DBT therapist has an enormous arsenal from which to select the next move.

CONTRIBUTIONS FROM
THE DIALECTICAL PARADIGM

Of equal value in expanding the imaginable options for eliciting commitment are principles from the dialectical paradigm. The first and most basic dialectical principle is that theses elicit antitheses, propositions elicit their opposites; *reality is composed naturally of oppositions*. If a therapist explicitly pushes for greater commitment, she may inadvertently elicit opposition to commitment. If a therapist lets go of the push for commitment (such as occurred in the example involving the dentist/tennis coach and his star player in the prior section), she may unwittingly elicit greater commitment. Where we see an adamant stance opposing commitment, we can presume that there is an implicit struggle between commitment and noncommitment already occurring in the patient, and we can act with that in mind. Assuming that commitment exists in a context of oppositions, we make explicitly and implicitly informed decisions about when to push, when to let go, how hard to push, how much to validate the causes of noncommitment, and so on. We act, and we observe. As we shall see, certain of DBT's formal commitment strategies are built on the understanding of how elements elicit their opposites. For instance, we alternate between asking for very little, to get our foot in the door, and asking for way more than the patient will be willing to take on, known as the door-in-the-face strategy. We highlight the patient's freedom to choose, with awareness that given the circumstances, there is a relative absence of acceptable choices. We move back and forth between asking the patient to enumerate the advantages of making a commitment to change, and the disadvantages, in what is known as the pros and cons of commitment. Going back and forth, pushing and pulling, highlighting opposites, whether using the standard commitment strategies, metaphors, or other dialectical strategies, often helps the therapist locate the right balance, the efficacious intervention, and creates an atmosphere of movement rather than stasis—all of which allow for the *discovery* of commitment rather than the creation of commitment. Working dialectically, we keep our eye on the ultimate goal, increased commitment, but engage in a process of searching, termed *dialectical assessment*, to find what is left out of the current equation. Perhaps the main point here is that when commitment is difficult to come by, it is more likely discovered in an atmosphere of searching, flexibility, and openness, while carefully observing and reinforcing any positive commitment-related influences.

A corollary of the reality-consists-of-oppositions principle is that within every commitment, even levels of commitment that appear to be strong, we will find the presence of opposition, perhaps best named as *ambivalence*. We find the same perspective in motivational interviewing. The pressures, so to speak, within the elements of commitment, are many and they can shift the balance toward or away from commitment in response to so many factors. One example was given earlier in this chapter, in which a young woman with anorexia appeared to be committed to learning behavioral skills, but in fact there was a tension within her between wanting to appear to be interested, which itself can influence someone toward a stronger commitment, and absolutely having no need for the skills given that her goals were antithetical to changing her eating patterns. So, what appears to be a strong commitment can unfold into a more complicated opposition between two "voices." What appears to be a weak commitment can obscure what is actually a strong one. In my inpatient DBT program, for instance, in our weekly community meeting, one patient raised her hand every week to put her item on the agenda: that "I am here against my will; I find nothing in this program to be helpful, and I can't wait to leave." Nevertheless this patient attended every group, diligently learned and practiced skills, and was engaged in psychotherapy. Watching what she was actually doing, rather than taking in her public pronouncements, helped us relax our temptation to push for greater commitment. There is the privately held commitment, the publicly stated commitment, and the actions manifesting commitment, and there can be hidden oppositions between them.

Commitment Is Interdependently Linked to All Systemic Factors

This perspective on commitment has been discussed in relation to the principles of Buddhism and acceptance, in that it is based on the idea that there are no boundaries and that everything is interacting all the time. Here the focus is on systemic thinking, emphasizing that commitment in any one individual can be seen as one element in a dynamic system with many interacting factors. For instance, commitment in one individual can be seen as being in dynamic interaction with influences from other family members. I once saw a family, two parents and their two daughters, ages

17 and 20. The presenting problem was that the 20-year-old daughter had made a decision, long considered and accompanied by constructive consultations, to enter into a transgender process that would result in transitioning to life as a male. The process was already under way. He had already undergone some hormonal treatment and had acquired some masculine characteristics. In addition he had chosen a male name and was asking his family members to use it and to use the masculine pronoun. The parents were enormously distressed. The mother had done research and had had several important conversations with her (new) son. She had moved in the direction of acknowledging the reality of the transition and had begun to accept it. She was willing to respect her son's request to use the masculine name and pronouns. But the father was unwilling to consider it, had been unable or unwilling to entertain the possibility that his daughter's gender change was for real, and he was stubbornly clinging to the image he had always had: that his talented and appealing little girl would grow into a charming, charismatic, heterosexual woman with her own family. The father found himself under attack in the first session, receiving crossfire from his angry, insulted transgender son. and his softer but change-oriented wife. It seemed that the pressure on him to change was eliciting a refusal in him to move in that direction. He was angry, stubborn, and refused to believe that his beloved daughter would follow through. No therapeutic interventions toward the father, mother, or 20-year-old son moved things forward.

Thinking systemically, knowing that everyone influences everyone, I wondered aloud what the 17-year-old thought of her brother's plans and requests. No one had asked her, and she had a quiet demeanor. Without any hesitation, she said, "There is nothing surprising about this. He's always seemed like someone who would be happier as a boy. It's actually a lot of what makes him as great as he is. So I'm just glad he can do it." I asked her how she reacted to the request to use the male name and pronouns. She said it made sense to her, but acknowledged and apologized to her (new) brother for sometimes slipping back to female pronouns. It was a poignant moment between siblings, completely reframing the whole process as a positive one, allying with her brother without seeming to judge her father. The father remained quiet. But in the next family session he said he had decided to work toward accepting the change in his (new) son, to use the requested name and pronoun, and he wept for several minutes, saying he was just so sad to be losing his older daughter, or his image of the future of his daughter. The 20-year-old seemed to appreciate his father's grief, and while looking right at him in a kind way, waved at the father and said, "Dad, I'm still here." The father's commitment to change, which seemed like a hopeless prospect, appeared spontaneously in the realignment brought about by his 17-year-old's comments.

Commitment Is Constantly Changing; It Is in Constant Motion

Here is another principle associated with dialectical philosophy that entirely overlaps with the Buddhist principle stating that everything is transient. Commitment is not really real, a thing, or solid. It is a construct we use to capture the confluence of moving, interacting elements that influence progress toward or away from a stated goal or task. The dialectical principles we are considering here suggest that commitment is not only a multifaceted construct, but also that this construct is itself always in motion. When I have found myself trying to elicit a stronger commitment but encountering a "brick wall" of noncommitment, it has been helpful for me to remember that what appears solid is actually not. That "brick wall," if I remain standing in front of it, trying various interventions, letting time and events happen, relaxing into moment after present moment, is likely to shift: perhaps to develop cracks, to soften, to crumble, or to change in nature, such that we can move forward. I am not claiming that this always happens—there are circumstances in which commitment, by anyone's definition, does not happen, at least within a tolerable or realistic time frame—but the stance informed by the awareness that commitment is always in motion moves me in the direction of endurance, patience, careful observation, and creative efforts to intervene over time.

Commitment Is Transactional (Just as Identity Is Transactional)

Again, this principle contained within dialectics captures the notion that it is far too narrow to consider commitment to be a property of the individual. It is a property of a transaction, or several transactions. My commitment may be dependent upon your support, or be a reaction against someone else's position. The strength of my commitment rises and falls in transaction with other people or factors around me. Keeping this in mind helps me to expand my focus beyond the behaviors of the "uncommitted" individual and to consider what kind of transaction is at work that elicits behaviors that go against commitment. If I can't elicit change from an individual by directly addressing him about his behavior, I might be more successful if I conceptualize the situation transactionally, between the patient and another person, and attempt to influence the transaction in a manner that influences the individual's commitment.

DBT'S FORMAL COMMITMENT STRATEGIES

DBT's commitment strategies themselves represent an interweaving of change, acceptance, and dialectical strands. In the most effective use of each strategy, the therapist radically accepts the patient's current level of commitment, and in that context pushes for a stronger and more specific commitment. This is the essence of the dialectical balance in DBT between acceptance and change. Most of the strategies represent a balancing act between acceptance and change: reviewing the advantages of a given problematic behavior alongside reviewing the disadvantages (pros and cons of commitment); asking for a tiny change versus asking for a huge one (foot-in-the-door and door-in-the-face); highlighting the patient's freedom to choose versus the reality of limited alternatives (freedom to choose in the absence of alternatives); and arguing in favor of noncommitment in a way that elicits greater commitment (devil's advocate). At other times, the therapist highlights the relationship between a current weak commitment and a prior strong commitment, hoping to catalyze a transfer of force to the current one (eliciting prior commitments).

Even in the use of a rather straightforward behavioral strategy, shaping, in the service of commitment, the therapist accepts whatever level of commitment is available and then reinforces the emergence of any small sign of increased commitment. In other words, the process of getting a stronger commitment is not a concise and linear approach to the patient, as if one could make a "direct hit" on the commitment dilemma. Commitment strategies, each of them a balancing act, are woven in and out of a dance between patient and therapist. The resulting conversation is filled with movement between patient and therapist, between opposing positions, between certainty and doubt. Done well, it is artful, weaving together all six/seven strategies in a fluid conversation that considers the values, the choices in front of the patient, and the consequences of different choices without "dragging" the patient toward commitment.

The artful application of strategies, with recognition of the movement inherent within each of them and among them, is the right antidote for the profoundly ambivalent patient whose emotional dysregulation comes with black-and-white thinking, with denial of interrelatedness, and with the fear of being trapped in yet another invalidating environment. Catalyzing commitment while in motion usually holds more hope than trying to get commitment from a dead standstill.

Now we turn to a consideration of each strategy from a principle-based perspective, not to review them since they are so well described in the treatment manual, but to enhance the therapist's ability to use them creatively and fluidly.

The six/seven, if the third strategy is counted as two) commitment strategies are:

1. Weighing the pros and cons: selling commitment
2. Highlighting the freedom to choose in the absence of alternatives
3. Foot in the door and door in the face
4. Eliciting prior commitments and connecting them to the present one
5. Taking the devil's advocate position
6. Shaping successive approximations to commitment

Weighing the Pros and Cons

The entire commitment conversation revolves around the weighing of pros and cons of making a commitment. It is far from a simple listing of pros on one side of the page, cons on the other side, and then weighing them. Ideally it is an artful weaving back and forth between advantages and disadvantages of making the commitment to behavioral change. My preference is to begin with the cons rather than the pros. I ask the patient to explain to me why she continues to use the problematic behavior, or why she does not engage in change. I enter into this conversation with a spirit of genuine curiosity, with the approach of truly wanting to "get it." My goal is to understand the reasons for the patient's persisting with the current behavioral pattern to such a degree that I myself begin to think I would make the same choice. As soon as I begin to notice that I am thinking, "Wow, if I were in that position, I would do the same thing," I feel that I have arrived at a potentially helpful place. From that position I can genuinely express understanding of the patient's rationale for not committing to change. I can articulate it to the patient and validate it, overcoming any judgmental reactions that I held before.

At that point I tend to switch to the pros of making the commitment. I ask something like, "Given how much sense it makes for you to persist in doing what you are doing, and how little sense it makes for you to change your behavior, are there any reasons at all that weigh in favor of committing to change?" If I have accurately recognized the cons of changing and have joined the patient in that position for the moment, I find that the inquiry about the pros of changing behavior flows much better. In a commitment session with a 40-year-old woman who was seriously victimized as a child, developed PTSD as an adolescent, began heavy polysubstance use as a teen, and then added severe self-cutting in her late teens, all of which had continued through her adult life, I got to the point of validating the cons of change, and then said, "Given how amazingly effective it is for you to cut yourself, unlike any other simple strategy in bringing immediate relief, and how well it has worked for you, perhaps even helping you to stay alive, is there any reason at all, anything you can think of, that would argue in favor of giving up the self-cutting behaviors?" At that point, she readily and genuinely listed several reasons for change: to stop adding to her scars, since they interfered with her interpersonal life; to stop "hurting other people," since she noticed that it hurt friends of hers to know that she keeps hurting herself; and to make it possible for her to get treatment for her PTSD, since most people wouldn't treat her for it until she was no longer hurting herself.

Perhaps the most salient point to make about using the pros and cons—which as I mentioned above, are already inherently dialectical—is to engage in this process with a dialectical spirit: moving back and forth, highlighting oppositions, searching for a synthesis that supports commitment, and remaining improvisational, flexible, and creative in considering interventions and timing.

Highlighting the Freedom to Choose in the Absence of Alternatives

I list this strategy second only to the pros and cons one because it is also a strategy that is woven, over and over again, throughout the discussions about commitment. In my opinion, the pros and cons and the freedom to choose strategies are the ever-present interventional pillars of the commitment conversation, with the other strategies applied as indicated. As mentioned, this strategy is also inherently dialectical, balancing freedom to choose with a functional lack of freedom to choose. Again, the best application is to continue to endorse both positions, weaving back and forth between them. Sometimes I highlight that the patient always has the freedom to choose to do DBT, or not; other times I highlight that there do not seem to be any good alternatives. Even if, from the patient's viewpoint, there is a lack of freedom of choice about what to do with his life at this point in time, making DBT the only viable alternative, the therapist wants to help him arrive at the place where his decision to enter DBT is voluntary.

Many DBT programs have been established in forensic inpatient settings with legally mandated patients, in prisons, and in residential programs for adolescents who are required to be there. In doing DBT, it becomes critical to structure the program and the commitment conversation in a manner that highlights that there *is* an alternative to engaging in DBT: either another treatment model altogether or variations to the framework of DBT as presented. Nothing will fuel anti-commitment sentiments more than being *made* to commit; such coercion creates resentment, pseudo-commitment, or open defiance. The therapist can acknowledge that a patient is mandated to be in treatment, and can validate the understandable resentment and passivity that follow. Furthermore, he can point out that treatment is likely to be useless, perhaps even counterproductive, if the patient goes through the motions while seeing no convincing reason to engage in it. He might suggest that DBT is only really useful if the patient has goals, freely chosen, toward which DBT can be applied. Sometimes this kind of statement will catalyze a conversation about that individual's goals in that setting and beyond. If the patient broadly insists on a total lack of interest or willingness to enter into the basic elements of DBT, the therapist can endorse that choice as the "free" choice of the patient, and then just highlight the consequences of that choice.

On my inpatient DBT unit, our treatment program was entirely based on DBT. Sometimes we had a patient who "refused" to do DBT, did not want to attend the groups, learn the skills, or go to DBT-based therapy. I would tell that patient that he always had a choice. He could enter into the DBT programming, or he could choose not to participate. "But what would I do if I don't participate in DBT?" I would answer that he would then receive something closer to "standard inpatient psychiatric care." "What is that?" he would ask. "That means you get up each day, you hang around the unit, you talk with nurses and other staff, you can watch television during acceptable hours, you will be seen by a doctor to receive a diagnosis and medication treatment if indicated, and we will monitor your progress until you get out." I was realistic, but it did not sound very appealing. The patient had the freedom to choose and a relative absence of alternatives. If the insistence on not participating in DBT went too much beyond the first weeks, we would look for another setting to which to refer the patient if possible.

Foot in the Door and Door in the Face

Of all of the commitment strategies, foot in the door and door in the face is the only one that guides the therapist to specifically ask for a commitment. As soon as the therapist asks the patient to commit to a change in behavior, therapeutic choices arise. Does she ask the patient for something more than what the patient seems to be willing to do, attempting to set the bar high?: "I want you to commit to completely abstaining from cutting, or drinking alcohol, using drugs, or bingeing and purging behaviors for the coming year!" Does the therapist ask for less than she actually hopes to get, in the service of eliciting and building upon the patient's willingness?: "I want you to commit to completely abstaining from cutting, drinking, using drugs, or bingeing and purging only for the coming week, and then we will review the week and consider whether to renew the commitment for another week." Or does the therapist begin by asking for something close to what she thinks is realistic and what the patient might be willing to do?

The success of this intrinsically dialectical strategy requires us to "feel" where the patient is with respect to commitment. Is it enough to just "hint" at commitment, and then "let it rest" for a time? Are we being too careful if we do not boldly insist on commitment, a door-in-the-face commitment? Are we being too timid, too bold, too warm and accepting, too pushy? There is no answer in the absolute. Without knowing the context, we can't say which route to take. What I find useful about the foot-in-the-door/door-in-the-face spectrum of options is the suggestion that we move back and forth across these positions, studying the patient's reactions all the while, finding our way to the highest available level of commitment.

For instance, I recently began therapy with a young man who, after 2 years of residential treatment for severe self-harm behaviors and suicide attempts, was entering college for the first time. His anticipatory anxiety was extreme, and he did not imagine that he could handle the academic expectations and the social life. As he put it, he was going to take it "one day at a time." Sensing that he might leave school at any moment, when his discouragement and anxiety peaked, I asked him to commit to me that he would finish the first semester (door in the face). He was incredulous, acting as if I were crazy. He said it was terrifying to even think that far ahead; it made him feel trapped. I told him that I thought his "one-day-at-a-time" strategy was a good one, but that if he were to commit for a longer period, in spite of whatever moods came about, it would give us a chance to work together on the challenges. It would give us breathing room. I asked if he could commit to the first month, 30 days. He said it still seemed like too much time to think about, but he would commit to make it through the first 3 weeks, 21 days, because that was the last date when he could drop out without paying the full tuition for the semester. I indicated a wish that we could look beyond 3 weeks, but praised his courage and settled on 3 weeks as an initial commitment. It was a dance, the art of negotiation.

Eliciting Prior Commitments and Connecting Them to the Present One

This strategy is a straight application of respondent conditioning, or classical conditioning, theory. The therapist attempts to establish a connection between the current stimulus situation, wherein the patient is being asked to make a commitment to something here and now, and a prior stimulus situation of a similar nature, wherein the patient made a commitment. There are two main uses of this strategy. As explained in Linehan's (1993a) manual, the first is to remind the patient of a commitment she made upon entering treatment and which has now weakened, trying to reelicit the previously made commitment, and in so doing, enhance her flagging commitment in the current moment. The other way, which if skillfully done can be very effective, involves locating some other commitment in the patient's past she once made to changing something—a commitment that resulted in a successful change—and try to connect the current challenge to that one.

I began working with a 40-year-old woman who developed behavioral patterns of borderline personality disorder after her husband left her for another woman, leaving her alone to care for her teenage children. She was angry and grief stricken, and the painful life episode awakened memories of having been profoundly neglected as a child when it seemed to her that her parents wished she had not been born. She began to drink alcohol every day and night, and made several moderately lethal suicide attempts. One result was the relative neglect of her own children, who began to show problematic behaviors of a rebellious nature. As a result, she was highly self-critical. In early sessions we formulated the target list. Second to eliminating suicidal behavior, to which she readily agreed, I suggested that she stop drinking. She was hesitant. She thought she did not have the strength to stop, since it was helping her to medicate away her grief and anger. Our discussion of her position regarding alcohol continued for three sessions. We used the pros and cons of abstaining from alcohol, I highlighted her freedom to choose whether to stop, and I wove back and forth between the foot-in-the-door ("If you could do it—if you weren't drinking—do you think your life and your kids would be better off?") and door-in-the-face strategies ("I want to you to commit, right now, beginning today, to 6 months of total sobriety"). As we continued, what emerged was her increasing estimation that it would be impossible for her to stop drinking. I asked her if she had ever done something in her life after thinking it would be impossible to do it. She volunteered that when her children were doing poorly in elementary school, and her assessment was that there was a poor match between her kids and the teaching style, she had made a really difficult decision to take them out of school and to home-school them. She said everyone opposed it, and she was not sure it would be possible for her to handle it. Once she did it, it turned out to be quite successful, and other families used her as a consultant. I asked her to consider what it took for her to accomplish that amazing life challenge, and whether she could see a connection and draw some strength from those memories now. This example helped her to see her choices in a new light and with greater confidence. Fairly soon she was flirting with the idea of abstaining, focusing more practically on the question, "But how will I do it?"

Taking the Devil's Advocate Position

This strategy of the devil's advocate position is possible because of the inherent presence of contradiction, in this case the contradiction between wanting to change and wanting not to change. Imagine that you and your patient are having a "commitment conversation" about some aspect of treatment, and the patient is reluctant to make the commitment. For example, you are asking the patient with an eating disorder to commit to eliminating binge-eating and purging behaviors. The patient shows some interest in changing, but is reluctant when directly asked for a commitment. As the conversation continues, perhaps you interweave other strategies such as pros and cons or foot in the door/door in the face, and finally the patient says, "All right, I'll stop my bingeing and purging." It may appear as if the patient has shifted to a committed position, but you have the feeling that it is a pseudo-resolution, that the patient might be just "giving in" to dissolve the tension, to appease you. It is exactly this set of conditions that sets the stage for the devil's advocate strategy. The formula includes:

1. The patient is ambivalent about committing, and the tension between the request to commit and the reluctance to commit is palpable.
2. In the course of the conversation, the tension seems to be lessened as the patient claims to have adopted the commitment.
3. The therapist does not trust that the patient's statement of commitment fully integrates the level of difficulty.

In this context, you then challenge the stated commitment by arguing against it. For instance, you might say, "I don't get it. Why are you signing on to stop your bingeing and purging behaviors when you have relied on them so heavily to solve your emotional problems?" The trick is to challenge the patient's commitment effectively enough to get the patient to think about it, but not so effectively or strongly as to talk the patient out of the commitment. In the best outcome, the patient will argue back something like, "I know it's going to be hard, but I can't see that I can go on just bingeing and purging to solve all my problems. I want a bigger life than that." Once the patient makes an argument like this in favor of commitment—one that sounds firm and genuine—you back off from the challenge and say something like, "OK, you need to remember that argument when things get tough."

In a challenging, ongoing commitment conversation, we are likely to weave in all of the strategies under discussion, in no particular order, and in practice they often overlap and blend in with one another. The shift from one to another should be subtle and smooth, woven in as part of a normal conversation. We should be focused not on employing strategies but on eliciting a commitment, exploring the ambivalence through pros and cons, creating movement back and forth with an effort to strengthen the argument, from the patient's standpoint, in favor of commitment. It's an artful task. I often find that my use of devil's advocate takes place in a matter of a few seconds, in a statement or two. While exploring the pros and cons, the patient might say, "I want to be in DBT because I know I have to change." I might say, "Yeah, I really like that about you, and it's why you are going to succeed. But let me ask you, just for a second. Do you realize that this is going to be one of the hardest things, if not the hardest, that you've ever done?" Just a touch, just a slight momentary challenge designed to test out the commitment, designed to strengthen commitment by eliciting a stronger statement from the patient.

Shaping Successive Approximations to Commitment

This is another commitment strategy used in the form of "brush strokes," quick comments to reinforce some evidence, even minor, of commitment. The patient says, "I really didn't want to come back to see you today; I have huge doubts about whether to enter your program." Wanting to reinforce the ember of interest in the context of ambivalence, the therapist might respond with warmth and sincerity, saying, "I'm really glad you came today, even with your doubts. It sounds like it took a lot of courage." The patient says, "I don't want to tell you I'm going to stop cutting myself, because I'm not sure I can stop it," to which the therapist might say, "I know you have your doubts; I just appreciate how honest you are about them. That way, I know that when you say something, you mean it." And when the therapist notices the reluctant-to-commit patient talking with slightly more comfort and confidence in the session, he might simply share the observation about the patient's growing comfort in the conversation, expressing admiration for the hard work the patient is doing to settle in. The therapist's readiness to shape the patient's responses, reinforcing successive approximations to a stronger commitment in any of a thousand ways, is ever-present.

CONCLUDING COMMENTS

When DBT therapists are themselves (1) committed to the treatment and to behavioral change, (2) committed to their patients' need to commit, (3) focused on specific goals or targets, and (4) have good connections with their patients, they stand a very good chance of eliciting sufficient commitment from their patients over time. To do so intelligently and artfully, it is helpful to grasp and implement the three paradigms and their principles, to maintain the "spirit of commitment," and to appreciate and make use of the complexity and richness of each of the commitment strategies.

CHAPTER 11

Behavioral Chain Analysis

THE NATURE AND FUNCTIONS OF BEHAVIORAL CHAIN ANALYSIS

Behavioral chain analysis has been described clearly and in detail in the treatment manual (Linehan, 1993a) and in many publications since then. Especially during Stage 1 in DBT, when problematic behaviors are being monitored, assessed, and treated, behavioral chain analysis serves as the centerpiece of most therapy sessions and functions in several ways:

- As the primary means of assessment for determining the controlling variables of the primary target behaviors
- As the initial step in the CBT-based problem-solving sequence (the subsequent steps being insight; solution analysis; change procedures such as cognitive modification, skills training, contingency procedures, and exposure procedures; didactic strategies; orienting strategies; and commitment strategies)
- As the organizing framework of the session—the platform of therapy sessions during Stage 1—within which data are gathered and organized, hypotheses are generated, solutions are considered and selected, and change procedures are implemented

Behavioral chain analysis serves several other purposes in DBT:

- *Case conceptualization:* As we saw in Chapter 10, the behavioral chain is the template for case conceptualization and treatment planning, a helpful graphic organizer upon which to visualize the problematic links in the chain and the possible remedies.

- *Missing links analysis:* In addition to serving as the primary tool for locating, considering, and treating the problematic links in the chain, the therapist can also use it for locating, considering, and treating the *absence* of effective links that might have led to better outcomes.
- *Strengthening of memory and attention:* The repeated microanalysis of links in the chain can train the patient to pay more attention to behavioral patterns and details before, during, and after problematic behaviors as they happen during the week. In fact, instruction in how to perform behavioral chain analysis is now included in the *DBT Skills Training Manual* (Linehan, 2015b).

At the same time, behavioral chain analysis can function in the service of other major DBT strategy groups:

- *Mindfulness:* Given that the procedure involves full engagement in the present moment, without judgment of whatever arises, and with a clear focus of attention upon getting the details of the story, behavioral chain analysis serves as an ongoing mindfulness practice, grounding the problem-solving approach in an accepting, mindful atmosphere.
- *Exposure:* Given that the chain analysis brings the patient's mind into contact with links in the chain that have been avoided and suppressed due to their power to elicit painful emotions, the procedure often serves as an exposure procedure, with the emotionally salient links serving as cues.
- *Cognitive modification:* Given that the review of the chain reveals certain dysfunctional thoughts in the sequence leading up to the problem behavior, and that the therapist can highlight that these thoughts are just thoughts rather than reality, the behavioral chain analysis becomes a mechanism for cognitive modification.
- *Skills training:* A review of the chain underlines the presence of skills deficits and serves as a real-time platform for skills training. The therapist is alert not only to skills deficits but also to adaptive behaviors that appear on the chain, which can be reinforced by the therapist.
- *Contingency procedure:* The conduct of the chain analysis often serves as a contingency procedure as well. The patient who is growing tired of the repeated microscopic chain analysis will sometimes refrain from the problem behaviors during the week in order to avoid spending session time on behavioral chain analysis. When I asked a certain patient how she managed to interrupt

her skin-picking behavior during the prior week, after months of daily picking, she answered, "I just thought, I'll be damned if I am going to spend another therapy session doing another analysis of picking my skin—it's so tedious!"

Everything is on the chain. There are manifestations of the biosocial theory: evidence of emotional vulnerability and the invalidating environment. In addition, there are the behavioral patterns discussed in Chapter 8, the dialectical dilemmas. We also find problematic cognitions, automatic intense emotional responses to cues, problematic contingencies, as well as functional cognitions and skillful responses. The patient's memories, implicit and explicit, appear on the chain; hence, developmental history is on the chain. Hopes for the future appear on the chain, and are sometimes the source of new growth and sometimes the trigger for negative emotions. Evidence of attachment to the therapist, and problems with attachment to the therapist can be found on the chain. Having practiced psychoanalytic therapy for borderline personality disorder for many years, I have the impression that everything found in psychodynamic therapy can also be found on the chain. Interestingly, behavioral chain analysis, the framework for assessment and treatment in DBT, is a horizontal framework, whereby the therapist looks for antecedents "to the left" and consequences "to the right," whereas the framework for understanding and intervention in psychodynamic therapy is a vertical one, with manifest content and latent content—"deeper and deeper" layers of defenses, fantasies, and internalized object relations. Most data points in each of these two models can be mapped onto the other model, often requiring translation of terms and concepts.

Progress in treatment is reflected in modifications of the typical chains of each patient. You could say that in Stage 1 of DBT, the therapist gets to know the patient through her chains, intervenes in her chains, and positive outcomes are reflected in transformed chains.

Recently a 37-year-old woman was addressing several target behaviors in DBT therapy with me. One of those target behaviors involved her yelling at her husband in front of her children, making highly critical comments toward him. Her yelling was accompanied by a sense of being out of control of her emotions and her judgment. It led to the emotion of shame, which had resulted in other dysfunctional behavioral patterns, and she worried that her yelling was having a detrimental impact on her children. She had little insight about why she was doing it, why she couldn't make herself stop doing it, and why it seemed to be out of her control. She had repeatedly attempted to dedicate or will herself to stop doing it, but had been unsuccessful. Every yelling episode further convinced her of her incompetence and her ineffectiveness as a wife and mother.

We specified the target behavior and started by using commitment strategies to strengthen her commitment to terminate the behavior. In particular, we reviewed the pros and cons of the behavior, and I highlighted the point that she had the freedom to choose whether to do it or not. I used the foot-in-the-door strategy to get her to commit to totally stopping the behavior for 1 week at a time, and I took advantage of opportunities to reinforce any evidence of her willingness and ability to interrupt the pattern (shaping). Her commitment was high, but once she was exposed to the aggravating circumstances, that commitment was overridden by her emotional dysregulation.

As the behavior repeated itself several times over the next few weeks, we had several opportunities to search for the most important controlling variables through chain analysis. Typically we began the chain with her description of the topography: exactly what she had yelled, how she had yelled, how it felt when she yelled, and what she noticed on the face of her husband and children as she yelled. We turned our attention to her vulnerability factors, which included high levels of stress in taking care of the kids and the house, and accumulated resentment toward her husband. In each chain we identified a prompting event. We detailed the links in the chain following the prompting event and leading up to the yelling behavior: her thoughts, her emotions, her actions, her husband's behavior, and her children's behavior, with special attention to the emotions she was trying to regulate throughout the chain. Then we zeroed in on the consequences of her yelling behavior in her and in the environment around her. In particular, we were searching for any consequences that reinforced yelling, and any consequences that may be leading to suppression of more effective behavioral strategies. We found a number of commonalities across the several chain analyses of her yelling behavior, as well as some features unique to particular chains.

We generated several hypotheses about the controlling variables of the behavior and brainstormed together about possible solutions. Regarding the vulnerability factors, we generated plans for her to take better care of herself with stress management techniques. Regarding the prompting events and situational factors, we identified choices that she could make to avoid or modify the most aggravating circumstances. Regarding links in the chain between prompting events and yelling, we identified and challenged cognitions that resulted in a sense of helplessness and deliberately practiced behavioral skills of observing her emotions, acting opposite the urges associated with her emotions, tolerating her distress with several techniques, and generally incorporating mindfulness skills throughout the more intense segments of the chain. We identified a number of consequences that reinforced her yelling: (1) It interrupted some of her husband's behaviors toward the children that she regarded as abusive; (2) it provided a vehicle for her to express her anger toward him and to "discharge" some of her accumulated resentment; (3) and it provided her with a sense of being in control, which reversed her painful sense of helplessness in these situations. Within her mind she was protecting her children from an abusive father, in contrast to her painful memory that as a child, her own mother had not protected her from a verbally and emotionally abusive father.

In spite of the potency and immediacy of these reinforcing consequences, the fact was that her yelling frightened her children, which triggered her into a cycle of guilt, shame, and helplessness. When we reviewed the possible effective behaviors that she was avoiding (missing links analysis), she realized quickly that her fear of her husband was causing her to avoid an assertive discussion with him about his behavior toward the children. Across the entire chain, her choices became clearer to her. She took better care of herself, made more judicious choices about how she related to her husband when with the children, and brought her husband into a session to discuss her fear of his irritability and anger. Having established more control and self-respect, having solved the "yelling problem," the focus of therapy shifted to long-standing marital problems.

As we see in this example, behavioral chain analysis can help patients move from chaos to order, from confusion to insight, and from helplessness to planful behavioral change. It provides a counterpoint to passivity and dyscontrol for both therapist and patient. It provides structure and direction in therapy, supplementing a mindful and compassionate, empathic and validating approach. It provides a ladder for descending into the patient's hell, and a ladder for helping the patient to climb out. It helps a therapist to think clearly amidst the chaos.

Doing behavioral chain analysis is a collaborative procedure in which the therapist and patient are building something together. Ideally it joins them together. And as they build the chain, link by link, it becomes possible to stop at any point, to interrupt building the chain and shift over to reflecting upon the chain up to that point: to deepen understanding of the current link, to step back and consider patterns that are emerging in the chain, to reflect upon the similarities between the current chain and other chains previously analyzed, and to think about possible alternatives to certain links or patterns.

In the course of identifying the links in the chain, the patient–therapist team will often arrive at certain links that could benefit from psychoeducational illumination. Right then and there, "striking while the iron is hot," the therapist can educate the patient didactically about the issue, whatever it might be. For instance, when treating a patient for substance abuse behaviors and arriving at the link of the chain in which the patient had urges or cravings to use, the therapist might briefly "step off the chain" and do a 3-minute didactic segment about urges and cravings. Similarly, while going over a segment of the chain, the therapist can invite the patient to "stand outside" the chain for a moment and consider a hypothesis about that segment. "Do you think it's possible that you were having a stressful day, that your kids were restless, that the disconnection between you and your husband set off more anxiety in you than you were aware of, and that your anxiety set off your anger?" Or: "Maybe yelling at your husband reduces your anxiety; what happens if you don't yell at him in that situation?" Again, alongside the construction of the chain is an ongoing reflective dialogue between therapist and patient. Early in learning to conduct behavioral chain analysis, therapists might wisely stick to the assessment function, simply spelling out a sufficiently detailed link-by-link chain, holding off on the solution analyses and other problem-solving steps until after the chain is completed. But more experienced clinicians can effectively weave problem solving in and out of the chain as it is illuminated. For example, amidst the conduct of chain analysis, the therapist might invite the patient into problem solving with statements such as these:

"Do you think there is any relationship between what happened in this chain and what happened last week?"
"Can you imagine how things would have proceeded if you had not taken his statement as personally referring to you?"
"Do you think it's possible that there may be a pattern here, where any reference to your body sets off terrible memories and shame?"
"Do you think you would have hurt yourself in the emergency room if you knew in advance that they would not be admitting you to a hospital?"

In a recent session, as we went over the links of the chain on the way to self-cutting behavior, another patient of mine acknowledged that she had thought of calling me for phone coaching when she felt like cutting herself. This had come up before, and I realized that she had never called me for coaching. Based on prior discussions, we had located a pattern of her not asking for help exactly when she most needed it. I highlighted the pattern, asking her if she thought the failure to call me was another example of not asking for help. Reluctantly, she admitted that it was true.

She went on to say that it was precisely when she feels at her worst that she does not want to reach out for help, since she thinks it will unnecessarily burden the other person.

We were hypothesizing "outside the chain" at that moment, reflecting on a pattern we had located on the chain. As we considered possible solutions, I suggested that we do a role play of a telephone coaching call. As is often the case, the role play combined several change procedures in one "package," including cognitive modification, skills training, and exposure to cues that she was avoiding. After briefly orienting her and setting up the role play, she "called me" on the telephone for coaching. She did it haltingly, reluctantly, as if she were not entitled to call me. We reviewed it, and I gave her feedback. I suggested some fine-tuning and we did the role play again. She came across as more "entitled" to ask for help, more effective in doing so. We reviewed the second enactment, considered whether she could do it "in real life," and I got her to commit to me that she would telephone me for coaching the next time she was in trouble. Then we returned to the chain where we had left off and continued our analysis.

When DBT is practiced competently, the therapist routinely moves back and forth among assessment, pattern recognition, solution analysis, and problem solving. The therapist must become facile about moving off the chain, engaging in solution analysis and focused problem solving, all while keeping the chain in working memory, then reorienting the patient to where they had been on the chain and jumping back on it. If this is done effectively, fluidly, and concisely, it need not feel disjointed, jerky, or forced. It requires practice to get to the point where moving on and off the chain, preserving the structure of the chain but conducting the session in a fluent way that works, feels more like a conversation and the unfolding of a narrative than the imposition of a procedure.

The clearer and more facile the therapist becomes in using the chain analysis in sessions, the more the use of the chain can also function to help the therapist regulate himself. Working with chronic and severe emotional dysregulation can be so trying. The therapist can "fall into the abyss" with the patient and not know what to do. The more he listens, the more he shares the patient's confusion and hopelessness. In behavioral chain analysis he has a friend: a systematic procedure, something of a ritual, as he explores and tries to recruit the patient to join him in figuring things out. Establishing and returning to the chain, again and again, can be something of a mindfulness practice for the therapist, and then for both parties. Rather than "back to the breath, back to the breath," it is "back to the chain, back to the chain." The chain is something to "grab onto," may have the effect of turning on a flashlight when groping in the dark. Even if the chain does not lead quickly to a remedy, it illuminates a path. As a "grounding" practice, it can restore order, reduce dysregulation, and generate hope for both parties.

THE "BASICS" IN DOING A CHAIN ANALYSIS

Readers who are familiar with the framework and practice of behavioral chain analysis are invited to skip over this section, but for those who are less familiar, this section may serve to introduce or consolidate your understanding of the technique. The DBT "chain" consists of five consecutive categories of elements, visualized from left to right. First are the vulnerability factors, the causes or issues that render the patient more vulnerable to the prompting event. Second is the prompting event, a significant moment for the patient that sets off the subsequent events in the chain, leading eventually to the problem behavior. Third are the "links in the chain," a category that includes all behaviors (thoughts, emotions, actions, physiological events) and events in the environmental context that follow from the prompting event and lead up to the problem behavior. Fourth is the problem behavior itself, described objectively and in specifics. Following the problem behavior is the fifth category, the consequences of the problem behavior, with a special focus on those results likely to reinforce future occurrences of the problem behavior, along with those likely to inhibit (extinguish or punish) behaviors that would be more adaptive than the problem behavior.

In doing the chain analysis, there is a typical sequence with many variations, depending on circumstances and clinical judgment. Typically, it begins with getting the specific account of the problem behavior, its phenomenology, without recounting the antecedents, consequences, interpretations, or judgments about it. This requires some discipline by the therapist, as it is natural to "move on" from the detailed description, especially because simply describing the behavior can trigger anxiety, shame, guilt, anger, disgust, and other negative emotions that the patient, and sometimes the therapist, would rather avoid.

Having gotten a satisfactory account of the target behavior, the therapist typically moves to the search for the prompting event. The therapist wants to locate a prompting event that is sufficiently "close" to the problem behavior (minutes, hours, maybe a day) to enable a meaningful recounting of events from the prompting event to the problem behavior within the time span of one session. One could argue that the prompting event in a given situation was the "day I was born," or the "moment my great-grandfather arrived in the United States from Europe." Although such a response may provide meaning, it does not provide information for a meaningful behavioral chain analysis in a session. The therapist looks for a prompting event that was an encounter between the patient and the environment (rather than a private event for the patient that was not set off in relation to the environment). There is something rather arbitrary about choosing a particular prompting event when there may be so many candidates. To elicit the prompting event, the therapist might use language such as the following:

> "If you were writing a script, and you wanted to pinpoint the event that happened that set things in motion toward the problem behavior . . . "
>
> "Try to think of a time when things were still going reasonably all right, and then think of the event that happened that changed the story . . . "
>
> "Try to think of the thing that happened in the chain that, if it had not happened, you would not have gone down that path . . . "
>
> "What do you think was the trigger, the turning point . . . ? "

Now notice that if you conducted a chain analysis as I have suggested up to this point, you would have characterized two "data points" along the chain: the prompting event and the problem behavior. I find it useful, in the back of my mind, or on paper, to envision the prompting event as existing about one-quarter of the way into the chain, and the problem behavior at about three-quarters of the way into the chain. This leaves one-quarter of the chain to the left of the prompting event for the discovery of vulnerability factors, half of the chain between the two data points to discover the links in the chain, and one-quarter of the chain to the right of the problem behavior for the search for consequences contingent upon the problem behavior.

Realize that the decision about the segment of chain that is chosen for analysis is to some degree arbitrary, since life is an endless and microscopic chain. We select a segment that will provide enough of a "story" to review, sufficient for the determination of some essential controlling variables of the problem behavior. It is important to realize there is no such thing as the "real chain," as if an expert would discover the "right" one. In fact, one senior DBT trainer has tested this point by role-playing a patient undergoing a behavioral chain analysis, presenting the exact same scenario to five different DBT experts, and finding that the five different behavioral chains were decidedly different.

Having named a prompting event, the therapist will typically either move "to the left," onto the determination of vulnerability factors, asking, "What do you think might have made you especially vulnerable that day to the prompting event?," or "to the right," asking, "After the prompting event, then what happened next?" Either choice can work perfectly well, and it is often simply the flow of the session and the direction of the patient's thinking that influence which way to go. After determining the vulnerability factors, the prompting event, the links in the chain, and the problem behavior, the last category to be investigated is that of the consequences of the problem behavior. Having reviewed the links in the chain leading up to the problem behavior, it becomes rather natural to ask, "And after you did X, then what happened?" Although this sequence may seem logical, in fact sometimes the flow of conversation will lead directly to the consequences from the description of the problem behavior. The patient might just naturally begin to describe the consequences, in which case the therapist can move in that direction too, getting the consequences "when they are hot," and then move back to the prompting event.

If a therapist is overly dogmatic about "getting the chain," including all of the details, which of course she wants to do, she must not do so at the expense of the relationship with the patient. The therapist should bring the chain into the relationship with the patient, not bring the relationship with the patient into the chain. In other words, the patient should not be "dragged through" the conduct of the chain, indicating to him that the chain is more important than he, himself, as the patient. If done correctly, even a rigorously conducted chain analysis should feel very natural.

If I want to fix a dripping faucet, I naturally think about the link-by-link antecedents of the problem as I consider how to proceed. When we take our car to a mechanic, the mechanic needs to know the exact nature of the problem (definition of the problem), the recent status and repair record of the car (vulnerability factors), the beginning of the problem (prompting event), and how things have proceeded from the initial awareness of the problem to the current situation (links in the chain). Behavioral chain analysis is a formalized version of a very natural human process of inquiry, and it will generally go better with a patient if it is conducted in that spirit. The therapist says, "Tell me more about it, and then tell me when it started; I want to know every step along the way so that we can figure out how to fix it." This type of phrasing typically works better than if the therapist begins with, "OK, let's do a behavioral chain analysis about that behavior." We want to invite patients to tell their story, to have a conversation about what happened, rather than to impose a therapeutic procedure onto the conversation. With some patients and therapists, it is helpful to do this on a whiteboard, diagramming every link in the chain, moving from left to right. This visual display makes the chain and the experience it is capturing very concrete and involves patients as collaborators, using their own pens. Commonly, therapists sit opposite their patients and diagram the emerging chain on a piece of paper as the data emerge. Sometimes therapists simply talk with patients, making no notes along the way; but it is often useful to write down the essential elements of the chain shortly after the session, for review at a later point.

I'm speaking here about finding a synthesis to the dialectic in which the therapist, on the one hand, is looking for a rigorously defined chain while simultaneously preserving a good relationship with the patient. In the back of the therapist's mind, he is disciplined, spelling out the narrative in a chronological, link-by-link fashion, filling in the template of the chain, while remaining fluid, attentive, and conversational, engaging the patient in a human encounter that makes sense to both parties. This is not dissimilar from the performance of a mental status examination, which requires getting a lot of "hard" data in a manner that is not simply experienced by the patient as an interrogation.

CONTRIBUTIONS FROM
THE ACCEPTANCE PARADIGM

Not surprisingly, the work of doing behavioral chain analysis with individuals who are chronically and severely emotionally dysregulated can be very challenging. We are served well by knowing how to conduct a chain analysis in a clear, sequential, and organized fashion, as a problem-solving technique described above. We can augment that behavioral approach with the use of principles from the acceptance paradigm and the dialectical paradigm of DBT. This augmentation will be especially needed in circumstances where the problem-solving work is interrupted by various manifestations of emotional dysregulation. The DBT therapist may benefit from integrating the following principles from the acceptance paradigm, as discussed in Chapter 3:

- Be fully present, entirely in the moment, 100% awake.
- Practice non-attachment to ideas or perceptions of how the chain should look and how the process should flow.
- Bring the perspective of no-boundaries, no-self, emptiness, and pervasive interbeing to the practice of chain analysis.
- Bring the perspective of impermanence to the practice of chain analysis.

Be Fully Present

Doing behavioral chain analysis is a complex cognitive task conducted with a goal in mind and impediments along the way. Earlier we described the challenge of maintaining a good relationship with the patient while conducting a rigorous behavioral chain analysis. As the therapist gets invested in the growing chain, figuring out the story, generating and testing hypotheses, trying problem-solving interventions on the platform of the chain analysis, summarizing the chain, getting "on and off the chain," it is easy for the destination-focused work of "doing" to override the present-oriented stance of "being." Therapy can get out of balance. The therapist's "doing" focus can be experienced as intrusive and disrespectful, with the patient feeling more like an object than a subject, more as a problem than a co-participant. Of course, the therapist's ideal stance would be to remain fully in the present moment while doing behavioral analysis and even while pushing for change. That is the central dialectic of DBT: to push for change in the context of acceptance.

Realistically, the implication for the DBT therapist is to begin the session fully awake and alert to herself, to the patient, and to the transaction between them, neither looking backward nor forward. The therapist might achieve this state by engaging in a brief mindfulness practice before the session: mindfulness of the body, the breath, the sounds in the room, or some other focus. Once rooted in the present moment with awareness, the patient enters the room and the session begins. The patient might notice that the therapist is truly there, with awareness, attention, compassion, and validation. Then, as the work of behavioral change gets under way, it will be natural (though unfortunate) for the "doing"—the review of the diary card, the determination of the session targets, the initiation of behavioral chain analysis—to interrupt "just being there."

At whatever point the therapist realizes that she has departed from "just being there"—being awake, aware, and present to the moment—she can return. In some cases this may be simple, beginning with acute awareness of having drifted, followed by a mental reminder to return to the moment, to the state of one's own body and mind, to the awareness of and interaction with the patient. At other times it is not so easy. Thoroughly caught up in the work of analysis and behavioral change, sights set on the target behaviors, and sometimes emotionally dysregulated by the work with the patient, the therapist is more "caught." Letting go of "doing," even for a momentary return to the present, is not so easy.

Under those circumstances, the key, once again, is to realize it has happened. Once aware of having departed from the present moment, the therapist may need to undertake a brief mindfulness exercise to "wake up." For me this often takes the form of noticing the sensations of my body sitting in the chair, which may lead me to become "embodied" again, or observing one or two complete breaths as a transition back to the present. Sometimes I will just let my gaze focus entirely on the details of the patient's facial expression. I might notice a previously unrecognized undercurrent of emotion as I study the patient's face. In each of these cases, the "mindfulness exercise" takes but a few seconds or perhaps a half-minute, and it does not interrupt my eye contact or focus. It is generally not noticeable to the patient. Importantly, it causes me to pause, however briefly. The pause is the manifestation of a transition from "doing" back to "being." At its best, this kind of transition leads to a softening of style and an opening of heart and mind. Minimally, it leads to a pause, an interruption of the change-oriented work just briefly, like "taking a break." It might allow the patient, or both of us, to simply be there with each other, for at least a moment.

Practicing Nonattachment

The essential point of nonattachment is to "take what comes," to radically accept that in spite of our best efforts and highest hopes, it is often the case that factors beyond our control will limit the kind of data we can get and the kind of process we can foster. We want to get a detailed analysis of links in the chain, sufficiently microscopic to shed light on the progression of links. But a hundred factors can interfere. The patient may have a poor memory for the links we seek, such as is typical in the context of episodes of self-injurious behavior, substance use, bingeing and purging, and antisocial and other problematic behaviors. Substance use can cloud the memory of entire episodes of behavior, and even result in confabulating explanations such that we don't know what to believe. Episodes of amnesia and other dissociative features can eclipse the memory of what happened. All experienced therapists have had patients who have said something like, "I have no idea what happened from X to Y." Often we are analyzing events that took place several days prior, and since those events the patient has been besieged by other stressful events that make it difficult to remember what happened several days ago. Avoidance can play a part, in that any one of us would often rather "forget" what happened, or even if we do forget, we would prefer not to bring painful experiences back to life. It is not unusual for patients to withhold or distort information in order to avoid displeasing the therapist or to avoid being disloyal to family or friends. In addition to all of these fairly common factors, and more, there are in-session episodes of poor collaboration, compliance, and cooperation. We have all experienced the disappointment of wanting to understand what happened yesterday, or what is happening in the session, but upon asking about it, the response is "I don't know," "I really don't want to talk about it," "I don't trust you—why should I tell you," or "Whatever!"

The Buddhist principle of nonattachment is meant to address the suffering brought about when we remain attached to outcomes that we cannot affect. By trying to "overcome the resistance," "get the data in spite of the patient," or otherwise hang on to our desire to get what we consider a requisite level of detail about what happened, we grow more frustrated, less flexible, less aware of the patient in the moment, and we can end up invalidating the patient. Fortunately, it is rare that we actually need an exhaustive, link-by-link analysis throughout the chain in order to problem-solve. By letting go of our attachment to getting a more detailed story and *genuinely* accepting what we can get, we can then apply the organizing technique of behavioral chain analysis to whatever links are available. Still we model a way of thinking, a way of investigating, of making sense of things. We can do that whether we have 4 data points or 14.

Earlier in my DBT practice, when I was convinced that I needed detailed behavioral chains, it was particularly frustrating when the patient had little to say. I remember once hearing: "I have no idea what happened during the evening, I just remember that I woke up with cuts on my arms." I wasn't sure whether I believed the patient. How could I get enough information to conceptualize and treat the problem? Whether I believed the patient or not, I had a limited amount of information. If able to let go of insisting that I get something I couldn't ever obtain, I could maneuver more flexibly, saying something like, "OK, what is the last thing you do remember last evening, before that point where you can't remember?" We get everything we can, leading up to the beginning of the forgotten links, and everything that follows, beginning with the first moment the patient can recall following the forgotten episode. In the course of treating the primary target of self-cutting, I thus may encounter another target, to decrease the patient's lack of memory, and try to assess that one as well. In other words, I push to get the chain of events to assess the target, and encountering poor memory or poor willingness, I shift gears and try to assess and treat the behavior that interferes. To summarize:

1. I try to get the chain of events needed to assess the primary target behavior.
2. I encounter a blockade of memory or collaboration.
3. I persist, perhaps trying another strategy to get the needed chain.

4. I find that the blockade is persistent.
5. I radically accept the reality of the blockade.
6. I then try to assess the blockade itself, as a behavioral target, in the service of assessing the original target.

The sequence is the same whether I am dealing with a dissociative episode, forgetfulness, or defiant noncollaboration. Ultimately, when necessary, I assess and treat the in-session dysfunctional behaviors that are interfering with our alliance. The spirit is captured in the Serenity Prayer in Alcoholics Anonymous. Applied to our clinical situation, it would read: "Give me the serenity to accept what I cannot analyze, the courage to analyze what I can, and the wisdom to know the difference."

Several other perspectives on behavioral chain analysis can help us, as therapists, let go of our attachment to the chain we wish we could get, and to accept whatever chain is possible to elicit. First, we can expect the process of chain analysis itself to offer benefits even when the data are scarce. Even if the chain has only three links, the patient can learn the skill of objectively and systematically reflecting on a behavioral sequence. Second, as previously mentioned, the practice of chain analysis can strengthen the patient's capability to pay attention during behavioral episodes and to register and recall more information. Third, if we use the behavioral chain analysis as a structured way of showing genuine curiosity in our patients' experiences, it can enhance the attachment between our patients and ourselves even if the quantity of data is minimal. Experts in another research-based therapy model for the treatment of borderline personality disorder, MBT, have described DBT's behavioral chain analysis as a form of mentalization, a way of expressing curiosity, engaging in open inquiry, getting to know the "mind" of the patient through the chains. Mentalization is thought to enhance the process of secure attachment. Finally, if we can let go of the attachment to more links of information, step back, and characterize the impediment to getting more information, we can refocus the session on an in-session dysfunctional behavior that is interfering with getting at the primary target. Once the impediment is assessed and solved, the therapeutic dyad can shift back to work on the primary target.

No Boundaries, No-Self, Emptiness, and Interbeing

The boundaries around a given behavioral chain are blurry. As mentioned, any given chain has an arbitrary beginning and ending, for practical purposes. The chain is actually one segment of an infinitely long chain. As difficult as defining where a chain starts and stops is the designation of whose chain it is. Is it the patient's chain, in which case the therapist's job has been to reveal it? Is it a joint product of patient and therapist, as they work together to construct a narrative that has a resemblance to what actually happened? Doesn't the chain represent an amalgam of a large number of individuals who have been in the patient's life? If you look carefully, in the patient's narrative, captured in the chain, are contributions from parents, friends, brothers and sisters, employers and teachers, and a multitude of events. A given chain also reflects all of the explicit and implicit dynamics that were occurring at the time the chain was constructed; if the therapist were to conduct a behavioral chain analysis of the exact same incident one day later, it would turn out differently.

All of this is another way of saying that the chain does not have a unique and static "self." The chain has no identity of its own. It is made up of history, present, future; patient and therapist and others who interact with them; thoughts, emotions, and actions of both parties; the context in the moment, even the physical surroundings; the imagination of both parties. It is more like liquid mercury than solid steel, more like a mirage than a body of water. Mindfulness practitioners argue that a thought is not the same thing as what it represents; it is not a fact; it is a thought and only a thought. We can consider the behavioral chain similarly. It is a representation of an episode in reality, but it is not the same thing as what it represents. It is not a factual narrative; it is a chain and only a chain, co-constructed in the service of assessment and treatment.

Still it is helpful if our "chain narrative" is as close to a real experience as possible, since we hope to grasp something about the relevant behavioral patterns, and we hope that our interventions in session will translate back into behavioral changes in similar sequences outside of sessions. So we relate to the chain in these two very different ways: We use it as a tool toward a goal: the assessment and treatment of a treatment target; and we recognize its insubstantiality, creativity, and flexibility. So, at the same time it is both a well-defined, substantial tool and simply a form with no distinct boundaries, no distinct self, made up of non-chain-related ingredients of many kinds. We can, on the one hand, use the chain in the process of "doing," and, on the other hand, we can *be with* the chain in the process of "being." To deeply grasp and use this duality offers us immense fluidity and freedom.

I was conducting a behavioral chain analysis with a 17-year-old boy who had been hospitalized because he was found to be using the Internet to find ways to murder his mother. We were reviewing an incident in which he had threatened his mother, ran out of the house, disappeared into the woods, and was eventually apprehended by police and brought to the hospital. As we were reviewing the links in the chain, and when we got to the moment when he threatened his mother, I asked him if he could describe what his mother had said, and how his mother's face looked just before my patient threatened her. He drew a blank. "I have no idea; I can't remember anything at that moment." Rather than push further for details "in reality," I asked him to make it up. "Just tell me what you think you might have heard, what you think you might have seen, given your knowledge of your mother." He rather easily recounted what she might have said, fully accompanied by describing his mother's likely facial expression, bodily posture, and tone of voice. For our purposes, including the assessment of his problematic behaviors, it was perfect as it was.

Impermanence

Inherent in the perspective of no boundary, no-self (no-chain), and interdependency is the further insight about the impermanence of the chain. As everything else in reality comes and goes, second by second and minute by minute, so does the chain. If one were to do a behavioral chain analysis at 10:00 A.M., and then analyze the exact same event again at 11:00 A.M., the analysis would turn out to be different. This is not surprising when you consider that 1 hour later, every molecule and subatomic particle in every cell of the brain and body of both parties will be different; the moods and thoughts of therapist and patient will be different; and intervening events will have happened. The analysis could not possibly be the same. This understanding can be distressing for the therapist who is searching for the "one true chain" of events. And yet again it is a liberating perspective. Chains change, perspectives change. The notion of impermanence can be especially helpful for the therapist and patient who conduct one behavioral chain analysis after another, session after session, about a problem behavior that is repeated every week, seemingly the same each time. The point here is that the behavior is *not* the same as before. It has to be different. Every antecedent, every consequence, every contextual event has to be different. The therapist can enter into each new analysis with a fresh mind, with "beginner's mind" as it might be called in Buddhist practice, curious about new descriptions, new links, new contexts, ready for new learning. Maintaining this posture can be modeled and transmitted to the patient, who has grown weary of "going over the same chain again and again." As soon as both parties are convinced they have traveled the exact same road before, the likelihood of being alert to a new link, previously not noticed or appreciated, or a new hypothesis, unexplored, is small.

Finally, the therapeutic attitude and interventions that flow from the Buddhist views of the chain will give rise to alertness, freshness, curiosity, stamina, compassion, and creativity. Being in the present moment, not attached to a particular outcome, aware of the emptiness and boundary- less nature of the chain, and mindful of the absolute impermanence of the chain, free the therapist to be wide awake, warm, and responsive, and to validate the patient quite naturally. In contrast to the sense of being stuck and burdened with the chain, it creates a feeling of openness, possibility, and hope.

CONTRIBUTIONS FROM THE DIALECTICAL PARADIGM

If the therapist did a behavioral chain analysis with a patient who showed a good capacity to regulate emotions, cooperate in the procedure, stay on track, and maintain a trusting attitude, the therapist could probably proceed with little use for the dialectical perspective. The two of them could assess the problem behavior, generate hypotheses and solutions, select and implement solutions, evaluate the outcomes, and adjust. In other words, they could stick mostly to pure problem solving. But with difficult-to-treat individuals who experience severe and chronic emo- tional dysregulation, the conduct of behavioral chain analysis is beset by a wide range of difficulties, some nearly paralyzing the problem-solving process. As discussed in Chapter 5 on the dialectical paradigm, the prin- ciples include:

- Reality is made up of inevitable oppositions; the "truth" is found through synthesis of the valid kernels of opposing positions.
- Our understanding of reality is holistic or systemic; everything is interrelated; everything is transactional.
- Change is constant; everything is in flux.

In addition, the dialectical stance is one that promotes improvisation, synthesis, "both . . . and" thinking rather than "either . . . or" thinking, and a sense of speed, movement, and flow.

Reality Is Made Up of Oppositions

The behavioral chain has to be a flexible, dialectical vehicle, inclusive of opposing forces, "holding" both sides of a conflict or opposition. In itself, the chain does not create syntheses from opposing forces, but as a structure and as a procedure that is "empty" of any bias or position of its own, it is inclusive and allows for work toward synthesis. The chain can provide the "playing field" upon which oppositions between therapist and patient can be represented and addressed. Within the chain we find oppositions that move toward synthesis, oppositions between the patient and others in her social and professional context, between the patient and the therapist, between the patient and her own self, between a biological and environmental perspective, and so on. The chain is dynamic, flexible, and can contain multiple oppositions at the same time. As I said at the beginning of this chapter, everything is on the chain; all sides are at the table. In that respect, the chain, well managed, is the ultimate integrative structure in DBT.

Having successfully reduced her life-threatening behaviors (suicide attempts and self-injurious behaviors) and a self-destructive quality-of-life-interfering behavior (shoplifting), a female college student was working with me on the next target behavior: to decrease behaviors that put her at risk of being mistreated by males, while increasing behaviors of a self-respecting and self-protective nature. After an incident of date rape, in which a good male "friend" had taken advantage of her, we were in the process of conducting a behavioral chain analysis to identify the controlling variables in her behavior and in the context. As we reviewed the antecedent links in some detail, it became clear that early in the chain she had acted firmly, self-respectfully, and self-protectively. But at a later point in the chain, at a point that she was aware of wanting to please him and not lose him, she had "let my guard down." She did not want to offend him by rejecting him and could not find a way to please him and respect herself at the same time. This was the tension, the opposing positions, at that point in the chain. Rather than trying to determine whether she should please him, or whether she should be self-protective and reject him, we tried to further illuminate this dialectical opposition. As we "jumped off the chain" for a few minutes, we identified the validity in each position rather than looking for the "right thing to do." We looked for a synthesis, wherein she could get what she wanted from male friends and at the same time respect and protect herself. It proved to be a "dialectical moment" that was productive for her.

Holistic, Systemic Thinking

In conducting behavioral chain analysis, it is essential that therapists remain aware that everything is interdependent on everything else, and transactional. Nothing happens in a vacuum. How one thinks affects how one feels; how one feels affects how one thinks. How one acts influences, and reflects, how one thinks and feels. How one is spoken to affects how one receives it. How one receives it will influence how one is spoken to.

In a family, how a father addresses the mother immediately affects each child, and how the children behave and speak affect the next interaction between the parents. How we think, even if we do not explicitly say so to the patient, affects our patients, and how our patients think affects us. The pervasiveness of interdependency and transactional influence at every moment is generally beyond awareness. But it argues in favor of therapists maintaining an open mind, always aware that we are missing something, ready to inquire about details, even seemingly irrelevant ones, the way a good detective would do at the scene of a crime. We should be generating hypotheses constantly, raising them and dropping them when they don't hold up, clearing the mind for another fresh look at the "data." The dutiful performance of a behavioral chain analysis can lead to a kind of sequential "tunnel" thinking, screening out a wide range of possible factors, thereby having a stifling, limiting, formulaic impact. As a transactional structure for us, the behavioral chain analysis provides a rational and productive way to organize information, allowing for the inclusion of a huge array of elements, including ones that don't seem pertinent at the moment. If we flexibly consider a wide range of variables and explanations, we model that kind of dialectical thinking for our patients. As Linehan (1993a, pp. 120–124) mentions in discussing the prioritized list of treatment targets, regardless of which target is being addressed, we are always addressing the pervasive target of increasing dialectical thinking and acting.

An interesting corollary to the concept that all behavior is transactional in nature is the proposition that all behavioral chains are transactional as well. While the therapist and patient are constructing the behavioral chain regarding the patient's behavior earlier in the week, they are simultaneously "creating" or "living out" another chain: the chain of events taking place between them in the session. Let's call the former the "out-of-session chain" and the latter the "in-session chain." Usually, while identifying the elements in the out-of-session chain, the therapist and patient are only implicitly aware of the in-session chain. When the links of the in-session chain become problematic, interfering with the analysis of the out-of-session chain, they become more noticeable and may require attention. In fact, the therapist may shift from the link-by-link analysis of the out-of-session chain to the link-by-link analysis of the in-session chain, during which the out-of-session chain remains "dormant," so to speak.

The therapist who maintains awareness of both chains, or who moves back and forth between them in awareness and attention, has added a powerful, dialectical tool to her repertoire. She may begin to notice the transactional influence between the two chains, noticing the intersections between the two: similar problem behaviors, similar prompting events, similar links in the two chains, similar vulnerability factors, and similar contingencies. This new awareness naturally turns into interventions highlighting the transaction:

> "What you are describing to me sounds pretty similar to what goes on between you and me, don't you think?"
> "Does that ever happen to you in here, with me?"
> "I notice that if I am a little too quiet, you pull back into your shell, and now I hear you are doing that with your girlfriend. I wonder what's going on?"
> "Have you ever noticed that you are more irritable on the days you get less sleep, because I think that happens when you see me after a poor night's sleep?"

This kind of regular cross-referencing between the two chains becomes another lens for assessment and treatment. To the degree that the therapist and patient can see that the same sequence of links, resulting in problematic behavior in external reality, goes on in the session, then the work that takes place in-session to solve the problem more adaptively can be generalized to the external reality. In my experience, if the patient is well oriented and the chains are compared accurately, this kind of cross-referencing heightens the sense of meaning and importance regarding the in-session work. This is also a core concept in psychodynamic psychotherapy, in which the problems the patient has in external reality are fought out on the battlefield of the transference in sessions.

I was treating an individual who would trash her apartment and destroy her own things whenever she became angry with her partner. Sometimes alcohol played a role. We reviewed several of these episodes with careful behavioral chain analyses, and although we succeeded in finding several variables that might be influencing the behavior, there was little evidence of behavioral change. I presented the problem, and my puzzlement, to my consultation team. After considering several alternatives about behavioral and contextual variables, one team member said, "I know it may sound crazy, but I wonder if you are doing something in sessions that is reinforcing or triggering the episodes." It did sound like a stretch; there was no obvious link that I could see. Another team member asked if I could provide a more detailed description of the atmosphere and the course of our typical therapy session. A certain pattern, almost a formula, came to light. She usually began those sessions with a shameful confession: "I know you're going to be mad at me; I did it again." She averted her eyes, lowered her voice, acted sheepishly, and communicated harsh judgments toward herself. I noted that I felt like some kind of interrogator as we went through the chain objectively, and she was the sinful, apologetic victim of the interrogation. In another metaphor, I mentioned that it was as if I were a priest and she were telling me her terrible sins in a confessional. In fact, she had been raised rather strictly as a Catholic and was very familiar with the procedure of confessions. As I talked with the team, I realized that our sessions always ended on a good note. We would do the behavioral chain, come up with solutions, she would commit to trying the solutions, we would both be hopeful about the coming week, and our relationship would have lost its tension.

I brought this perspective to her in the next session. She immediately agreed that she felt like she was confessing sins, receiving absolution (through behavioral treatment), and feeling cleansed, connected to me again, and hopeful. I wondered aloud whether this procedure, this sequence, between her and me, might be reinforcing the "sinful" episodes. She could lose control of her impulses, knowing (in the back of her mind) that she could come to her psychotherapy "confessional" and receive absolution. There was something satisfying and complete about the overall process. She was willing to consider the possibility, but she was not so sure. I suggested that things might go differently if we did not reach such a happy conclusion at the end of these sessions. Instead we could notice our urge to find a comfortable ending, but remind ourselves that the real resolution would come if the behaviors stopped. From the perspective of stylistic communication strategies in DBT, rather than shifting from an irreverent (change-oriented) style during the session to a reciprocal (acceptance-oriented) style at the end, I would remain in the irreverent style until the actual behavioral changes took place. Almost immediately this change in my behavior made a difference. It seemed to heighten her awareness of our in-session chain as she engaged in the out-of-session management of her anger toward her partner. Ultimately, we were cross-referencing among several chains: the external, out-of-session, reality chain; the in-session chain; the chain as it evolved in my consultation team; and the "confessional chain" that she had learned in her Catholic upbringing.

As this example shows, it is often productive to refer back to prior behavioral chains to add explanatory power and the credibility that comes with recognizing repetition. To complete the consideration of how many chains are actually at work during the review of one out-of-session chain, we might consider that another (usually silent) chain comes from the therapist's prior experience either in personal life or in sessions with this patient or other patients. Something done or said by the patient activates the therapist's prior behavioral chains, which could bias his way of listening to the patient and responding to her. We could understand this process as a behavioral version of the way the psychodynamic psychotherapist discovers and manages his countertransference as he implicitly responds to the patient.

Of course this process of keeping multiple chains in mind takes center stage in the treatment of the adolescent and the family in DBT. The therapist and the teenager might construct a chain of events in an individual session, as filtered through the teen's perspective. Then, in a family session involving the teen and his parents, the focus may turn to the even more complex matter of constructing a "family chain," in which everyone contributes a review of his or her own behaviors and a perspective on everyone else. As the family members construct a chain of events combining several perspectives, the explanatory possibilities multiply, and the therapist can help all family members recognize that the adolescent's behavioral outcome had contributions from all of them.

I was conducting a family behavioral chain analysis with a young man who was addicted to multiple substances. Although he had "made sense" of his behavior in an individual session in building a chain, and even though his own chain analysis had included the impact of interactions with his parents, the family chain in a subsequent family session opened our field of observation and explanation to a wider set of factors. Unbeknownst to the teen, who formulated that his mother's harsh criticism of his "laziness" was a prompting event leading to that instance of substance use, the mother had just emerged from a painful encounter with the father who had criticized her for being too lenient with the son. Coming out of this family session, everyone in the family had work to do and solutions to generate. The pressure was not only on the "identified patient," and in fact one result was several individual meetings with the father about his own sense of isolation and loneliness, which indirectly seemed to help his son commit to reducing substance use.

Change Is Constant; Everything Is in Flux

Discussed above as "impermanence" in the context of doing behavioral chain analysis, the recognition that everything is constantly changing, including every element brought into the chain, can set the stage for hope for the therapist and patient who are stuck repeating the chain analysis of a repetitive target behavior. I have often reminded myself, "This too will pass; this too will change." Similar to the Buddhist recognition that "one never steps in the same stream twice," the DBT therapist can recognize that one never conducts the same chain twice. The perspective that change is occurring helps to combat the sense of stuckness and paralysis that attends some therapies. And it promotes an approach to the chain that is itself characterized by movement.

In spite of the fact that the therapist might think she and the patient are covering old territory, simply repeating what was identified before and therefore hopelessly stuck, this dialectical perspective helps her (1) realize that things are changing and (2) maintain a sense of movement and flow in conducting the chain analysis. This can be done in so many different ways. The therapist can shift back and forth in focusing on different chains. For example, an adolescent patient might show little willingness to review her own chain of "misbehavior," but she might be willing to engage in recounting a chain of events within the family, or within one of her friendships; or the therapist might sequentially bring up one or another perspective from her own learning history that might relate to the patient's situation. The therapist is wise to keep therapy moving, intervening with anything, almost anything (within DBT's limits), to avoid prolonged and repetitive interactions such as:

"And then what happened?"—"I don't know."
"Do you have any ideas of how to explain what she did?"—"I don't know; isn't that your job?"
"I don't want to talk about that." [repeated again and again]

Fortunately, within the strategic repertoire and stylistic stances of the DBT therapist, there are many options to keep things moving. When "stuck" at a certain point in the chain, or mired in getting the patient's cooperation with the procedure, the therapist can shift back and forth between validation strategies and a huge number of change strategies. He can similarly shift between an irreverent and reciprocal communication style. He can take a step back and generate hypotheses and test them with the patient out loud. He can move among dialectical strategies, such as metaphor, making lemonade out of lemons, extending, and balancing different treatment strategies. He can zoom back and forth between different segments of the chain; jump on and off the chain for careful assessment alternating with hypotheses, solutions, and didactics; zoom in and out between views of the "big picture" of the chain and the fine details of certain segments; and shift back and forth between validating the patient's experiences and pushing for behavioral change. I find over time that the more respect I have for the chain and its purposes, the more clarity I have about its evanescent and changing nature. The more ways I have to maintain my balance and freshness, the more effective I am at sustaining movement by shifting, improvising, and sometimes just sitting back and watching for possible openings.

OTHER TECHNICAL MATTERS
IN DOING CHAIN ANALYSIS

In this final section we consider two technical matters in the conduct of behavioral chain analysis: (1) the conscious use of language and tone to enhance the impact of the procedure, and (2) the ongoing selection of "where to work on the chain." Given that behavioral chain analysis is an assessment that requires the patient to retrieve detailed events from hours or days prior, the procedure is usually enhanced by trying to bring the memory to life in the session. First, it will be easier to recall relevant details while recounting a "hot" memory than a "cold" one. Second, if solutions are found to elements of the chain during the process of review, those solutions are more likely to be integrated in the patient's mind if the recalled story is "alive" rather than "dead." Finally, the lively and detailed recall of a memory during the session creates the opportunity to use the process as an exposure procedure, helping the patient to approach rather than avoid, to remember rather than to forget. In spite of the advantages of bringing the story alive during the behavioral chain analysis, at other times it may be indicated to go over the story with less intensity, to help the patient review something painful that happened without fully rekindling the painful emotions.

To bring life to the story, the therapist can use language and tone that promote activation of the episode. She might use the present tense even though discussing a past episode. "OK, now you *are* in the kitchen, and you *haven't yet considered* taking the knife you use to cut yourself. What *are* you thinking about? What emotions *are* you experiencing? *Are* there any things you could do to manage your desperate feelings other than turning to the knife to cut yourself?" In addition, to enhance the sense that this "reenactment" is taking place in the presence of the therapist as witness and supporter, the therapist might use the pronoun *we* rather than *you*: "OK, now *we* are in the kitchen, and you haven't yet considered taking the knife you used to cut yourself. What are you thinking about? What emotions are you experiencing? Let's consider what you can do to manage your despair." These subtle uses of present tense and the pronoun *we*, along with a tone of voice that fosters a sense that "this is happening now," can heighten the relevance and strengthen the uses of the chain.

As soon as a therapist enters into a chain analysis with the patient, questions arise about "where to work on the chain." As mentioned, we are likely to start with an explication of the problem behavior, then move on to the prompting event. From there we are likely to move either "backward" to consider the vulnerability factors, "forward" to consider the links in the chain from the prompting event to the problem behavior, or "jump forward" on the chain to consider the reinforcing consequences of the problem behavior. Although these broad guidelines are useful, they still leave a huge number of choices for the therapist. Should he try to get an "overview" of the entire chain, a kind of summary of the behavioral episode, before homing in on certain segments to get more detail? Or should he just proceed link by link, getting the detailed story, getting as far as possible into the entire episode? Sorting through these choices requires finding the right balance between the overview, from which the therapist can make an informed decision about the most immediately relevant segment of the chain to address, and the value of spending the finite time getting at the details of a particular segment. In most cases, I try to get a brief overview of what happened before zeroing in. This approach helps to avoid the situation in which the therapist spends the entire session on one segment of the chain, only to learn at the end that there was another segment containing high-risk behaviors.

Beyond getting a brief overview, how does the therapist decide where on the chain to bring attention during the session? The therapist could focus anywhere from the "left end" of the chain, addressing problematic vulnerability factors or the prompting event, to the "right end" of the chain, addressing antecedents close in proximity to the problem behavior or consequences following the problem behavior. I operate with four guidelines in mind, respectively related to:

1. The imminence and severity of the target behavior.
2. The level of detail in the patient's memory.
3. The patient's willingness to work on a certain segment.
4. My hypothesis of what is functionally most relevant to the problem behavior.

First, I consider the imminence and severity of the target behavior. If risk is high and the repetition of the behavior seems imminent, I am likely to focus in on the right end of the chain, assessing the factors promoting high-risk behaviors and finding solutions to them. To "stabilize the right end of the chain" is consistent with targeting the highest-priority risk behaviors before moving on to others. Common interventions to address problems at the right end are distress tolerance skills and contingency procedures.

Second, if the imminence and severity do not necessitate prioritizing the right end of the chain, the level of detail of the patient's memory for some segments over others might influence the direction in which I focus. In other words, I might get started by assessing an area where there are more data, then moving on to ones with fewer. Third, if the patient is more willing to work on some parts of the chain than others, I may go along with those preferences to enhance our collaboration as long as it does not violate the order of priorities in the target list. Earlier in this chapter I referred to a young female patient who was working with me to assess an incident in which she had been raped by a "friend." I prioritized a review of the segment of the chain where she "let her guard down," in order to generate solutions that would make her safer in the near future. Her preference would have been to avoid that segment of the chain altogether, because it elicited feelings of shame in her. She wanted to focus on her "need" for a boyfriend, which in her opinion rendered her vulnerable to predatory males. We "made a deal" early in the session to work on both segments; and of course they were interrelated.

Finally, in choosing where to work on the chain, I am influenced by my up-to-the-minute hypotheses about which elements of the chain are most functionally related to the problem behavior. Naturally, if I am correct, addressing and changing those functionally related links are more likely to have an impact on changing the behavior. In one case, this could lead me to focus intensively on factors in the environment that reinforce the patient's problem behavior. In another instance, I might work on the deficit in emotion regulation skills that promoted emotional dysregulation and eventually led to the problem behavior as a "solution." In any case, I try to make these decisions in a collaborative way if possible, and to be transparent with the patient about my reasoning.

CHALLENGING SITUATIONS
FOR BEHAVIORAL CHAIN ANALYSIS

Best-laid plans can go awry. We could learn everything about behavioral chain analysis, the CBT fundamentals, and principles from the acceptance and dialectical paradigms, and still run into difficulties. Whereas some of these difficulties may relate to problem behaviors in the therapist, many will relate to challenging behaviors in some patients. Next I consider five such situations.

First, there is the patient who provides little verbal data with which to work. The patient might forget entire episodes or significant details, dissociating during the session when asked to recall certain segments, generating very brief responses with little memory-based information, or be entirely silent for stretches of time. To reiterate and expand on a comment earlier in this chapter, my approach is typically to take what I can get, analyze what I can, and assess and address the factors interfering with providing the story. This process is different, of course, with each case, so there is no general formula. If I think there is a memory blockade in a relatively willing patient, I will try to elicit more memories of a crucial event if I can, or simply work with the paucity of memories I've got. I might ask the patient to manufacture some likely details of what is forgotten, so that we can practice behavioral chain analysis, with the hope of strengthening the patient's memory of his experience. If I think there is a willful component, and I cannot determine how to increase the patient's collaboration, I will try to name the willful behavior standing in the way and elicit the patient's help in assessing it. In particular, I am interested in what emotions are involved. The fearful, anxious patient might avoid discussion of emotions and retreat into the cognitive details of the story. The shamed, embarrassed patient might try to hide the humiliating details. The angry patient might present a blockade with a sense of defiance to maintain control over the situation. Each requires a different approach. If I have few clues as to how to understand the blockade, including the case in which the patient is entirely silent, I may use every approach I can think of, noticing whether any one of them elicits a better response from the patient. Using trial and error is sometimes the most productive means of assessing a blockade.

Some patients present with such a high degree of emotional sensitivity and reactivity throughout the conduct of the behavioral chain analysis that I find it nearly impossible to bring their attention to details, hypotheses, and solutions. In such cases, I typically let go of my plan to do behavioral chain analysis in any detail, do what I can do without causing hyperreactivity, and use in-session strategies for the reduction of the emotional sensitivity. Usually this begins with my validation of the patient's emotions as accurately and effectively as possible—which may take a good part of the session. These are opportunities to prompt, teach, or reinforce emotion regulation skills, mindfulness, and distress tolerance.

Third, sometimes a patient's level of distractibility interferes profoundly with "getting the story" of the chain. As the patient's attention jumps around, she cannot elaborate with detail on any one link, thereby blocking any chance to assess the chain in detail. Typically this type of patient response will require attention to the "therapy-interfering" behaviors of shifting attention, distractibility, and impulsivity. These need to be named and assessed, with a goal of finding solutions. In the treatment of adolescents and some adults, these behaviors may by a symptom of ADHD, so the therapist needs to learn strategies and skills for working with these problems.

Fourth, I have worked with many patients who seem compelled to provide an excessive level of detail to the behavioral chain analysis, making it nearly impossible to get the big picture of the problem. It is hard not to get frustrated, and the therapist's efforts to push the patient forward through the story tend to heighten the patient's anxiety and worsen the problem. In this case, I will often step back and assess the patient's tendency to provide excessive detail, bring it up in a straightforward way as a factor interfering with "getting the big picture," and see if it is possible to come up with solutions. With one of my patients presenting this way, who carried diagnoses of obsessive–compulsive disorder (OCD) and hoarding disorder, we made more progress when I could bring his attention to the problem and get his agreement to accept my judgment about how much detail was needed. I found ways to reinforce him for compliance.

Finally, all DBT therapists have worked with patients for whom the very imposition of a structure or procedure such as behavioral chain analysis triggers intense emotional responses resulting in anger, defiance, and willfulness. Such patients may judge the therapist as intrusive, pushy, simplistic, or insensitive, and they might feel that they are being "hit" or "punished" with a behavioral chain analysis. They might "just want to talk," not be forced into a structured exposition. Again, this kind of behavior requires an assessment of the unique individual factors involved; there is no formula. The general rule is to identify and nonpejoratively specify the factor interfering with the chain analysis procedure, and to try to solve it. Sometimes the therapist magnifies or triggers the problem by proceeding in a rigid manner. The essence of a behavioral chain analysis is a very natural and conversational thing to do, familiar to most people in how they are approached by their medical doctor or their auto mechanic. It simply requires getting the story. One need not use the term *behavioral chain analysis*, or any synonym, or act as if there is anything special or different about this part of the session. One can simply start by saying, "What happened?" Then something like, "How did that happen?" Or, "Tell me about it." As DBT therapists doing behavioral chain analysis, we can simply try to learn about the story, and in the backs of our own minds we can frame or structure the story in the form of a behavioral chain. There are such advantages to doing so!

CHAPTER 12

Validation

Y ou take a walk with a 3-year-old child. You have a destination. Noticing a potato bug in the dirt, the child stops. She crouches down on her heels and is completely absorbed in the bug. She picks up a sliver of a stick she finds in the dirt, and as gently as she can, she touches the bug with it, watches what the bug does, and pushes the bug around. You stop too and quietly crouch down. Were it not for the child, you never would have noticed this bug. You observe everything about the bug, what the child does, and how the bug responds. You notice that the child is immersed in "bug reality," and you let yourself be there too. It's a wonderful moment. You have dropped everything else in the world, including the direction you were walking with her, momentarily forgetting the destination. You are completely there, with the child, with the bug, in the moment.

In so doing, you embrace and endorse the child's existence, her pace, curiosity, and fascination. She matters, what she does matters, and you convey, with no words at all, that what she does makes sense. You enhance the child, implicitly support her instincts and choices, and reinforce her interest in the world.

Validation in psychotherapy has this quality. It asks you to stop and be with your patient in the moment, seeing what she sees, hearing what she hears, stopping along the path with her, completely letting go of the change-oriented agenda for the time being. This presence enhances your patient. Her agenda, her interest, her pace are embraced and endorsed. She feels connected, substantial, and meaningful. She has been recognized, appreciated, and confirmed. Even before a word is spoken, this is validation. When validation takes a verbal form, the same spirit flows into the words.

Defining validation is a bit like defining breathing. On the one hand, we already know what it is. It's a familiar term and concept. We do it all the time. "No wonder you are upset after what he said to you"; the individual feels understood. "It makes complete sense that you mistrust that guy; he's been acting unpredictable"; the individual feels that you "get it." "You show a lot of courage by going to the party without a date"; the individual feels recognized, confirmed, enhanced. Just listening, looking, being there with and for someone else is validating. These are all validating moments and they strengthen connection between any two people. We need not know that validation has certain features, complexity, and certain boundaries until it fails us. It frequently fails us when we are treating an individual with a high degree of emotional sensitivity and reactivity, a long history in a pervasively invalidating environment, and therefore a strong tendency toward self-invalidation. We try to validate; it doesn't work. It doesn't go as we expect. We don't make the kind of connection to which we are accustomed. Not uncommon in DBT, these circumstances require that we develop a deeper, sharper, and more variegated understanding of what we mean by validation, especially because validation plays a crucial role in the treatment.

Linehan (1997) proposed the defining features and technical requirements of validation—the what, why, whether, when, and how to validate—in her 1997 article on the topic. I begin this chapter by revisiting many of the salient points from that article and illustrating them with clinical examples before discussing how it is that principles from the change, acceptance, and dialectical paradigms can expand our validating capacities. I cover the following topics: .

- The functions of validation in DBT
- What is validation?
- Valid versus invalid
- What are the targets of validation?
- When do we validate (and when do we not)?
- What are the six levels of validation?
- How do the change, acceptance, and dialectical paradigms enhance our applications of validation?

THE FUNCTIONS OF VALIDATION IN DBT

During the development of DBT, validation was added to the cognitive behavioral core of the treatment to balance the dysregulating impact of pushing for change. As Linehan expressed it in her early workshops and seminars in the 1990s, validation provided the "sugar coating" that helped the "distasteful medicine" of cognitive-behavioral strategies go down, or it is "the oil to lubricate the machinery of problem solving." So the first function of validation was to assist the patient in maintaining or regaining emotional balance during problem solving. Since then validation has proven to have several other functions in DBT. It strengthens clinical progress by functioning as reinforcement for improvement. It strengthens the therapy relationship. It is one of the factors that hold the patient in therapy. This function was noticeable in a randomized controlled research trial in which standard DBT was compared to a specially designed control treatment, comprehensive validation therapy (CVT), consisting only of DBT's validation strategies (Linehan et al., 2002). CVT did reasonably well at reducing symptoms, but it's most remarkable impact was noted in the 0% rate of dropout from treatment.

As one might expect from DBT's biosocial theory in which invalidation plays such a central role, validation helps to reduce self-invalidation while increasing the capacity to self-validate. Given that validation strategies are considered the purest acceptance-oriented strategy group, it is interesting that validation plays a role in changing emotional responses. Typically, an emotionally salient prompting event elicits an aversive primary emotional response, such as criticism eliciting shame. For the individual with borderline personality disorder, shame might be intolerable and will set off a secondary emotional response, such as anger or sadness, or a dysfunctional behavioral response such as self-cutting or substance use. If the therapist can identify and validate the primary emotional response (in this case, shame), and in so doing can help the patient remain in contact with that emotion, he begins to learn new ways to modulate the painful emotion. In this respect, validation serves as a step in an exposure procedure, one of the four change strategies in DBT.

When I was once teaching a workshop along with Marsha Linehan, a participant posed an intriguing question. "Marsha, if you were one of two survivors of a shipwreck, and you and the other sole survivor ended up on a small remote island, unlikely to be rescued for many years, and the other person was diagnosed with borderline personality disorder, and you were only allowed to bring one DBT strategy to use on that island, what would it be?" Marsha liked the question, saying, "So you want to know the aspirin of DBT." Fairly quickly she answered: "Validation. Validation would help our relationship, which might be the most important thing. It would help my island companion to regulate her emotions. It might even make her a better problem solver without teaching her any problem-solving strategies. Sometimes we can be pretty confused, and if we just get validated, we figure out what to do." Validation: the aspirin of DBT!

WHAT IS VALIDATION?

Validation is the act of substantiating, confirming, or sanctioning what is. Consider how we use the term outside of psychotherapy. We *validate* research findings, passports, election results, arguments, and logical proofs. There are three steps involved in validating. First, we have to "get it": We must recognize and understand the phenomenon being validated: the research findings, the passport, the election results, the formal argument or proof. Second, we check for validity: Do these research findings, does this passport, do these election results, does this argument or proof meet some kind of standard? Do they make sense in some context, using some method of reasoning? We are trying not only to recognize and understand, but also to certify that the phenomenon has some kind of "truth value." Actually, only the second step is validation, but the first step is a prerequisite. The third step involves communicating the validity . . . of the research findings, certifying or stamping the passport, and so on. *Validation* is a transitive verb. We validate *something*.

Step I: Recognizing and Understanding a Behavior

The first step, recognizing or understanding the phenomenon, is synonymous with empathizing in our clinical context. To empathize is to recognize and understand someone's predicament, experience, and behavior, to be able to "put oneself in her shoes." We can empathize with someone's experience without trying to locate the "truth value" in her experience or behavior. Empathy is a prerequisite for validating, and many failures to validate hinge on a failure to empathize. If I have no idea what is meant by *disappointment*—if I didn't know what it felt like—my efforts to validate someone's disappointment would fall short, would sound phony (unless I were to acknowledge my unfamiliarity in the process). As we will see shortly, there are certain clinical circumstances in which we may empathize but may choose to stop short of the second step, identifying the "truth value" of a behavior.

The validity of a behavior is already present (or not) before we validate it. We validate what is already valid. We simply confirm its validity; we don't create validity by validating. This point may seem obvious, but some therapists seem driven by a mandate to validate even if they don't yet know what to validate. We recognize and understand a thought, an action, an emotion, perhaps a capability—we empathize with it—and then we may choose to validate that phenomenon. In DBT there is no absolute value placed upon validation; it is used for certain purposes, mentioned above, the ultimate goal being to accomplish the treatment targets leading toward a life worth living. At times we recognize and understand a behavior, and we strategically withhold validation. I was consulting with a seasoned DBT therapist about her treatment of a sensitive, reactive individual who often felt shortchanged in life. The therapist explained that her patient was unhappy with her best friend. The therapist wanted to validate the patient, and thought she should validate her, but something was interfering. She asked me if I could help her figure out how to validate her patient.

I asked her if she could role-play the situation in therapy with me, where she played the patient and I played the therapist. I would try to validate her. Playing the patient, the therapist began to complain to me. "My best friend is not returning my calls or my texts. She is ignoring me. It hurts my feelings. I'm so angry at her!" I asked, "Do you know why she is not returning your calls?" She replied, "Just because her husband is dying of cancer, and is in the final days or weeks of his life, that is no reason to ignore me. I need attention too!" "Oh," I thought to myself, "now I realize why it is hard to validate the patient." Although her disappointment was recognizable and understandable, and I felt like comforting her, her response actually was off base. To validate her disappointment with her friend at that moment would also have validated her belief that her friend should attend to her even though the friend's husband was dying. My instinctive response in the role play was irreverent, not validating; change-oriented rather than acceptance-oriented. Continuing the role play, I said:

"If you think you need your friend's attention as much as her husband does, maybe you should tell her that you are dying too."

"Why would I do that?"

"Maybe your friend pays more attention to people who are dying." Still playing the patient, the therapist was confused for a moment, but then she said, "but she *should* be upset about it—he's been her husband for 25 years! I think I might be expecting too much from her, or maybe my timing is bad." *That* I could validate: "I see what you mean, that makes complete sense." And then I could validate her initial response, her disappointment: "You're right, but you know, I can also see how you would be disappointed."

Step 2: Determining the "Truth Value" of the Behavior

Linehan (1997) proposes three contexts within which we determine the validity of a behavior, and five methods of reasoning with which to do so. Although these might not be exhaustive, they do provide a kind of menu for determining validity, and within that menu different people might find different ways to validate the same behavior in a given individual. It all is part of what Linehan calls "finding a nugget of gold in a bucket of sand," referring to those frequent instances in DBT where it is not so obvious what is valid about a given behavior. The three contexts are time perspectives: the past, the future, and the present. Is this behavior—in this case, the patient's disappointment, valid with respect to her past? Is her emotional response valid with respect to her future, her "ends-in-view"? Is it valid with respect to the current context? The five methods of reasoning involve different types of logic: Is this behavior valid with respect to some accepted authority or with respect to a meaningful consensus? Is it valid based on inductive (empirical) reasoning or deductive reasoning? More unique to DBT, is this behavior valid based on "wise mind" reasoning? Later, in the section on dialectics in validating, we consider the tricky situations in which a behavior is valid in one context but not in another, or with respect to one type of reasoning but not another.

Validation with Respect to the Past

We consider a behavior valid if we can understand that it is aligned with the individual's unique learning history or biological constitution. When I stand before an audience on a stage, I automatically and instantaneously experience fear, and I move back from the edge of the stage. This is not valid behavior in the current context; there is nothing obvious of which to be afraid. But if you know of my learning history when standing on stages, the instinctual fear and the moving away from the edge are easily understood. In high school, 48 years ago, I was playing a lead role in a Shakespeare play at my school (I was the Duke of Orsino in Shakespeare's *Twelfth Night*). I was wearing a fake beard and an excessively long purple robe. With my friends sitting in the front row, having vowed to playfully distract me during the performance, and in the middle of a famous soliloquy ("If music be the food of love, give me excess of it . . . "), I stepped on the robe, my knee buckled, and I fell to the floor and then off the stage! I got up, walked back up on stage, and finished my performance. I recovered in the sense of completing the job, but my brain changed forever. I had been startled, hurt, and humiliated, and my current "stage fright" is valid with respect to my one-trial learning history.

My patient, who had been raped by a friend the previous year and whose PTSD had worsened, was using several locks to secure her apartment, even though the perpetrator lived far away and showed no signs of returning, and the town in which she lived was small and relatively safe. Her actions were not valid in the current context, but they obviously were valid with respect to her past. She was ashamed to be taking such extreme measures; she recognized that they were not aligned with current reality. But her shame was lessened as I empathized with her position and validated her behaviors with respect to the past. I could honestly communicate that many individuals would be taking the same actions if they had the same history and if they had developed PTSD.

Behaviors that are valid with respect to the past will often be valid with respect to current and future contexts as well. In the first session of a new skills training group, a young woman arrived wearing sunglasses and a heavy coat, and when she sat down she turned her chair away from the group toward the wall. She spoke to no one and didn't respond to my questions or comments. Although I found her behavior odd, it did not interfere with my capacity to teach and for the patients to learn, so I made no effort to challenge her. After several weeks she changed: She took off the sunglasses, faced the other group members, and began to participate verbally. She seemed to have learned all the skills we had covered. As I learned more about her, it became easy to recognize the validity in her behavior based on the past: She had a social anxiety disorder and had been painfully excluded many times in her life. She was trying to avoid that experience. But her behavior was interestingly valid in the current context, in that it "worked"; her peculiar behavior made it possible for her to function in the present and to achieve her goal of learning skills. Her behavior was also valid with respect to her future, in which she envisioned learning more skills that would allow her to participate in life. This is a good example that even if a behavior is odd and unconventional, triggering disapproval and disagreement, and does not lend itself quickly and easily to empathy or validation, it may be valid in every respect.

Validation with Respect to the Future

We consider a behavior valid with respect to the future if it is aligned with, and makes sense in relation to, the individual's view of the future, his ends-in-view. A colleague of mine was unhappy about the school attended by her three children, ages 6, 8, and 10. She tried to improve matters at the school and with the teachers, but remained dissatisfied. She didn't want to remove her children from the school, and to home-school them meant that they would lose valuable social opportunities and would complicate her home life. Moreover, it would go against the chorus of opinions of teachers and school advisors. But her alignment with her view of the future of her children's educational development led her and her husband to withdraw them from school and embark upon home schooling. Her choice, controversial for many around her, dysfunctional from the school's point of view, and not aligned with her own distant and successful history in school, was valid with respect to the future, with respect to her ends-in-view.

Several years ago I assessed a 23-year-old man whose life had taken a tragic turn 1 year prior. Due to an accident he was quadriplegic, and he entered my office in his wheelchair. By the time I began working with him, he was enraged, depressed, and suicidal. He refused to accept a life with such severe physical limitations. He refused to take part in various vocational programs for the disabled. His family members and friends grew frustrated with his refusal. They assumed that it was based on anger about what had happened to him, which would never change. His behavior seemed invalid to them, and in fact their responses invalidated him. What they were missing was that his anger-fueled refusal, by that point in time, was based not on the past. It was based on a future image of himself as walking. He could not understand how it was that a society that could get humans to the moon and beyond could not build a better wheelchair. He wanted a wheelchair that could be reconfigured and motorized in a manner that helped him to ambulate. As he explained his view to me, it made complete sense. His image of the future was understandable, was valid; and his subsequent anger at the world was understandable. He and I went on the Internet to investigate the current state of bio-robotic wheelchair technology. We communicated with a professor at the Massachusetts Institute of Technology (MIT) and another one in Oxford, United Kingdom, each of whom had worked on projects exactly like the ones he envisioned. Even though the technology was not yet available, the validation of his viewpoint—his anger based on his ends-in-view— encouraged him, alleviated his rage, and allowed him to move forward.

Validation with Respect to the Present

Of enormous clinical importance is the fact that behaviors can be valid with respect to the current context. In that sense, the behaviors are normative and functional. It is a high priority in DBT, with individuals whose history of invalidation has resulted in their own conviction that they are not normal and not functional, to validate their behavior in the current context: "You are indeed capable of valid, normative behavior in the present." Those therapists who are trained to rate adherence to DBT in individual therapy sessions "require" at least one instance per session in which the therapist validates the patient with respect to the current context (as we shall see below, this is known as a *Level 5 validation*).

But it can be complex. How do we decide if a behavior is valid in the current context? For instance, is it valid for someone to deliberately and loudly fart during a highly controlled and somber church service? It depends. When a patient walks angrily out of a group meeting in a therapeutic setting, is it valid behavior in that context? It depends. If an adolescent patient smokes marijuana every day before and after attending school, is it valid behavior in that context? It depends. We need more information in each of these cases. And this brings us to the five different methods of reasoning through which we determine validity. These are of particular value in considering validity in the current context. Behavior can be considered valid with respect to:

1. *Accepted authority*: Is the behavior aligned with accepted authority?
2. *Consensus*: Is the behavior something that others would do in that context, either everyone or a relevant subgroup?
3. *Empirical reasoning*: Is the behavior valid through empirical or inductive reasoning, reasoning based on a number of past trials?
4. *Deductive reasoning*: Is the behavior valid through logic, or deductive reasoning?
5. *Wise mind*: Particular to DBT, is the behavior valid in that it is aligned with the individual's wise mind, even if it is not aligned with any of the above criteria?

Reasoning with Respect to Accepted Authority and Reasoning with Respect to Consensus. Although a suicide bombing may be objectionable and disturbing, it may also be valid in the current context in that it may be aligned with mandates or values held and perpetrated by certain radical *accepted authorities*. In a clinical example, a patient might stop all psychiatric medications even in the face of apparent success. This choice might not seem valid in that most people in the treatment community might disapprove. With respect to empirical reasoning, it may seem like an invalid choice in that previous attempts to stop medications led to symptomatic relapses and hospitalizations. It may not seem logical to stop psychiatric medications, since the predominant clinically accepted argument is that the medication corrects chemical imbalances and allows higher functioning. However, when we learn that the patient is devoted to the fellowship and the teachings within a given Alcoholics Anonymous (AA) meeting that opines strongly against the use of psychiatric medications, we realize that the behavior is valid in the current context based on *accepted authority*, within AA, and based on the *consensus of the subgroup* of people in that AA meeting. Even if we would like the patient to take the medications for proven clinical reasons, we are wise to begin by recognizing the validity of the patient's position.

When I was directing a DBT inpatient unit within a large psychiatric hospital, I was strict in expecting meetings to begin on time. The routine lateness of my therapy staff to some on-unit meetings struck me as invalid behavior, not aligned with my expectations, with what would be most functional from an empirical standpoint, and with the consensus among the rest of the staff. When I inquired further into their lateness, I learned that they were accustomed to being late in hospital-wide meetings for therapists, where the leading clinical authority in the hospital was never on time. For me, the "current context" was my meeting of staff on my inpatient unit. For the therapists, their "current context" included the conduct of meetings in the hospital as a whole. Once I could see their situation and validate their behavior on the grounds of *accepted authority* within the hospital, and *consensus of their peer group* in the hospital at large, I then was able to explicitly request that they join me in establishing an on-time culture within our program. Having felt understood by me, they were very willing to join me.

Empirical Reasoning. In working with individuals with addictions, we might fail to see the validity of lying even though it is not uncommon in that population. We tend to invalidate lying. We disapprove, we can feel betrayed, and it certainly interferes with treatment. But as soon as we take an objective look, we can see the *empirical validity* of the behavior. Through trial and error the patient has learned that the negative consequences of telling the truth about substance use, across both treatment and personal contexts, are more profound than the negative consequences of lying.

Deductive Reasoning. I once watched Marsha Linehan interview a suicidal woman who would visit her mother's grave, cut her wrists, and bleed on the grave. We were disturbed by her behavior. We could not see the validity of it at first. It did not seem to be valid with respect to any *accepted authority*. Certainly there would have been no *consensus* in that others did not do it. We couldn't see it as *empirically valid*, as being based on her learning from prior trials of this behavior. But on further inquiry, we came to see the underlying *deductive* logic. We learned that she missed her mother terribly and constantly, and the idea that she could mix her blood with her mother's body brought her a feeling of comfort. The logic was a strange one, but it was logical nevertheless. Once we validated her with respect to this way of thinking, she opened up further about her suicidal intentions. Beyond the concept that she was mingling her blood with her mother's blood, she held the "logical" conviction that she might be united with her mother in death, lying side by side, close to each other. The more we could see the validity of her thinking, the more effectively we could ally with her and begin to challenge her logic.

Wise Mind Reasoning. We have considered examples of behavior being valid based on accepted authority, consensus, empirical reasoning, and deductive logic. Finally, behaviors in the current context, even the ones that seem invalid by most methods of reasoning, might be valid in that they are aligned with the individual's *wise mind*, as taught as the centerpiece of the Core Mindfulness Skills module of DBT. The behavior is valid because it represents a creative and integrative intersection between emotional and rational thinking, intuition, and what simply feels "right" for that person. Not long ago I was working with a 35-year-old woman who was doing reasonably well in her life until a tragic event ended her relationship with the woman she loved, the woman with whom she wanted to spend her life. She worked hard to maintain her functioning and to understand and grieve her loss, but the grief overcame her and set off a major depressive episode with psychotic features, a series of hospitalizations that further traumatized her, and a growing conviction of hopelessness about her future. She was unable to work, unable to socialize, she was agitated nearly every minute, and psychiatric medications helped only insofar as they reduced the intensity of her psychotic symptoms. She desperately wanted to die.

She came in to see me for a session after I had been away for 1 week. She was smiling and seemed relaxed for the first time in months. She informed me that she had decided to move back to where her life had been interrupted 3 years earlier, that she had found an apartment, that she had been hired for the job she used to have, and that she was ready to begin life again. I was shocked by this amazing turnaround, was taken by a feeling of disbelief about such a sudden and bold plan, and I could only imagine a terrible outcome after a brief surge of optimism. Her family and friends tried to dissuade her, thinking it was "a flight into health." But I quickly learned that her determination was solid and that she was moving within a week. She agreed to follow up with me, traveling some distance to see me every other week.

Her choice seemed to be invalid in several respects: with respect to accepted authority (mainly me at that point); with respect to empirical reasoning (there was no evidence in 3 years that she could simply "will" her way back to functional improvement); with respect to consensus (neither she nor I knew of any cohort of individuals in her kind of condition that would be likely to succeed in this scenario); and with respect to deductive logic, it was a stretch ("If nothing else is working, why not go back to where things went bad?"). But she told me she knew, in her wise mind, that this was the thing to do. She felt that she "had to do it," that she could see a "ray of sunlight" coming through the clouds for the first time in a long time, that she knew it would be hard but that she felt "grounded." Although I was not convinced about her reasoning, since she was just barely removed from an episode of psychotic thinking (how could I distinguish wise mind thinking from psychotic thinking?), she was determined to do it anyway. As it turned out, it was a huge and positive step for her, and even though she was not able to sustain the life she had resumed, it marked the turning point in her course, and the beginning of a several-year upward trend that led eventually to a wonderful outcome. Her behavior, as I think of it now, was *valid with respect to wise mind.*

Step 3: Communicating the Validity of a Behavior

Having recognized and understood a behavior, leading to empathy with the person, and having determined the truth value of a behavior, the final step in validation is to communicate it to the individual. This can take place nonverbally or verbally, in action or in speech. No matter the form, the therapist essentially communicates that he grasps the essential nature of the individual's predicament and the grounds for the particular behavior in question. Successful communication will depend not only on having "gotten it right," but also on understanding how to speak that individual's "language." This may require soft speech, even silence but with a certain facial expression. It may require very direct, almost irreverent communication for some to experience validation. It may require slowing down or speeding up speech. It may even be difficult to validate some individuals unless it is spoken in their language.

It is useless to be "accurate" in our determination of validity if the communication of it is not "received" by the patient. I was treating an adolescent girl who told me that she had gotten upset after talking with her mother on the phone. Thinking I understood and intending to validate, I said, "So you were upset after talking with your mother." Forcefully, she said "NO!" I didn't understand. She said, "You don't get it—that's not what I said!" I apologized and asked her if she would tell me again what had happened. "I spoke to my mother on the phone; she said some stupid things that made me angry." I said, "So your mother said some stupid things that made you angry." She fired back, "NO!"

From my point of view I was simply trying to understand the source of her anger and then see if I could grasp the validity of her reaction. From her point of view, I was completely missing the mark. I didn't get it; it didn't seem that complicated (how wrong I was!). Her "validation receptor" seemed to me as if it were impossibly small. I shifted gears: "So I guess I'm not understanding you very well." She seemed relieved: "Yeah, you got *that* right!" She felt validated. It took extra work to find a way to validate her, and then in fact it did make a difference and allowed us to do some problem solving. When we validate we have to consider the patient's age, cognitive style, culture or subculture, vocabulary, and particularities of rhythm and tone. Most of all, we need to notice whether our attempt at validation was received. Sometimes we need to return again and again, sticking with the effort to validate.

Finally, at the foundation of any "type" of validation is the deeper concept: *functional validation.* We accurately appreciate the patient's predicament, and we act accordingly. Sometimes that involves verbal validation, as is the case in the examples already given. But at other times, we validate through our actions. Rather than commenting on the individual's tears, we might just offer a tissue. Rather than sympathizing with a colleague's overwhelmed circumstance, we offer to make some phone calls for her. Rather than verbally validating our children's extreme sense of thirst during a long and hot car ride with no rest stop in sight, we engage them in a game that serves to distract. Once we understand that functional validation means that our actions reflect and communicate an understanding of the validity of the individual's behavior in the context of the predicament, we realize that all validation is functional. It is just that sometimes we validate with words, sometimes with action.

Typically the three steps of validation take place in a matter of seconds, with no time for deliberate thought. At other times we get stuck at one or more steps, and the validation may require more work and more time. We might not recognize or comprehend what the patient is communicating; we might not be able to empathize, to put ourselves in the other person's shoes; we might not be able to see the wisdom or truth value of the behavior; and/or we might be ineffective at communicating our understanding to the patient. If we run into difficulty validating a patient for a particular behavior, we can break it down into these three steps in order to assess the failure to validate.

Our understanding of validation is sharpened by understanding what validation is *not.* Validation does not necessarily signify agreement. Validating someone for something is separate from one's own personal attitudes, perceptions, or preferences. We might indicate our agreement with something the patient has said. But this is not the same as validation. The distinction between agreement and validation can get lost in the heat of the moment. We may try to validate a patient ("It is understandable that you felt attacked by him"), but the patient feels invalidated because she actually wants our agreement ("I agree, you were attacked by him").

Sometimes the therapist confuses the two, thinking that in order to validate someone's behavior, she must agree with it.

The patient may feel very much alone in his version of his history, perception of individuals or events, or intended plan of action. We might be able to validate his version, his perception, or his plan—that is, to see the wisdom or validity in light of his past, present, or future contexts. But if he can't get our personal agreement with his version or his plan, he remains distressed. We might feel pressured by the patient to agree with his version of events, but it is important to maintain the distinction. Some therapists fall into a trap of acting as if the solution to patients' distress is to agree with them; although doing so may bring immediate relief to patients, it may also reinforce an unhealthy dependency on therapists' willingness to agree. This dependency can interfere with efforts to help patients tolerate distress and validate themselves.

Therapists, too, can be confused about the distinction. A DBT therapist in supervision with me said, "But how can I validate my patient's unilateral decision to go off his medications? I totally disagree with it." To reiterate: To *validate* a patient's behavior is to find the valid grounds for it, of one kind or another. It is an entirely separate matter to personally agree or disagree with it.

The same kinds of confusion sometimes arise in the distinction between validation and approval. The patient may want our approval, not just our validation. Patient: "Before I decide to move out of my family's house, I want to know if you approve." Therapist: "I think you know that in my opinion, it is going to be difficult, but that your reasoning makes complete sense." Patient: "I know, but I want to know if you are in favor of it." The patient here is asking for something more than validation; she wants the therapist's personal approval before she acts. In some situations, the therapist may convey approval of the patient's choice, which could be effective and appropriate. But there are other times that therapists disapprove of patients' decisions but can still validate them. On my inpatient DBT unit, the patients could enter the dining room in the evening on the condition that they cleaned up after having their snack. One of the evening staff members came to me one morning with a question. "Charlie, last night the patients didn't clean up after they used the dining room. I wanted to tell them that they would lose the privilege of evening snacks if they didn't clean up, but I didn't say anything because it didn't sound very validating." This staff member, trying to learn the treatment, evidenced confusion: He was merging the essence of validation with the essence of approval. As we discussed, it was fine to highlight the negative consequences of the patients' behavior, while validating it. "No wonder you guys don't want to clean up the dining room;

no one likes to do that. But you know you will lose snacks tomorrow night if you don't clean up tonight."

Finally, we are wise to remember that validating someone does not require a warm communication style. We can communicate to a patient that his behavior makes sense with either a warm or cool style. Communication style is an independent variable, not linked to whether we validate or not, even though it is more typical to communicate warmth along with validation, since they are both in the larger package of acceptance strategies in DBT.

VALID VERSUS INVALID

Experts in DBT often instruct therapists to "validate the valid, and invalidate the invalid." This statement can be rather confusing, given that, theoretically, every behavior has validity. Every behavior has been caused by all events up to that point in time. As I said in an earlier chapter, the world is perfect as it is. We can take this to mean that every behavior is valid with respect to the past. So, what do DBT experts mean? If everything is valid, why do we consider some behaviors to be invalid? Why do we choose to validate some behaviors and not others? The short answer is that we sometimes choose to invalidate behaviors because they will interfere with progress toward the patient's previously stated goals. They are invalid with respect to the stated ends-in-view.

Let's say that our patient abuses heroin and has agreed to enter treatment to get clean. It is a high-priority treatment target. If the patient then goes on to use heroin, is there validity in this behavior? Yes, clearly there is. The behavior is valid with respect to the past and the individual's biology; she has an addiction and we can see that, given this history and this biology, the use of heroin is valid. And it may be valid with respect to current context, in that it may be the one and only means through which she can alleviate her distress in her current context, and she may in fact function more effectively after using. The problem arises if we take validation to the final step of communicating the validity to the patient. Because validation usually also functions as reinforcement, we would probably be reinforcing her heroin use—obviously, not a good idea. If we validate in this context, we are opposing very important goals of the treatment. So we choose not to validate the heroin use even if we do validate the cravings for heroin in light of the past, or validate the distress in the current context, the distress that leads to the cravings. We may even *in*validate heroin use, challenging it and pushing against it, to pursue the goals of behavior change. So when DBT experts say to invalidate the invalid, we do not mean that it would be impossible to find validity in the behavior. Instead, we mean that certain behaviors in certain contexts are *clinically invalid*. Since the clinically valid and invalid often lie together in the same intricate tangle of behaviors in the moment, we need to exercise accuracy and agility in using validation effectively in those situations. I return to this dilemma in an upcoming section on using validation with dialectical principles in mind.

WHAT ARE THE TARGETS OF VALIDATION?

Now we take on the question, what exactly do we validate? There are five different categories of validation targets: emotions, thoughts, actions, capabilities, and the person-as-a-whole. Although we rely on the same three steps in validating each target category, different considerations arise with respect to different categories.

Emotions

DBT's biosocial theory begins with the proposition that patients have a higher-than-average degree of emotional sensitivity and reactivity, and a slow return to baseline from an emotional response. These patients' emotional responses were invalidated in childhood by a pervasively invalidating environment, and over the course of time, they have come to respond to their own emotions by invalidating them. It has become automatic for them to respond to their own emotions by judging them, hating them, and maybe even hating themselves in their entirety. They have acquired the tendency to avoid emotional cues, suppress emotional responses, and escape from current emotions through actions or secondary emotions.

Given the confusion and suppression that attend emotional experience for many DBT patients, it is important and validating simply to notice them, inquire about them, listen carefully to them, and encourage them to communicate with us. We notice when their emotions are suppressed or obscured, minimized or maximized. We empathize, imagining ourselves in our patients' situations, imagining what it would be like to have the same emotions, looking for the "sense" in the presence of a given emotion, and communicating these understandings to patients. DBT needs to be an emotion-focused therapy in order to strengthen each patient's capacity for emotion regulation.

One patient said to me, "Last night I was texting with my friend while she was driving and I was at home, and suddenly she stopped responding. She had driven off the road, hit a tree, and she was killed instantly." She told me this shocking news in a brief, controlled, clipped manner, suppressing any and all emotions. I instantly found myself emotionally dysregulated. I felt like crying, and I asked her if she could say more about how she felt. She said, "These things happen in life; she shouldn't have been texting." I was struggling between my intense emotional response and her brisk dismissal of emotions. I said, "But this was your best friend." She said, "Yeah, but you can't control who lives and dies." I stepped back within myself, took several conscious breaths, looked at my patient carefully. She was physically restless but seemed uncharacteristically quiet. There were so many things that I wanted to say and to ask, but realized that these would have been more for me than for her. I stayed silent for an unusually long time, perhaps 3 minutes, wanting to create space for her to think, feel, and communicate. I was trying to get out of her way but to stay connected. Suddenly she said, "I think I've had enough." It sounded like she meant she had had enough of the session and wanted to leave. I asked, "Enough of what?" "Enough of life," she responded. "Enough of hurt, enough of doing things right and then getting hurt, enough of doing things wrong." Her tears started to flow. "She was my best friend, almost my only friend—I don't know what I'm going to do. I killed my best friend." It was almost too much to bear. My task was to bear witness to her painful thoughts and her emotional expressiveness. This is what we mean by emotional validation. In the coming minutes she was able to express a complex and disturbing tangle of sadness, anger, and guilt. It allowed us to come closer rather than distancing from each other to insulate the pain. It allowed her to have her feelings, to see where they went, and to feel understood. Eventually it was the beginning of the process, to continue for months, of untangling the impact of what happened, how it happened, who had responsibility, and what to do. It was, for this patient, a huge step toward emotional regulation.

Validating emotions can be very hard to do. It requires remaining focused on the importance of an emotion, letting it emerge at its own pace and run its course. We often need to consciously avoid the thousand things we do as therapists to spare ourselves, and our patients, from the full impact of emotions. We sometimes fail to recognize the presence of an emotion, sometimes underestimate its intensity, sometimes fail to understand how the emotion fits the circumstances, and, as I suggested, we sometimes simply cannot regulate our own emotional response, which then interferes with the patient regulating his. Mindfulness of emotions, which evolves into validation of emotions, is a prerequisite for accomplishing the overarching task of DBT: patients' improved emotion regulation.

We do not validate all emotional expressiveness, however. Sometimes the expression of an emotion is done in the service of escape from a prior emotional response; that is, the secondary emotion serves as an escape from the primary emotion. For example, I might escape from unbearable sadness or shame through an intense expression of anger. If my therapist and I take anger as the primary emotion, failing to see its role in my escaping from sadness or shame, we will reinforce the escape and miss the opportunity of enhancing my capacity to regulate the primary sadness or shame. A DBT therapist needs to be alert as to whether a given intense and repetitive behavior represents a secondary emotion, while simultaneously considering what the primary emotion is.

Thoughts

We validate thoughts. Again: We recognize a thought; we understand a thought; we imagine what it would be like to have that thought; we listen for or seek the valid grounds for the thought in the past, present, or future contexts; and we communicate all of this. Most of the time this process is easy and automatic. The patient says, "I'm embarrassed about what I said to my boyfriend yesterday. I'm afraid he's going to end the relationship." The therapist might validate the patient's thought that the relationship might end: "I can understand that you think he will end it over this; it wasn't your most balanced moment. No wonder you are afraid." The patient feels understood; the therapist validates the thought as understandable in the current context. He may also know that the patient has lost important relationships, and he can validate that her thinking may be valid with respect to the past. With respect to the patient's future, he knows that she has hopeful dreams about her life with this man, and it is valid for her to worry about losing him. So, with respect to past, present, and future contexts, the therapist can validate her thought about losing her boyfriend. Having validated her thinking, he can then pivot to problem solving: "Given what you know about you and him, and how you guys have managed misunderstandings before, what do you think is the likelihood of his breaking up with you over this?"

Inherent in the validation of thoughts is the understanding that they are just statements about reality; they are not facts. It is so easy to forget this major point. We want to help our patients notice and acknowledge their thoughts, elaborate on them, and find what is valid about them. At the same time, we want to convey, implicitly or explicitly, that thoughts are just thoughts, and that whereas a thought may have some validity, in other ways it might not be so valid. In the above example, it is valid for her to regret what she said to her boyfriend, valid for her to have the thought that he could leave her, and valid for her to experience fear of loss; but given the history and trajectory of the relationship, and given how they have handled previous problems, it is invalid to expect him to end it over this. Although we start with validating the valid, we move into problem solving, which sometimes includes invalidating the invalid.

Among the more challenging scenarios in DBT are those moments when the patient gives voice to intense suicidal thoughts. The therapist may be reluctant to validate the presence of suicidal thoughts, fearing that doing so will somehow validate suicidal action as well. The thought of suicide is likely to be valid in the context of a life of suffering, invalidation, self-hatred, and maybe a lack of improvement over previous weeks or months. The therapist may be tempted to insist that the patient "take suicide off the table," by which she implicitly communicates that she does not want to hear any more about suicide. The patient may feel that he cannot bring his suicidal thinking to his therapist, and thereby feels further invalidated. Precision is important here. We want to validate suicidal *thinking* as a response to the context in which it developed; validate suicidal *thinking* as making sense in response to an impossible current context and in the absence of a vision of a viable future; and yet sharply invalidate the *action* of suicide. We cannot take emotions "off the table," and it is unrealistic to take chronic suicidal ideation "off the table," but DBT therapists, even recognizing that there is validity in the act of suicide from various perspectives, do not validate the plan, the imminent intent, or the attempt. In my experience, finding the right balance in this frightening area is helpful to the patient who is "stuck" with suicidal thinking as the natural outcome of life circumstances and brain chemistry, who benefits from being able to express that thinking in an empathic context, and yet who benefits from the therapist's unambiguous stance against the act.

Actions

Validating actions can become rather complicated. If we say to a patient, "No wonder you came late today; you were stuck in traffic that would have been difficult to anticipate," it is usually not complicated. But consider this scenario: A child comes home with a report card on which she got a bad grade in a class. She is a youngster who ambitiously seeks to get all good grades. She says to her parent, "I can't believe I did so badly—I never should have gotten a grade that bad, and I will never get into college." Of course, this one sentence includes actions (how she performed on the test), thoughts ("I should never have done so badly"), and emotions (anger at herself and fear that she will not get into college). In trying to validate the action, the parent says, "But you had three other exams this week, you played in a tournament on the weekend, and we had to attend a funeral on Monday. It's not surprising at all that you didn't do as well as usual since you couldn't prepare the way you usually do." For one child this response might suffice; it might be received as accurate and empathic, as underlining the validity within the poor performance. But for a different child, this response may be off target. She might protest, saying, "It doesn't matter! Life happens and you still have to get good grades. I should have been able to do a lot better." The more you validate the poor performance, the more the kid is distraught. In truth, the parent is locating validity in the performance but at the same time is invalidating the child's high standards about his performance. She has high standards, possibly harsh standards; nothing "should" stand in the way of total success. It is one of many ways (more later in the chapter) in which validation can be difficult and may require a dialectical approach. There are two phenomena intersecting in this scenario: the poor performance and the high standards. To validate the former might invalidate the latter. Perhaps the parent would be more successful to validate both together: "I know your standards are very high, and we are proud of you that you work so hard. Given how high your standards are, it must be just terrible to get a lower grade than you are capable of."

This is the problem that can come up in validating the actions of individuals who tend to have a rigid or self-invalidating stance. You validate the action. The patient rejects the validation (which means, essentially, that the intended validation is not validating), highlighting that he should do better. The therapist then is wise to discover the grounds for the "should" and validate it. If that can be done successfully, the patient may be able to move toward the understandable emotion of disappointment, which the therapist can then validate. All of these validation examples are in the service of reducing the belief that thoughts are reality; reducing the degree of rigidity in a patient's thinking, feeling, and/or acting; and facilitating emotional experience and regulation.

Capabilities

We validate capabilities—which we also call *cheerleading*. In parallel with the validation of the various behaviors we have discussed, we validate the individual's capabilities by (1) recognizing them; (2) understanding what it would be like to have those capabilities and appreciating their significance; (3) seeing how those capabilities are valid given the past, given the present context, and given the future; and (4) communicating that we notice the capabilities and see them as valid. Since the patients that we treat in DBT often doubt their capabilities, or don't recognize some of their accomplishments as capabilities, it is both crucial that we recognize and validate them, and important that we understand that our attempts to validate might not be accepted.

After 3 years of hospitalizations for suicidal and other problematic behaviors, one of my patients had grown convinced that she was incapable of building a life. Everything seemed to come to naught; everything seemed like evidence that she should just give up. From her point of view, even though she had shown promise earlier in her life, it was gone and she had nothing to offer. I could see how she came to that conclusion. I think almost anyone would become convinced of lack of capabilities if they lived the same 3 years that she had lived. I could recognize and validate her despair and her pessimistic beliefs, and there were many opportunities to do so. I had to look hard to find a way to validate her capabilities, which I thought would be important. So many ways to do so might have seemed false to her. Just as she was going on about how useless she had become, I realized that I genuinely regarded her as one of the most compassionate people I knew. I said, "I know these years have just stripped you of the experience of being useful. I'm sorry that's happened, but I want you to know that you have a really unique quality that has not gone away. I know that if I were having some kind of difficulty, and I were in need, and if I asked you, you would help me in a second. I wouldn't do it, but only because it would be inappropriate in my role with you, but if I did, I know that you would help me. You are simply that kind of person, and it is still there even though you have been through hell." She knew I meant it, she knew that it was true, and she thanked me in a completely genuine way.

It may be misleading to use this example of personal self-disclosure in the service of validating her capabilities. In fact most often, validation of capabilities is more ordinary: The therapist recognizes and highlights capabilities as they occur during the session, or as they emerge in the patient's story. Unlike the validation of actions, thoughts, and emotions, usually the patient does not bring her capabilities to the therapist's attention; they are recognizable if the therapist is alert but could easily remain out of the conversation. There are so many opportunities to validate capabilities, to simply note them, and it is my impression that we underutilize this helpful intervention. A patient completes her diary card, clearly having given her full attention to each rating; I highlight her strength in self-monitoring and cooperation with the treatment. A patient who has seemed dysfunctional in managing her life announces to me that she is planning a cross-country trip with a friend. She has taken the lead in figuring out the logistics. Although certain aspects of her plans may worry me, I comment on her previously hidden strength in planning a trip like that.

Because patients sometimes worry that if they are seen to be capable in one domain, they will be expected to be capable throughout life, they shy away from the recognition or acknowledgment of capability. This stance poses a technical challenge. First, the therapist might be wise to highlight capabilities using only brief "brush strokes" and a matter-of-fact style. Second, the therapist may want to accompany the validation of capabilities with the validation of the fear that if seen to be capable, too much will be expected of the patient. I used irreverence while validating one patient: "If I didn't think it would scare you, I would tell you that you are really capable."

Person-as-a-Whole

Validating particular behavioral responses does not necessarily validate the person-as-a-whole. For instance, I might validate my patient's reluctance to attend a skills training group, given his social anxiety, in a manner that inadvertently also suggests that he is a person who gives up too easily. By validating the person-as-a-whole we are treating our patient as someone of substance, relevance, meaning, and intrinsic worth. In speaking of this type of validation, we are referring to something very close to "unconditional positive regard" as described in Rogers's (1951) client-centered therapy, or in what Buber describes in *Ich und Du* [*I and Thou*] (1923). We need to maintain our deep regard for the patient, sometimes in spite of problematic behavioral responses, communicating that our patient is traveling alongside us on the path of life as someone who is no less deserving of respect and compassion than we are. Anything less undermines our mission.

WHEN DO WE VALIDATE
AND WHEN DO WE NOT VALIDATE?

First, it may be important to state that we do not always look for opportunities to validate. Because validation is emphasized in DBT, some therapists mistakenly think that validation is the goal or essence of treatment. It is not. The ultimate aim is the pursuit of a life worth living through specified goals. Validation is one of the interventions that can be instrumental in getting there; it is a means to an end, not an end. I sometimes have shown videotapes of Marsha Linehan conducting individual DBT sessions. Not uncommonly the first question from the audience is, "Why didn't Marsha validate the patient more?" There are two problems with that question. One is that the videotape may not reveal the presence of validation even if it is occurring in the room. It can be a subtle transactional process recognized only by the two participants. The other problem is that the questioner may be thinking that Marsha should have validated the patient more. Deciding whether, when, and how much to validate are complicated assessments and should be based more on whether the patient is progressing toward her goals than on some moral mandate to validate.

Having said that, it is also true that ideally we use certain levels of validation all the time. In the next section, I outline the six levels of validation in DBT. Level 1 and Level 6 should be present consistently throughout treatment. Level 1 prescribes that a therapist be "wide awake" and alert while listening to the patient. Level 6 is described as "radical genuineness," a stance in which we remain our genuine selves as we engage the patient in treatment. If we are wide awake, listening carefully, and genuinely being ourselves, we tend to create a validating atmosphere in which patients feel that they are substantial, meaningful, and worthy of respect. Layered on top of this baseline, we engage in more specific validation strategies, outlined below, as examples of the other four levels.

Validation is a stance that accompanies assessment, is a set of strategies that balances the push for change during problem solving, and is the purest set of acceptance-oriented strategies in DBT. Although there is no rule requiring the use of validation during behavioral assessment, often this stance is the most conducive to discovering the links in the chain and the controlling variables of the target behavior. The patient who finds that we are interested in the rationale behind her various behaviors is more likely to be forthcoming about details of all kinds. Still, probing into the detailed circumstances of emotionally triggering events can set off emotional reactivity and lead to avoidance and withdrawal. And of course, during behavioral chain analyses, even careful efforts at behavioral change can provoke similar responses.

When we are pushing for change and using one of a multitude of problem-solving strategies, we can easily underestimate the patient's difficulty in tolerating our best-intended interventions. As we push forward toward change, we usually need to validate emotional pain and the difficulty of trying new behaviors. When working with a suicidal woman with borderline personality disorder, panic disorder, agoraphobia, OCD, and anorexia, there was a moment when I was convinced that if she could learn to use progressive muscle relaxation and diaphragmatic breathing exercises, she could reduce her tension and anxiety without self-injurious behaviors or eating disorder behaviors. As I oriented her to these skills, her anxiety unmistakably intensified in front of me. She said she didn't want to try them, she knew they wouldn't work. To push her further would have been counterproductive, but I still thought she could benefit. I didn't want to give up. I paused to consider what had just transpired and wondered aloud, in a nonaccusing manner, what had happened. "It seemed like you were interested in some techniques for tension and anxiety, but now it seems like I have scared you off. What happened?" She quickly responded, with obvious fear and caution: "I don't want to focus on my breathing, change my breathing, or do anything about my breathing!" I asked, "What is it about your breathing?" Her response: "If I focus on it, it will stop—I know it will." Rather than challenging the scientific likelihood that her breathing would stop if she attended to it, I looked for the validity in her statement. She certainly was not the only person with panic disorder who experienced "suffocation anxiety." I said, "I get it; no wonder you don't want to do it. Lots of people with panic disorder think the same thing. Why don't we put aside the focus on breathing and just do the muscle relaxation? It can be really effective in its own right." She was willing and eager, and in fact found it to be a helpful technique.

We use validation strategies to convey understanding and acceptance. At times during several consecutive sessions, I have pushed the patient to change behavior, and, despite the patient's hard effort, the process has been wearing on both of us. Realizing that I have been pushing for change without balancing it with acceptance, I enter the next session with the plan to "just listen," essentially to just check on how my "partner in problem solving" is doing, what she is thinking. It is something of a "heart-to-heart" exchange about how things are going, and functions as a breather for both of us. It reinforces hard work and can be effective in restoring balance and strengthening our bond. On the other hand, using validation through a heart-to-heart talk when a patient has not been collaborative or effortful runs the risk of reinforcing passive problem-solving behavior.

Sometimes we want to validate one behavior of a patient, but at that very moment he is engaged in a simultaneous dysfunctional behavioral pattern that might be reinforced by the validation. I recall on my DBT inpatient unit, a particular patient was remaining in bed at 8:30 in the morning when it was time for all patients to attend groups. A nursing staff member went to her room with the intention of prompting her to get to group. Nurse: "OK, it's time to get up and go to group." Patient: "I'm so tired. I was up really late after a really bad phone call with my father. I hardly got any sleep." Even on biological grounds, it was valid to want to remain in bed. The staff member, having learned to validate, said, "I understand. It's very hard to get going after you get hardly any sleep. What made the phone call so bad?" The staff member was doing fine until that final question, which opened up several minutes of explanation. Her initial validation based on poor sleep was enough and her next sentence should have been something like, "I get it; but now come on, you have to get up right now!" Instead she was almost certainly reinforcing the patient's stalling behavior.

THE SIX LEVELS OF VALIDATION

Linehan (1997) has articulated the six levels of validation as six guidelines or strategies that build upon one another; these constitute her most concise statement of how DBT therapists validate. The three steps of validation that we discussed early in the chapter—(1) recognizing and understanding a behavior, (2) finding the truth value in the behavior, and (3) communicating that understanding—map onto these levels. The first three levels provide guidelines for how to implement the first step, understanding the patient's behavior (and empathizing with it). The next two levels provide guidelines for finding the validity in the behavior. And the final level provides guidelines for validating the individual as a whole being. We review these levels here so that we have all the technical aspects of validation in our minds as we move on to considering how the principles of the acceptance, change, and dialectical paradigms influence or modify our use of validation.

Validation Level I

Level 1 requires that the therapist remain "wide awake," fully present, listening with full attention. Ideally the therapist uses Level 1 constantly, throughout every session of therapy, including during episodes of problem solving. By being truly present, he creates an atmosphere that conveys to the patient, "Your behavior has substance, meaning, makes sense, and is worthy of my attention." As discussed above, it is one of the levels that contributes to a validating environment and sets the stage for all other levels. To offer a patient one's full presence is of immeasurable value. It's the most natural thing in the world if you care about someone, and yet it's very hard to do. The therapist must be grounded in the moment and current reality, wide awake to what is influencing the patient, and sufficiently emotionally regulated to really listen. In this respect, doing psychotherapy in DBT is itself a type of mindfulness practice, with the objects of awareness being the patient's communications, behaviors of interest, and person-as-a-wholeness.

A young woman entered my office and sat down. I had canceled her previous session with only 1 day's notice due to an emergency, and could not offer her a makeup session. I apologized to her on the phone, and she seemed to accept it. As she walked into the session, I said "Hi." With a sing-song voice, sounding completely phony and perturbed, she responded with a drawn out "Hiiii." Because I was present, in the moment, balanced, and ready to listen, I was alerted by her tone of voice and the subtle aspects of her timing, her body posture, and her lack of eye contact. I wasn't sure exactly how to read her, but I knew that something was wrong. I guessed that her removed yet perturbed state was related to the cancellation. I brought it up: "I'm sorry I had to cancel last time." She responded quickly with a tone that was decidedly annoyed and sarcastic: "Yeah, thanks a lot! Great timing! I'm sure you had something more important to do than to see me." This quickly led to a review of what had happened and what her interpretations had been. We were able to repair the rift in less than two 2 minutes, and in fact it strengthened our relationship. Had I not been present, not been alert and awake, I would have missed the subtle cues, would probably have become defensive, and the matter would have festered.

Factors That Interfere with Level 1 Validation

So much can go wrong with validation before we utter a word to the patient. We can mishear her or misunderstand her verbal and nonverbal communications. We can have blind spots and fail to recognize what really matters. We might not detect her emotion, and our subsequent comments would indicate that we "missed the boat." We might notice the emotion but underestimate its intensity. The presence of the syndrome of "apparent competence," brought about in the patient in reaction to invalidating environments, can make her emotions difficult to "read." Even if we accurately perceive the emotion and its intensity, it is easy to misunderstand that the patient feels her emotion is nearly out of control. It is almost impossible to validate accurately if we don't detect the emotion, its level of intensity, or the patient's experience of being nearly out of control.

We might fail to appreciate that an assignment we give to the patient, which may seem rather straightforward, might feel nearly impossible to him. If we do recognize the level of difficulty as experienced by the patient, we may still assign the task, but we would know to acknowledge the patient's experience and validate the difficulty. If the patient feels recognized and understood, his willingness to engage in the assign-ment may increase. We can easily underestimate the magnitude of the patient's attachment to us, or the degree of insecurity associated with that attachment. We might assume that our patient feels as we do, that our solid bond will outlast any minor differences between us, when in fact our patient fears that the slightest hiccup could lead to the end. And there are so many ways that we can fail to notice that we are "going in one direction" when the patient is actually going in a different one. In workshops Linehan has called this a failure of "location perspective." We think we are one place in the work and the patient thinks we are somewhere else. A 16-year-old girl was referred to me for psychotherapy due to her multiple episodes of self-injury and her recent physical attack of her father. She was pleasant, and in taking a history, she was coopera-tive and engaged. I had the impression that she was quite interested in learning what DBT had to offer. Things seemed to have gone well. At the end of the session I pulled out my appointment book to schedule the next appointment. She stood up rather abruptly and announced that she had to leave right away to meet her friend. I said, "So, should we schedule the next session by phone?" She responded in a businesslike manner: "No, I only wanted one session, and obviously you don't understand me." Obviously, I had missed some cues and misread her "location." About a week later, she left a voicemail, very matter-of-fact, asking when our next session was. During the next session, I knew to "check out her location" and was surprised to find that her cooperative style was completely out of synch with her hopelessness. Knowing that, I was able to read between the lines, recognize her hopelessness in spite of her upbeat presentation, and validate her reactions.

Validation Level 2

Level 2, which involves reflection, is a natural extension of Level 1. By already being awake, aware, and listening, we are more likely to detect something in the patient's words or gestures. We check it out by restat-ing it, even using the patient's words. A patient said to me the other day, "Charlie, in the last session you really disappointed me." I took it in, restated it: "Oh. I didn't realize that. I really disappointed you." Patient: "Yeah, you came on way too strong." The patient communicates it, I receive it and restate it (to confirm that I got it), and then we can move on. On the other hand, by restating it, the patient may hear that I did not really receive it or understand her accurately. The patient says, "My husband doesn't understand me." I respond, "Yes, I know, you've told me many times, you don't feel understood by him." The patient hears that I didn't "get it": "No, I don't think you get it. It's not that I don't feel understood by him. He doesn't understand me, he never has." If I am alert, awake, and I hear her correction of my reflection, I can try again: "Oh, I guess I misunderstood. You are saying that he just doesn't understand. Right?" "Right." The process of reflecting back what the patient actually says plays an important role in getting in synch with each other. It's a back-and-forth dance that ensures mutual understanding or that lays bare a gap, which can then be acknowledged and addressed. It fosters attunement and attachment.

Factors That Interfere with Validation Level 2

When we see our reflection in a pond, it resembles us most accurately when the pond's surface is still. Similarly, when we reflect something back to our patient, even using the patient's words, we are most likely to be accurate if we are still. Our own emotional dysregulation can interfere with validation at this level. If we hesitate, shift around in our chair, avert our gaze for an instant, or voice our comments in an inappropriate tone, we distort a perfectly accurate reflection. I was treating a patient who repeatedly presented with dire but ultimately unfounded medical conditions. Our treatment was punctuated by crisis after crisis. During a medical hospitalization, she told a physician, who later communicated this conversation to me, that she was deliberately causing her own medical conditions and was reinforced by receiving hands-on medical care. In our next session I spoke about these behaviors. I wanted to understand and assess them, with an eye to adding them to our list of treatment targets. I thought I was listening carefully and objectively. She interrupted: "Are you fed up with me?" I was surprised by her question, but quickly realized that I was more "fed up" with her than I had realized. Her dishonesty and her deliberate creation of medical problems, resulting in crisis after crisis, had gotten to me. My lack of emotional self-awareness had interfered with my reflective capacities.

Validation Level 3

Level 3 is a close cousin of Level 2. Whereas Level 2 involves reflecting what has been explicitly communicated, Level 3 involves reflecting what has been *implicitly* communicated. The patient might say he is fine, but his facial expression and subtle gestures communicate otherwise. The therapist notices and reflects it back: "You say you are fine, but you don't seem fine." The patient may then feel recognized and deeply seen, or instead might feel exposed and insulted. As with Level 2, Level 3 involves making a statement that may or may not be accurate from the patient's viewpoint. For instance, if we continue with the example "You say you are fine, but you don't seem fine," the patient may then clarify, "No, I really am fine, but I saw the dentist just before coming here, and my face feels distorted." The interplay between Levels 1, 2, and 3—listening, reflecting, finding common ground, finding differences, correcting errors, repairing ruptures—goes on almost constantly in a good psychotherapy relationship. It is the dance of listening, recognizing, and empathizing. As the interaction between the therapist and patient unfolds, the therapist tries to hold the other person's mind in her mind, hold her own mind in mind, and hold in mind the interaction between the two of them. It's a finely honed skill, which, in attachment theory, is seen as the core skill for forming secure attachment relationships. It involves careful listening, sensitive responding, attunement, regular reflection, reading between the lines, and getting an increasingly elaborated narrative of the patient's story (Bateman & Fonagy, 2004).

In describing validation, and especially Levels 1, 2, and 3, Linehan (1997) does not emphasize the process of eliciting an increasingly accurate, rich, and elaborate narrative while listening and inquiring. But that process, highlighted by those who practice MBT and psychodynamically oriented psychotherapy, fits well with validation in DBT. The patient feels understood and validated not just because we hear and reflect this or that element of communication; it is also because we increasingly understand the story behind the elements. To validate effectively, and especially as we move on to Levels 4 and 5, we need to "get" the patient from the inside— her history, the implications of her culture and subcultures, the way she experiences current contexts, the hopes she has for the future, and so on. Levels 1, 2, and 3 are the building blocks of understanding.

Validation Levels 4 and 5

When we get to Levels 4 and 5, we communicate to the patient our understanding that his behaviors make sense in two ways: (1) with respect to his history and biology (Level 4) and (2) with respect to his current context (Level 5). In the section in this chapter where I described how to determine validity, I distinguished between validity based on past context/biology, versus current context, versus future context (ends-in-view). Here we are talking about how to put our understanding of what makes a behavior valid into action, while communicating with the patient in a session.

Let's use an example to distinguish a Level 4 from a Level 5 validation, and see some of the technical challenges of each. My patient had been raised by a mother who placed an exaggerated focus on her daughter's appearance. The mother made comments reflecting her fear that her daughter would get fat, even though she remained at a healthy weight throughout her childhood. By the time she was 20 years old, my patient was preoccupied with her weight and began to alternate between bingeing, purging, and restricting her intake. By the time I treated her in her 30s, she had overcome the symptomatic actions of her eating disorder, but remained highly sensitive about her weight and her appearance. She was dating a man and was hopeful about the relationship, though any time he complimented her appearance, she wondered if he really thought that she was too fat.

For the first time in years my patient reengaged in bingeing and purging. In her session the very next day, we were conducting a behavioral chain analysis of the target behaviors. As the narrative went, she and her boyfriend had been having dinner with another couple at a restaurant. After they had ordered their meals, bread was brought to the table. As she reached for a second piece of bread her boyfriend said, "Honey, do you really want that?" She described that, internally, she exploded with emotion while externally trying to hide it. She felt angry that he commented on her eating and humiliated that he did so in front of their friends. From her perspective, she now had evidence of her deepest fears, that he didn't like her body. As she recounted this story in the session with me, her male therapist, her emotions were intensely activated. By using Validation Levels 1, 2, and 3, I was able to hear and understand her emotions and thoughts at dinner. Once I grasped the story, I realized that her emotions and thoughts could be considered valid at both Levels 4 and 5. They were valid at Level 4 based on her history with her mother, which had left her vulnerable to almost any comment about her appearance or her eating. They were valid at Level 5 based on the context of sitting at dinner with her boyfriend and another couple, since most people would have felt embarrassed and angry if their partner commented publicly on their eating (validation based on consensus). If I had used a Level 4 validation at that moment when a Level 5 was also available, even if I had used it accurately, it would most likely have been invalidating to her rather than validating. Imagine if I had said, "Of course, you were upset. After all, with your history with your mother, almost any comment about your eating would have led to embarrassment and anger." Although technically correct, it would have the effect of ignoring her boyfriend's inappropriate behavior and would have been upsetting for almost anyone. It would highlight her pathology and ignore the normative nature of her reaction.

As a guideline, if the therapist is aware that the behavior is valid with respect to the past, as well as valid (and normative) in the current context, the first move should be a Level 5 validation. In this case, it would then be best to say something like, "No wonder you were angry with him and humiliated—he was really out of line. Almost anyone would have been angry and embarrassed." You start by highlighting the patient's accurate and normative recognition of reality. She might then feel understood. Often the Level 4 validation will then naturally emerge, initiated by either the therapist or the patient. For instance, she might have said, "I'm glad you see that he was out of line, but you know, it's also true that I have kind of an exaggerated response and then I get in a really bad state of mind." Or I could have followed the successful Level 5 validation with a Level 4 one: "I wonder if it made things even worse because of your history with your mom?"

Validation Level 6

I mentioned that validation at Level 1—present, awake, alert—is ideally operating throughout therapy. I would say the same about validation at Level 6, which is termed *radical genuineness*. In other words, we always want to be present, listening, and genuine. But what does it mean specifically for a DBT therapist to be *genuine*? It means that in responding to our patients, we allow our genuine responses as a person to show and to be part of the conversation. We embed our manualized interventions in the context of our genuine responses. As I have sometimes put it, we want to bring DBT into a relationship with the patient, not to bring the relationship into DBT. Sometimes therapists "act" therapeutic, use the language of the therapy model, follow the guidelines, but don't act like themselves. To practice radical genuineness means that the way the therapist interacts with the patient will look similar to the way she acts with friends and family, except she will also be doing therapy. Sometimes in the effort to be technically proficient, we depart from our natural responses, which could have had a healing effect on the invalidated individual.

VALIDATION AND THE ACCEPTANCE PARADIGM

Validation is considered the purest of the acceptance strategies. Yet, this doesn't mean that it is used only in the service of acceptance. As we will see, it is also used in the service of behavioral change and dialectics. But we begin with considering validation as the purest form of acceptance-based strategies.

The acceptance paradigm is based squarely in present-moment awareness. The therapist locates his awareness entirely in this very moment, letting go of any attachment to the future or the past. As such, present-moment thinking is without destination and is focused on just "being," not "doing." When the therapist can succeed in entering into and staying in the present moment, using both the mind and body, the patient is likely to explicitly or implicitly notice that the therapist is truly present—in that moment, and in that space, awake and alert. This kind of presence already validates the whole being of the patient. Level 1 establishes a platform from which the therapist uses the other five levels.

As I pointed out in Chapter 3, the acceptance paradigm involves awareness that reality, in all its elements, is impermanent. Everything that exists in this moment will not exist in the same way in the next moment. Everything changes; everything is transient. This moment is unique; things will never be the same again. Although the recognition of transience can be unsettling, it can also be liberating because it makes each moment precious. To the degree that the therapist, sitting with the patient, maintains awareness of the impermanence of reality, she will treat each moment as full and unique, and the patient is likely to experience the therapist as completely present and genuine, noticing and reflecting the reality of the patient in the moment. This enhances Level 1 validation (awake, alert), Level 2 validation (accurate reflection), Level 3 validation (articulating the unarticulated), and Level 6 validation (radical genuineness). If the moment is full and alive for the therapist practicing awareness of impermanence, the patient also feels that the therapist is present, with her, in that moment.

Next, the acceptance paradigm involves cognizance that everything and everyone is profoundly interconnected. No one is separate and unique, and everyone is made up of everyone else. *Emptiness* refers to this property: that any form (e.g., one's body, one's ideas) is entirely made up other elements, derived from elsewhere, and therefore there is no unique identity, no unique self, no boundaries between different phenomena and different individuals. Accordingly, the therapist maintains an awareness of the profound interrelatedness between the patient, himself, and other contextual entities. The therapist is made up entirely of nontherapist elements, including elements that come from the patient. The patient is made up entirely of nonpatient elements, including elements coming from the therapist. Recognition of this principle weakens or dissolves the boundary between patient and therapist and creates a sense of the two being one. The patient and therapist are not simply fellow travelers on the path of life, next to one another; they are actually intertwined, interdependent, and operate as one as they work together. Validation strategies delivered from this perspective are natural. The patient experiences the therapist as compassionate, concerned, and feels that the therapist "gets it." This deepens the experience of Levels 2 (accurate reflection) and 3 (articulating the unarticulated) validation.

Finally, the acceptance paradigm involves awareness that everything is "as it should be," and that the "world is perfect as it is." The response to everything is "Of course!" This sense of rightness about how everything unfolds deepens the therapist's communication that the patient's behaviors make sense—they make sense based on the past, biology, and on the current context. "Of course" it is this way—it has to be! Validating the person-as-a-whole in this way, or validating any particular behavioral responses, helps the patient to accept himself: "I'm OK," "I can make sense," "My behaviors are understandable," "I'm not the terrible person I thought I was," and "I'm not too fragile to build a life worth living."

As we can see in this brief discussion, the therapist who engages in the principles of acceptance—entering into awareness of the present moment, recognizing impermanence, embracing interrelatedness and emptiness, and maintaining the sense that things are perfect as they are—tends to create a context that is, in itself, validating. Validation strategies, and all levels of validation, flow naturally from this position.

VALIDATION AND THE CHANGE PARADIGM

Validation fits neatly into the acceptance paradigm, flowing naturally from its principles, as we have seen. What is initially not as obvious is that the use of validation in therapy is also crucial when engaging the patient in the principles and strategies of the change paradigm. As discussed previously, validation balances the interventions of the change paradigm in that it "oils the machinery of change." In addition, there are times when validation itself is used to push for change.

Classical conditioning, as discussed in Chapter 4, focuses our attention on a cue, an intense emotion, and a behavioral escape. This model gives rise to strategies to modify or avoid the cue (stimulus control) and to reduce the emotional response to the cue (exposure procedures). These procedures can be transformative but also painful for the patient. Validation of the patient's emotional pain and the difficulty of changing her response are critical to help her engage in the procedures. The therapist who is present, alert, and validating during an exposure procedure fosters a sense of safety and control. And in the special case wherein the therapist validates an aversive primary emotion, leading the patient to stay in contact with the emotion rather than escaping, she may succeed in helping to enhance the patient's ability to experience and modulate that emotion.

Operant conditioning focuses our attention on the stimulus context, a particular behavior, and its reinforcing consequences. During sessions, the therapist is mindful to use validation when the patient is using adaptive behaviors and to avoid validation at the moment the patient behaves maladaptively, because validation typically functions as a reinforcer. In this respect, validation is used a change-oriented strategy, as a contingency procedure to reinforce some behaviors and not others.

The model of cognitive mediation focuses our attention on the way in which certain beliefs or assumptions, in response to an antecedent event, set off certain emotions and actions. We can change the chain of events by identifying and changing certain repetitive cognitive elements. When we validate a particular belief or assumption (e.g., "No wonder you believe that; lots of people do"), we are hoping to strengthen that cognitive element, hoping to modify the patient's cognitive responses. At other times, we deliberately fail to validate a thought, or even deliberately invalidate it, highlighting that it is not credible or useful, hoping to weaken a thought in that person's repertoire. It pays to be mindful of the power of validation to enhance some elements of the chain and weaken others, and this includes the thought elements.

Similarly, as we address skills deficits in the patient's behavioral chain, we validate the causes and conditions of those deficits. Otherwise, highlighting deficits can generate shame and self-hatred. By validating, we help the patient to have a balanced appreciation of the deficit and the need for skills. In that respect, validation can increase motivation and commitment. Furthermore, especially given that we are working with individuals who invalidate themselves due to their prior environments, our validation of their behaviors teaches a nonjudgmental approach by using one. If the patient can adopt a self-validating stance as a result, we have brought about behavioral change through the use of validation. Finally, validation itself is taught as an important interpersonal skill in DBT, used by the patient as one of several skills that help to maintain good relationships, as well as within the teaching of the middle path, in which validation is directly taught as a practice among family members.

VALIDATION AND THE DIALECTICAL PARADIGM

In using the dialectical paradigm to address and resolve opposition and rigid positions, validation plays a vital role. Having found the opposing positions amidst tension, the therapist works to validate the valid kernel of each side. This sets the stage for finding a synthesis of the two sides. While working with the family of a teenage girl whose target behaviors included self-cutting and substance abuse, the sessions were nearly paralyzed by tension. The girl adamantly insisted that her mother was judging her, disapproving of her, in spite of her mother's "proper" behavior in session. The mother was indignant to be accused of being judgmental when she saw her suggestions to her daughter as helpful and supportive. As the therapist, I could see the validity on both sides: The mother clearly intended her suggestions to be objective and helpful, but just as clearly, her tone was subtly and persistently judgmental. When the therapist can see both sides, it is still challenging to find the way to move them toward synthesis. Because the girl was the most distressed, I began by validating her perceptions, saying to the mom, "I don't think you can hear it in your own voice, because you are truly just trying to help, but I hear a distinct tone of restrained disapproval. When you told your daughter that her behavior was different than the other girls at the party, you were probably right in some way, but at the same time it sounded judgmental, as if you were telling her she had done the wrong thing." The girl clearly felt validated by me. She sat up more confidently, and her emotional dysregulation decreased. Meanwhile, her mother looked a bit defeated. I shifted to validating the mother when I spoke to the daughter, saying, "As much as I can hear the judgment in your mother's voice, I really don't think she realizes it. It looks to me as if she just wants to help you avoid painful reactions from your friends." Finding the validity on each side and articulating them moved the conversation toward a possible synthesis: The mother was doing her job as a parent to help her daughter behave in more effective ways, but she presented her observations in a tone that sounded judgmental. The daughter was trying to establish greater independence and self-respect, and understandably challenged her mother, but while doing so she dismissed the mother's constructive intentions. From there we could work toward a way of interacting that honored both sides.

This process works the same way when there is tension between patient and therapist. The therapist, taking an objective view of the interaction, tries to validate the patient's position, opposed as it might be to that of the therapist. Once the patient feels understood and is likely to be better regulated, the therapist can move to identify the validity in his position: "Knowing what I know about you [Levels 1–3 validation], I can certainly understand your urge to refuse completing the diary card. It makes complete sense to me [Level 4 validation]." Beyond that, it's pretty common for patients to want to avoid the diary card, for lots of reasons (Level 5 validation): "If I were you, I might want to refuse it too. At the same time, I need the information that comes to me from the diary card. There is no other way to get it as accurately, and it all goes to making a better therapy." The stage is now set for the two parties to find a synthesis.

Dialectical thinking is systemic and holistic, recognizing the complex interaction among all parts. Every entity is part of a larger whole, interconnected with other entities. Every entity has within it smaller parts, which are interconnected as well. When we validate one individual in a group or family, we may unwittingly invalidate another person in the same meeting. It is almost inevitable. Similarly, when we validate one phenomenon in an individual patient, such as his thought, emotion, or action, we may be simultaneously invalidating another thought, emotion, or action. For instance, if a child is bullied at school and runs away crying, we might validate her for leaving the scene. It makes sense. However, in some cases, we may be simultaneously invalidating another aspect of the child. By validating and reinforcing the urge to flee, we may be invalidating the child's capabilities for staying and standing up to the bully. This is actually not so unusual. There are always so many trends running in parallel, that to effectively validate one we may need to remain cognizant of others that coexist. This could lead to validation of one phenomenon, then another, in sequence.

Dialectical thinking promotes the awareness of transactions. There is no such thing as a person or a behavior outside of a transaction. There is no such thing as an intervention that solely and purely targets one entity. A change in one thing causes a change in another. If I am in a relationship with you, and I change, then you change. If I am feeling that my life is terrible, and then something worse happens to you, my life might not feel as bad. When we validate one individual, it will have an impact on other individuals. When we validate one aspect of a person, it will have a ripple effect on other aspects.

I was seeing a mother and her two boys in family therapy. Life had been unkind to them in recent years. When I saw them, each one seemed to be harshly judging the others. None of the three seemed to be able to validate either of the other two, as if each one were fighting for his or her life. When I validated one of the boys, immediately the other boy pointed out that I was not seeing his brother "for who he really is." When I validated the mother regarding the difficulty of parenting under undue stress, each boy countered what I had said by explaining that his mother was exaggerating her problems to get my sympathy. To be effective I had to take the transaction into account. In fact, I decided to meet each of them individually, to find the validity in the perspective of each before bringing them back together. And I tried to find ways to validate each of them that would not in some way invalidate the others. It was a challenge, and it was also an excellent example of the importance of seeing the dialectics of validation.

In validating, we are wise to remain aware that everything is always in flux. Everything just changed, and everything is about to change. Validation is an intervention for the moment, recognizing something valid right now and communicating it. The entity to validate might not be present in the same form a minute from now, and once validated, the validated entity is no longer the same. If we plan on validation in advance, which is a reasonable strategy in many cases, we still need to adapt the timing and nature of our validation to the circumstances of the moment. A given validation belongs in this moment, and we cannot expect that moment to last. And we need not forego an opportunity to validate due to our fear that we will be reinforcing something that happened earlier. On my inpatient DBT unit one morning, a patient lost control of her anger and threatened to hurt another patient. It was a dramatic and frightening moment. Later on the same day, that patient was noticeably kind to another patient in a meeting. The staff member in that meeting wanted to validate the patient's ability to accurately understand and help a fellow patient, but she withheld that intervention, fearing that if she were to validate the patient she would somehow be condoning the patient's threatening behavior earlier that day. In fact, it is best for the patient if we address the problematic behavior with interventions, including consequences, when it happens, and then be open and ready to respond to later behaviors with appropriate interventions, including validation.

Most therapists are convinced that they understand how to validate. But in all of my experience as a trainer and a supervisor, the most common shortcoming of therapists when validating is the failure to give 100% acceptance while validating. In other words, the therapist tries to validate a patient's response, but fearing that it will somehow undermine the push toward behavioral change, will be slightly withholding. Validation is most effective when it is done all the way. For that moment, the therapist should give the "pure gold" of validation, total acceptance, and then if behavioral change is needed, to give 100% to that agenda in another moment. To try to balance the two dilutes the efforts toward both. Dialectics is not the same as a compromise; it involves a commitment to the act of acceptance, all the way, and a commitment to change, all the way. It is the essence of dialectics in DBT.

CONCLUDING COMMENTS

Validation is the purest manifestation of the principles of the acceptance paradigm in DBT. Whereas most people think that validation is a completely familiar concept and practice, in fact it is much more complex. Its complexity becomes obvious when we use it in psychotherapy to treat individuals with emotional dysregulation, a history of pervasive invalidation, and a tendency toward self-invalidation. In this chapter, I have reviewed and illustrated many technical aspects of validation—functions, definitions, targets, and levels—and then considered the ways in which validation plays a role in the implementation of all three paradigms in DBT. Maintaining awareness of the principles of all three paradigms leads to greater appreciation of the opportunities and constraints of validation, and to a higher level of accuracy, fluidity, and effectiveness.

CHAPTER 13

Dialectical Strategies

To set the stage for this discussion of using DBT's dialectical strategies, it should be stressed that the three core paradigms each provide a unique source of power that can be harnessed in concert to help the patient change her life, to get a life worth living. The change paradigm provides the *power of purpose*. Guided by this paradigm, we identify the goals and targets that we want to increase or decrease; secure a commitment to the goals, targets, and treatment methods; assess the controlling variables of each target behavior; and arrange for the patient to self-monitor the target behaviors. We teach new skills, reinforce old skills, structure treatment to reinforce functional behaviors, extinguish and punish dysfunctional behaviors; we modify problematic assumptions and beliefs; and through exposure procedures we help the patient approach cues and emotions that have been avoided. The therapist relies on discipline, direction, accountability, and discrepancy monitoring to make use of the change paradigm. Irreverent communication strategies support the change paradigm, as does the therapist's bias toward using consulting-with-the-patient strategies rather than intervening in the environment on behalf of the patient. As we have discussed, however, the change paradigm is necessary but insufficient to succeed in the work with chronic and severe emotional dysregulation.

The acceptance paradigm adds the *power of presence*. We fully utilize the riches of being in the present moment, seeing and accepting things as they are, without judgment, without destination, noticing the interdependency and the impermanence of all phenomena, and understanding that because everything is caused by all that came before, all is as it should be. By seeing things fully in this present moment, our awareness sharpens, compassion flows naturally, and patience expands. From this paradigm flows DBT's strategies of validation, reciprocal communication, and under certain defined circumstances, intervening in the environment on behalf of the patient rather than simply consulting the patient. By combining change and acceptance paradigms, the options for intervention are multiplied. Still, treatment can often grind to a halt. Pushing for change often aggravates, frustrates, and invalidates the patient, resulting in pushback, stalemates, and relationship disruptions. Communicating only acceptance, however, could spawn hopelessness and despair in the patient who feels that the therapist is not helping him to change.

Augmenting and potentiating *the power of purpose* and *the power of presence* is the dialectical paradigm, which adds the *power of improvisation*. Bolstered by the understanding that this moment, however terrible, is but a brief moment in a never-ending flow of time; that the current painful and stubborn phenomenon, however consuming and depressing, is dynamically interdependent with a multitude of contextual factors; that the current trajectory, however destructive, is but one trajectory in transaction with many others; and that truth comes about through the synthesis of opposites rather than the triumph of one; the DBT therapist has access to a range of improvisational strategies. The dialectical strategies exponentially multiply the avenues for intervention toward synthesis, movement, speed, flow, and creative solutions. Dialectical strategies provide a range of maneuvers that can help break the logjam of the moment and get things moving again.

The therapist can employ the specific dialectical strategies in a flexible, fluid, and creative manner if she simultaneously remains aware of the principles of the dialectical paradigm. She can combine these strategies, since in principle they overlap one another. She can float among them and even develop new ones for the same purposes. We can see an analogy in language acquisition in humans: Because of children's intuitive and biologically based grasp of the deep structure and rules of language (cf. the principles), they can create verbal constructions that adapt to the moment and that they have actually never heard before. As we consider each of DBT's designated dialectical strategies, and an additional two that I find useful, we can note the relationship to the principles and the overlap with one another, still recognizing that each strategy provides its own unique dialectical "flavor" that might be best suited for a particular stalemate in treatment. While considering the various strategies, keep in mind that these are not intended as behavioral change strategies; instead, they augment the problem-solving enterprise by creating movement, speed, and flow and by shifting trajectories and creatively unbalancing certain rigid predicaments. After listing all of the dialectical strategies from the treatment manual, I begin with the most straightforward application of dialectical principles, the strategy of balancing treatment strategies.

1. Balancing treatment strategies
2. Making lemonade out of lemons
3. Eliciting wise mind
4. Playing devil's advocate
5. Extending
6. Entering the paradox
7. Allowing natural change
8. Using metaphor
9. Using dialectical assessment

BALANCING TREATMENT STRATEGIES

We begin with the most straightforward application of dialectical principles: balancing treatment strategies. In particular, this strategy refers to the pairing of an acceptance-oriented strategy with a change-oriented one, either simultaneously (in parallel) or sequentially in close temporal proximity. We utilize the natural opposition between acceptance and change that is inherent in reality. Beyond this specific strategic maneuver, the synthesis of pure acceptance with pure change is the underlying theme throughout all of the dialectical strategies.

I once worked with a patient who, upon entering my office for each session, would stand near the door and refuse to sit down until announcing that she was enraged with me, that she hated something I had said or done (or not said or not done). Typically, she concluded by insisting that she could not go on working with me until the disruption was resolved. Although her anger was often understandable given the incidents she mentioned—I could imagine that what I had said might have offended her, hurt her feelings, or disappointed her—the extreme nature of her response often seemed disproportionate with the relatively mild severity of my offense. Her comments were dramatic. It felt "over the top," dramatic, and did not offer the kind of angry expression that could lead to discussion. Her manner blocked engagement or resolution.

I first used several change-oriented strategies sequentially. I highlighted the problematic nature of her communication and clarified that even if she were technically correct about me, her behavior, rather than opening a door to dialogue, was closing it. I invited her to start over and express her feelings but with a more skillful approach. I tried to ascertain what her objective was in shouting at me. I sharply insisted that she stop talking to me that way and asked that she sit down and tell me how she felt. I tried to reinforce any effort she made to engage with me in problem solving. I wondered aloud what kinds of thoughts or assumptions informed her intense presentation. I asked her to observe and describe her feelings as accurately as possible. These efforts produced almost no increase in collaboration, skillful communication, or self-reflection. She was not open to inquiry or change; she expressed her conviction that I had injured her, which made her response entirely appropriate, and suggested that I should never do it (whatever it was) again or else she could not work with me.

Making no progress in change-oriented problem solving, I pivoted decisively to the principles and strategies of the acceptance paradigm. I temporarily "let go" of the change agenda; I tried to validate her responses to me, and I communicated with warmth, genuineness, compassion, and a measure of self-disclosure. I just listened to her, tried to remain present, and paid careful attention to her words, gestures, facial expression, tone of voice, and my own private responses. I made sure not to counter her or suggest that she needed to change anything in her approach. I did what I could to allow her to express herself from beginning to end, with the hope that if she felt heard and understood, her emotional reactivity would decrease and she would act more skillfully. Instead, her hyperbolic statements continued, as if she were impervious to validation. It seemed to me almost as if her emotions were intensified. Then she suddenly withdrew into a shell, sitting quietly and hopelessly opposite me.

Pushing for change had aggravated her further. Letting go of change and using several levels of validation had aggravated her further. I was stymied. This is the kind of circumstance that had led Linehan to import dialectical thinking and strategies into DBT. Acknowledging that we were stuck, I tried to find a synthesis of the use of change and acceptance strategies in the moment, improvising as I went. I find it difficult to name the steps by which one weaves together acceptance and change in a moment like this. I have no formula other than to remain attuned to the patient, truly accept the patient's reactivity without judgment, maintain the conviction that things have to change, and proceed with an open mind. I continued this stance for another two sessions, both of which began in the same dysfunctional way. Finally, at the beginning of the third such session I found, by trial and error, the "sweet spot": an intervention that synthesized acceptance and change and that was more fruitful. I began the session in a more relaxed state of mind, perhaps more willing to improvise, and without a script in mind. I had arrived at a place in my feelings about her that was both compassionate and firm. As she stood in the doorway, raging at me again, seeming to be utterly exasperated with me and at the same time somewhat removed or detached, I spoke to her sharply. "I want you to sit down, right now, and listen to me. I have something to say to you." She acted as if caught by surprise, perhaps even a little frightened by me. She stopped her rant and sat down. I continued. "You are doing it again. You enter the session, having had no contact with me since last session, you stand at the door, and you vent at me. It's almost like a cartoon of rage. You do it in a kind of detached way, as if you and I don't have a real human relationship. You know what? We *do* have a relationship, and apart from these episodes it's a really good one. I treat you like a person and you treat me like a person; you are really smart and really likeable, and it's just really good. But when you get upset with me—which is fine—and you start the session like you did today, it's like something totally different, something almost unreal. Do you know what I mean?"

She was stunned and did not speak at first. Then she asked, "Is it really like a cartoon?" I answered, "It really is. When you talk to me that way it's as if you are talking to me like I'm some kind of inhuman object. You talk *at* me, not *with* me. I know there are plenty of reasons to be upset with me—I'm not denying that, and I'm not telling you to suppress those reasons, but I am just asking you to recognize that there is another person here with you, someone who feels, thinks, cares, and reacts. I just want you to talk with me that way."

We then proceeded in a more human and connected way. Over time we were able to assess her "cartoon-like rage," which, as it turned out, helped her to escape from persistent shameful feelings that something was really very wrong with *her*. As I reflect on my intervention, I think it worked because I found a way to ask firmly for behavioral change while at the same time remaining human, genuine, and caring. I was able to insist on improving our relationship in the context of highlighting how good our relationship already was.

More often than not, *balancing treatment strategies* is simpler than this example, fortunately. For example, the therapist might say, "I realize that you feel the way you do, and it makes a lot of sense [validation]; but I want you to express it in a different way, in a way that works [asking for change]." The rapid or simultaneous juxtaposition of acceptance and change is often all that is called for and helps to find that middle ground that speaks to the individual's need for both acceptance and change simultaneously. Whether it is a challenging example or an easier one, I am convinced that the secret to this strategy of *balancing treatment strategies* is that the therapist has one foot solidly grounded in acceptance, the other foot solidly grounded in change, and remains in good contact with the patient.

MAKING LEMONADE OUT OF LEMONS

Even before therapists study DBT, most are familiar with this dialectical strategy. *Making lemonade out of lemons* is a ubiquitous proverb in our culture, referenced when we look for the opportunity in a crisis; other metaphors for this same idea include finding the silver lining of a dark cloud, or the saying that "when one door closes, another one opens." Whichever the metaphor, it represents a spirit of hope by reframing a negative experience or seeing it from another angle. Given the transactional nature of reality and the systemic point of view that is part of dialectics, we can always see that one phenomenon is in transaction with another. A negative perspective is in transaction with a positive one; a narrow perspective is in relationship to a broader one.

In DBT, opportunities abound for *making lemonade out of lemons*. With the patient who refuses to fill out a diary card, the therapist might begin with assessment, move on to validation of the desire to avoid the diary card, and then move on to problem solving the controlling variables associated with diary card noncompliance. If the pattern remains, the therapist might "go dialectical," making *lemonade out of lemons*: "Actually, it's just perfect if you continue to not do the diary card, because we can just do 'diary-card-therapy' as long as necessary. Since doing diary cards is so similar to so many other uninteresting but essential tasks in life, any progress we make on the diary card problem might help you in other areas." Notice that in this strategy, the therapist conveys acceptance and endorsement of the patient's problem behavior along with a patient but relentless insistence upon change.

So often the impasse, roadblock, or paralysis takes place within a constricted, narrowed, and stifling view of momentary reality, as if the individual were in a very small room with no doors or has crawled down a tunnel and gotten stuck. The therapist recognizes and "accepts" the patient's constricted view, but then communicates a broader perspective on space, time, and/or context. The therapist might feel what it is like for the patient to be in the small room with no doors, or stuck in the tunnel unable to move further, but the therapist is not actually limited to that perspective. He can maintain the awareness that this moment is just one passing moment in time, however terrible. He can realize that there are actually a number of doors through which the patient could get out of the small room. As convinced as the patient may be about her constricted view of reality, the therapist realizes that she is in transaction with him, and that he (and others) thinks quite differently. He knows that there are many ways to get out of the trap, and he trusts that the patient's narrow view will be altered as it interacts with a wider view. When the patient gets to the point of seeing only "lemons," the therapist can imagine a number of varieties and recipes for "lemonade."

Solving painful problems with patients—suicidal behaviors, dissociative episodes, therapy-interfering behaviors, substance use behaviors, and so on—always has a silver lining in that it encodes the memory of solving a difficult problem, which can serve as a platform or template for future problem-solving efforts. Repairing a terrible disruption in the therapeutic relationship can augur a stronger therapy relationship and an enhanced skill set for solving other relationship problems. Arriving late to therapy offers the opportunity to solve lateness or to learn from it. The painful experience of losing a boyfriend or girlfriend can open up the possibility, in some cases without precedent, of learning how to cope without relying completely on another person. The list goes on and on, and if a therapist has a *lemonade-out-of-lemons* mentality, it can be interpolated naturally, fluidly, almost seamlessly into the therapeutic interaction in a way that allows for continued movement and improvisation.

A potential problem with this strategy is that it is too easy to use. The therapist can become facile in pointing out the potential "lemonade": It can sound almost trite and therefore prove to be less effective. Sometimes this strategy serves a self-protective function for the therapist, who finds a way to frame and deflect the patient's pain, without really having absorbed the degree of the pain. Two deliveries of the same exact words in applying the lemonade-out-of-lemons strategy, used in the same context with the same patient, but by different therapists, can come across completely differently. In one case, the effort to extract opportunity from crisis blocks the therapist's appreciation of the suffering; the patient then feels as if the therapist is treating him in a trivializing and dismissive fashion. In the case where the therapist clearly has "gotten it"—has "crawled into hell" with the patient and can see how bad it is—she can deliver the same "opportunity-from-crisis" intervention, and the patient, sensing the compassion, is more willing to consider another angle. In using dialectical strategies such as these, which have the potential of leaving the patient feeling "tricked" or dismissed, much depends on the depth, the genuineness, and the integrity of the therapist's relationship with the patient—most of which is communicated implicitly and over time.

Some of the most effective uses of the lemonade-out-of-lemons strategy happen without an explicit statement about this approach. The patient might be sharing the depths of her despair, possibly the conviction that suicide is the only way out or that taking street drugs is the only way to survive. The therapist is listening compassionately, nonjudgmentally, serving as a witness to the dark side of the patient's experience. The underlying essence of this strategy is based on the fact that even while taking in the patient's terrible circumstance or despair, the therapist maintains the ability to have a broader perspective, a more hopeful attitude, and a conviction that some kind of meaning or progress can emerge from the circumstance. He believes that successfully navigating the despair could bring the patient valuable tools. In a sense, the therapist is practicing the lemonade-out-of-lemons strategy in his own mind; he opens his heart and mind to the patient's despair but retains the capacity to imagine and to find the lemonade. The lemonade-out-of-lemons strategy need not be spoken as such; if the therapist can experience the "lemonade" while in contact with the patient's lemons, it may provide a wordless dialectical opening that synthesizes despair with possibility.

ELICITING WISE MIND

In a popular American television quiz show, when the contestants are faced with a challenging question and are uncertain of the answer, they can use a "lifeline" and call a friend for help. In DBT, *eliciting wise mind* is the equivalent option. When both the patient and therapist are stuck and don't know which way to turn, the therapist can direct the patient to access his wise mind for a wiser perspective (of course, it is also the case that the therapist can, and should, try to elicit wise mind in himself). Of course, the prerequisite is that the patient has acquired and practiced the skill of *eliciting wise mind*, which is taught in the skills training group and can be taught in individual therapy. The therapist might say something as simple as, "What do you think wise mind would say about this?"

In the middle of a difficult session, my 34-year-old female patient grew very frustrated with me. Nothing seemed to help. She began to stand up, and it was clear she was intending to walk out of the session. Aware that her urge to leave was strong, and that I was not likely to change her mind at that moment, I used *eliciting wise mind* to bring about a brief pause and catalyze further reflection in the moment. I said, "I can see that you are leaving, and I am not going to try to stop you, but can I ask you one thing before you go?"

She shouted back at me, "What!?"

"I just want to know, in deciding to leave, are you in rational mind, emotion mind, or wise mind?"

She was definitive: "You know damn well that I am in emotion mind!"

"Can I ask you one more thing then?"

Again, "What!!!"

"If you were in wise mind, what do you think you would do?"

Her response was immediate: "I would just sit right here and tell you what a fucking asshole you are!"

I just thanked her, and she walked out, albeit with a moment of hesitation. It didn't stop her from walking out of the session, but from my point of view it was a significant step forward, helping her to directly express her anger. We could build on that step later.

This skill is such a perfect antidote to the narrow, rigid, black-and-white thinking process that can easily accompany the mounting pressure and conflict between opposite poles. Dysfunctional behaviors arise out of this kind of stalemate, and eliciting wise mind provides a structured way to "hit the pause button" and invite patients to reach into themselves and find a more complex and thoughtful response. It is as if the patient were saying, "My emotions are very intense, the choices are few, it is an emergency, and I need to shut out complex information and bypass careful thought." And it is as if the therapist is saying, "I understand that your emotions are intense, and your urges are strong, but I want you to pause for just a moment and consider what your 'wise mind response' to this situation would be."

In the middle of a family session, a 15-year-old boy named "Josh" felt himself to be backed into a corner. His mother sat quietly, but his father was angrily accusing him of sneaking out of the house at night to smoke marijuana with his friends, and threatening to ground him for the entire school year. Although there was some truth to his father's suspicions, the boy felt that his father was being unfair. From Josh's perspective, the father was controlling, abusive, and made it nearly impossible to relax at home in the evening. He said that he tried to behave at home, so that his father would not yell at him, and then he needed a "stress outlet," which he found by smoking marijuana. Though Josh's argument was somewhat reasonable, his father grew more incensed, pushing for Josh to reveal where he got the marijuana and where he hid it. Josh escalated as well: "You are a hypocrite! You don't want me to use the one thing that gives me some relief at night, but you drink beer every night!" Each party was escalating, the tension was mounting, and Josh and his dad stated increasingly rigid positions. Dad: "You are going to be grounded for the whole year." Josh: "If you don't want me here, just tell me—I'll just move out and live on the street!" I found myself stuck, unable to find a helpful intervention.

Things were getting worse. I intervened. "Guys! Time out! We're not getting anywhere. These aren't good solutions. They're extreme. I want all of us to pause. You all know what wise mind is from the family skills training. I want us to take a break. Go your separate ways for 5 minutes and do whatever you need to do to contact your wise mind. Then let's come back to this."

It was a difficult intervention to make. I had no idea what the outcome would be. Both the father and son seemed angry with me for blocking their argument. They both looked at me as if the idea of stopping, and locating wise mind, was stupid. These kinds of interventions require that we jump in with both feet and proceed boldly and hopefully, not knowing if they will help, tolerating the doubts of the patient(s). Once we jump into such an intervention, it is best to try to do it "all the way."

Josh asked if he could go for a walk, and I agreed as long as he came back in 5 minutes. The parents each sat silently. The mother looked wistfully out the window. Josh returned in 5 minutes. I thanked him. We resumed. I thanked all of them for trying to make this work, and said that I knew all of them wanted things to work better. I asked if anyone of them had gotten a wise mind perspective. For the first time since the session began, Josh's mother spoke. She was filled with emotion. "I am so sad about how this turns into a fight. I just think we are all scared. We are scared that Josh is making some bad decisions. We just don't want him to ruin his life. We are worried and we don't know how worried to be. And I think it's natural that Josh doesn't want to be controlled; he just wants to make his own decisions. I don't think he really wants to leave home, and grounding him for a year is just too much." She turned to her son, crying: "Honey, we love you so much. I'm sorry things don't feel comfortable at home. We just don't want you to make bad decisions. And I am just so sad that we are in a battle like this. So sad." Her honesty was disarming. She turned to her husband. "Honey, I know you love Josh, but sometimes I think you are trying to control him a little too much. You and I had way more independence when we were his age; no one was watching us that closely. We made our mistakes. He needs to make some of his own mistakes." While the disagreement continued, the pause and the mother's balance and genuineness cooled the flames and set the stage for a more productive negotiation.

Although we usually emphasize what the intervention can do to help the patient find balance and synthesis, it is at times just as valuable for the therapist. By trying to *elicit wise mind*, allowing some time and space in the middle of a stuck moment, therapists also get a chance to pause, step back, and try to locate their own wise minds. Mindfulness is pervasively valuable in DBT for the regulation of both patients and therapists, and *eliciting wise mind* is the dialectical technique to insert mindfulness into the present heated moment.

PLAYING DEVIL'S ADVOCATE

With this strategy, the therapist surprises the patient by advocating for the "devil's position." Just as the patient is advocating for the pro-treatment position, saying what she thinks the therapist wants to hear, the therapist takes the opposite position. It commonly comes up when the therapist and patient are discussing whether the patient is willing and ready to commit to the treatment program or to a particular expectation within treatment. Frightened and daunted by the prospect, the patient initially refuses to commit. The therapist uses commitment strategies to win a commitment from the patient. Suddenly the patient appears to overcome her doubts, saying something like, "OK, I'll do it, I'll commit to treatment for the next year to give up self-harm and suicide. OK? I'll do it." In spite of the apparent momentum in the direction of commitment, the therapist has her doubts. After all, isn't this the patient who, just minutes ago, could not imagine making a commitment? Isn't this the patient who, in spite of claiming to commit now, has in the past been unable to stick to such intentions? And doesn't it feel a little bit like the patient is just saying the words in order to get the therapist off her back? The therapist turns the tables. She jumps to the other side and challenges the patient's stated willingness. "Are you really sure you want to get into this? Are you remembering that this is going to be difficult, one of the hardest things you've ever done? Are you sure you don't want to take some more time before signing on to something like this?" If it works, the patient then says something like, "I have to do it—things are really bad in my life and I have little choice." The therapist has strengthened the patient's commitment by playing the *devil's advocate*.

This dialectical strategy must be used with subtlety and savvy. The therapist, recognizing that the patient is superficially resolving ambivalence by claiming to commit, divides herself in two: the part that wants to reinforce any flickers of commitment, and the part that challenges the depth of the commitment. The therapist would be unwise to accept the patient's statement of commitment if it seems overstated. On the other hand, if the therapist simply argues successfully against commitment, she might convince the patient it will be too hard. The therapist has to find the middle path between these two positions. The patient must perceive that the therapist is arguing against making a commitment, but at the same time sense that the therapist is on the side of promoting commitment.

Although commonly used in the service of strengthening commitment, *devil's advocate* can also be used in other contexts. I saw a young man who lived with his parents and had never lived on his own; one of the targets of treatment was to establish an independent life. He repeatedly claimed that he wanted to be autonomous of his parents, but he did not take the needed steps to make it happen. Following his lead, I worked with him to solve the problems, but we made no progress to get him to live outside his parent's home. I validated his fears of independence and avoidance of the steps he needed to take. Still, there was no movement. Meanwhile, his parents were in conflict with each other about their son's dependence on them, and they were often arguing. Realizing how stuck we were, I switched over to the *devil's advocate* strategy. I argued that he should put aside his hopes of independence for the time being. "I have come to realize that your intentions to move out come at a bad time for your parents. They are arguing a lot, they seem unhappy together, and I think they need you at home to mediate their conflicts. Their problems could take years to resolve, if ever, but as their son it is your job to help them out."

He immediately argued back: "But you are asking me to put off my life to help them, and we don't even know if it will help."

I kept advocating for the "devil": "Yeah, I hear what you are saying, but can't you just stay with them at least another couple of years so they can get their feet on the ground?"

He responded, "but that's 2 years of my life, and I've already been there forever." By turning the tables, arguing against independence, his resolve to move out was strengthened. He was then in the position to convince me that he *should* move out, which provided more momentum than before. One might raise a question about this kind of paradoxical intervention in DBT. After all, as his therapist I actually did not want to have him stay with his parents for another 2 years for their sake. It sounds as if it is antithetical to the radically genuine stance that characterizes DBT. The problem is relatively minor if in fact (1) the therapist cares about and respects the patient, (2) sees the outcome as very important, and (3) has run out of other interventions to effect the outcome. It is a manipulative intervention, turning the tables to get the patient to reconsider his avoidance of moving toward independence. Any damage to the integrity of the relationship can be repaired after the fact if the therapist's heart is in the right place. Occasionally there is a tension, a dialectic, between two priorities of DBT; in this case the priority on accomplishing the agreed-upon goal is in the service of building a life worth living, and the priority of being radically genuine. The synthesis is to be radically genuine in *playing the devil's advocate* based on deeply caring about the patient's life.

Having reviewed four of the dialectical strategies, it is clear that each offers a different flavor of the same intervention. In each case, when we get stuck in the therapy, we recognize that current reality is made up of opposing, contradictory elements. Any energy toward therapeutic movement is cancelled out. By shifting our position, where we stand in relation to the polarization—by *balancing treatment strategies, making lemonade out of lemons, eliciting wise mind,* or using the *devil's advocate*—we disrupt the rigid polarization, liberating energy and movement, which then can hopefully result in a new and more workable reality. I continue to demonstrate this formula in different ways in the remaining dialectical strategies.

EXTENDING

It is but a short step from *devil's advocate* to *extending*. Both of them are applied to a situation in which the patient is stuck in a nonproductive or destructive pattern. In both of these dialectical strategies the therapist jumps to the unexpected side of the argument. The therapist uses *extending* when he is working with a situation in which the patient issues some kind of threat to engage in a problematic behavior. For example: "I want to quit treatment right now"; "I don't want to go to work any more"; "I want to kill myself"; "I should just stop fighting my cravings and let myself get as addicted as I want." But the therapist has the impression that the patient is not actually, deeply committed to those pathological positions. His hunch is that the patient is using threats as a way to express strong feelings. The patient says, "I want to quit therapy," but the therapist senses that this is not the true intention but is a dramatic communication of displeasure with the therapist. The patient says, "I think I need to spend a few days in the hospital," but the therapist senses that this "threat" is a way of asking the therapist to take his distress more seriously. The patient is challenging the therapist and expects the therapist to oppose, or at least to question, the threats: "You don't really want to quit therapy" or "I don't think you need to go into the hospital—let's work on some other way to build security." But having already tried straightforward problem solving and validation, the therapist takes a surprising stance, *extending* the patient's threat beyond what was stated. "Oh, you want to quit therapy with me? OK, I have a list of referrals; let's find you a good therapist." Or: "You need to spend some time in the hospital? Let's look at a long-term setting—maybe that is the way to get your needs met." If the therapist has accurately assessed the situation, the patient is likely to object to the therapist's proposal of extending the threat beyond the patient's comfort zone. "You know I don't want to quit therapy with you! I'm just really angry at you." Or: "I don't need to spend a long time in the hospital! I need to have more support in my life!" If the therapist finds the right balance, accepting and *extending* the patient's threat while implicitly challenging that threat, taking a more dysfunctional position than the patient takes, it may result in the patient's arguing for a more functional position. By shifting the alignment of forces between dysfunction and functionality, new opportunities might come into view. As I addressed regarding the apparent sacrifice of radical genuineness in the use of *devil's advocate, extending* is also manipulative. Again, the manipulative aspect seems necessary if other interventions do not help, and if done with heartfelt concern and respect for the patient, the negative consequences to the relationship are easily repaired.

Extending is not always an appropriate response to threats or dysfunctional intentions. If the patient is not ambivalent about the threat, then *extending* it might just reinforce the dysfunctional response. In the context that calls for the use of extending, the therapist should be aware of two elements: (1) the patient communicates a manifest threat or dysfunctional intention, but (2) the manifest threat functions to communicate yet disguise a latent agenda. For instance, the manifest threat might be to quit therapy; the underlying agenda might be the communication of anger at the therapist. Or, the manifest threat might be a 15-year-old patient's announcement that she is leaving home to live on the streets; the underlying agenda is to communicate that she is not being taken seriously or cared for at home. If the therapist simply works with the manifest threat with problem-solving strategies, she misses the latent agenda and perpetuates the stalemate. If she tries to address the latent agenda directly—"I guess you are angry at me and that is why you are threatening to leave me"—the patient denies it and strengthens the manifest threat. By *extending* the threat, the therapist is appearing to support and even amplify the manifest threat, but is actually precipitating an imbalance by turning the tables. If it works correctly, the patient can now state the underlying agenda. The therapist says, "Yes, let's get you out of that house and on your way; shall we look at some homeless shelters where 15-year-olds can live?" The patient is caught by surprise, stops arguing for leaving home, and might counter, "I don't really want to leave home! I just hate it there!" Now the therapist and patient can shift to problem solving about the home environment.

If the therapist is understandably frustrated with the patient and has become emotionally dysregulated and out of balance, *extending* can misfire. The suggestion to the patient that she do something even more pathological than she is threatening to do can feel like a rejection and a trick by the therapist. This strategy, like other dialectical strategies as well as DBT's irreverent communication strategies, should be used by a therapist who is grounded in compassion and regard for the patient, feels emotionally balanced at the time, and can accurately read the patient's ambivalence.

ENTERING THE PARADOX

The preconditions for effectively using this next strategy are that (1) the patient is stuck in a rigid pattern of thought, action, and/or emotion; and (2) the therapist, looking from a broader perspective, can see an alternative, even contradictory, way to understand the patient's rigid pattern. Then the therapist reframes the patient's rigid pattern, usually in a matter-of-fact manner, without further explanation, which strikes the patient as absolutely wrong or impossible. For instance, I worked with a hospitalized patient who, although determined to give up her self-cutting behavior, was unsuccessful in doing so. In explaining why she could not give up the behavior, one factor she cited was that she could not bear the loneliness of managing life independently. Her rigid conviction was that she "should" be independent, which would mean handling everything all by herself. I said to her, "Your courage is admirable, but don't you know that in order to be truly independent, you have to be able to depend deeply on others?" She was quiet, and looked rather puzzled or confused. As tempted as I was to explain what I meant, I remained quiet. The value of this strategy depends in part on allowing patients to sit with their confusion during that moment. I had not really said anything confusing, startling, or paradoxical; it is simply true that we all become more independent after having been successfully dependent on others. But to the patient, it seemed paradoxical in that moment. She was stuck in the commitment to doing something totally by herself, and my statement reframed her belief in a surprising way.

The therapeutic intervention does not create a paradox; it creates an awareness of already being in one. To reiterate, part of what makes this intervention work to unbalance the situation and create movement is that the therapist delivers it in a matter-of-fact manner, without further explanation. The point is not to teach the patient some piece of information; the point is to create imbalance and movement. And the dialectical principles from which the therapist draws are that (1) reality consists of oppositions, (2) everything is transactional (i.e., one person can undermine another person's interpretation by reframing it), and (3) change is constant.

In another example of *entering the paradox*, let's say that the patient, following the therapist's instructions, telephones him between sessions for skills coaching in the face of crises. The calls have become frequent and extreme in number. Furthermore, the patient uniformly ignores all of the therapist's suggestions during telephone coaching. The therapist becomes frustrated and points out the problem to the patient. The patient, realizing that the therapist is asking her to be more cooperative, feels insulted. Realizing that he has hurt the patient's feelings, the therapist makes an effort to validate the hurt feelings. Still, the patient remains angry, continues to make frequent phone calls, and does not change the problematic behaviors. Things are stuck. Realizing this, and turning toward a dialectical intervention, the therapist can use *entering the paradox*. Conveying a mixture of acceptance and change at the same time, the therapist says, "I care too much about you to let you continue to make the phone calls the way you do, so I am asking you to stop making the calls." Of course, there is no deep contradiction here: The therapist does care about the patient, and he does need to limit the rather ineffective phone calls in order to preserve the relationship. But the fact that the patient is immersed in the conviction that she needs to make all of the calls, and is momentarily unaware of the broader perspective, means that it is a paradox for her: "If you care about me, how can you take something away?" She is confused, puzzled, off-balance; there is a disequilibrium, and something different can happen. One way to think about dialectical interventions is that they catalyze or allow a change in the usual (stuck) script.

ALLOWING NATURAL CHANGE

This strategy provides yet another (potentially) therapeutic response to the moment when opposites are colliding. We typically use this dialectical strategy when there is disagreement or tension around the conditions of treatment. Perhaps the patient feels the sessions are too long, too short, too infrequent, or too frequent. The patient, especially an adolescent, may find that sitting in an office, facing a therapist and talking, is oppressive. A patient may want to give the therapist a gift, the therapist may refuse the gift, and the patient feels painfully rejected. The patient might want to deviate from the typical agenda of sessions, and the therapist wants to stick to that agenda. I once worked with a young woman whose target behaviors included shoplifting, self-cutting, and the use of hallucinogenic drugs. She acknowledged that all of them were bad for her, but she did not want to talk about them. I insisted that we assess the factors maintaining each of these behaviors. She thought that my methods were "old school," based on "limited concepts" about how she functioned, and she insisted that she would do what she needed to do to stop the behaviors. She wanted to talk about her music and her interest in "dark arts." Our struggle persisted for a couple of sessions. I felt that she might be too stubborn to treat; she felt that I was too rigid and controlling. She revealed her secret conviction that she was an oracle and that she could cure herself; she just needed me to listen to her. We were in a stalemate. I decided to *allow natural change*. I told her that she could determine our session agenda, and she could report her findings as an oracle, as long as she reported to me each week about her shoplifting, self-cutting, and drug use. She was willing to fill out a diary card that included these targets. In fact, she totally and immediately interrupted the shoplifting and self-cutting; the drug use persisted and we discussed it repeatedly; she was unwilling to see it as a problem behavior: "It opens the doors of my mind to new insights."

I once was working with a 45-year-old woman with borderline behavioral patterns and significant problems with executive functioning. Taking care of her apartment, her car, her dog, and keeping track of her medical and psychiatric appointments was overwhelming for her. She had no job and was living on disability payments. She was forever forgetting and losing things and it made her life nearly impossible to manage. I met with her for the usual once per week for 50 minutes and she attended a DBT skills group. Much of her session time was devoted to the chaos resulting from her self-management problems. It felt to both of us as if once per week was insufficient, but she could not afford twice per week with me even at a significantly reduced price. I suggested that I might be more helpful if we met twice per week, for 25 minutes each time, and focused on helping her to stay on track. She was not happy about signing on for briefer sessions, but agreed to the change. Both of us were surprised how helpful it turned out to be. She was able to use 25 minutes much more efficiently than 50 minutes, and we were able to make progress on her self-management skills with more frequent monitoring and problem solving.

In *allowing natural change,* there is a risk of violating other important principles of DBT, and these factors should be weighed into the decision to do it. Importantly, there is the risk that by resolving conflict through allowing natural change in the conditions of the frame of treatment, the therapist might be reinforcing avoidance. For a therapist to insist on consistent timing, location, and conditions of sessions is reasonable. If these structures trigger negative emotions in the patient, the therapist would usually be wise not to "remove the cues" in order to alleviate distress. The ideal position for a DBT therapist is to hold to the frame and the treatment model, acknowledge the patient's negative reactions, find the validity in the reactions, and help the patient to adjust to the frame. For the patient to come to grips with realistic expectations can provide a valuable learning opportunity that can be generalized into many life circumstances. So it is important to consider whether we are reinforcing dysfunctional behaviors or providing short-term relief at the expense of long-term avoidance. I have no formula for deciding when to hold to the frame and when to allow natural change; awareness of this potential dialectic allows the therapist to consider the priorities and to make a "wise mind" therapeutic decision. For instance, it was such a decision for me with the aforementioned patient with severe self-management problems to bypass the usual time frame in therapy and to flex toward a different kind of schedule. While I would not want to make a regular practice of altering the frame, this struck me as being in line with her manner of functioning and the immediate treatment targets.

Allowing natural change, although a formally defined dialectical strategy used in certain circumstances, also represents a process that goes on more subtly throughout treatment. In nearly every session during the first stage of treatment we encounter challenging moments, oppositions, contradictions, and moments of rising tension. These commonly pose a momentary challenge, requiring adjustments by the therapist to maintain flow, resolve conflict, and preserve collaboration. The therapist is always deciding about the degree to which to "go with the flow" versus to challenge behavior. The whole treatment is based on the therapist's capacity to define conditions of treatment, hold to those conditions, push for change, accept things as they are, and to find the synthesis of the two in the moment. *Allowing natural change* as a crystallized strategy and as a subtle in-the-moment set of decisions is part of that dialectical enterprise. While relentlessly pushing for change, we also incorporate the message from the Beatles: "Let it be, let it be, let it be, let it be, whisper words of wisdom, let it be."

USING METAPHOR

Another dialectical response to a stalemate is to embed that dialectic in a metaphor or story, in such a way that it catalyzes further thought, movement, and improvisation. Linehan's (1993a) manual is filled with metaphors, and the use of metaphor is an essential part of practicing DBT. Done well, it allows for a more creative and playful process to take place regarding a conflict in which the possibility of solution and movement seems to have ground to a halt. Metaphorically reframing a rigid opposition that depletes both parties can transform and energize. One of my patients was suffering through one emotional crisis after another, and in each case she was insisting that I go beyond my usual practice to rescue her and help her through the moment. She left me messages threatening that if I didn't take further action, such as to come to her, call someone, spend lengthy times on the phone, make special arrangements to see her at hours when I was not available, cancel vacations, and so forth, she could not survive. I told her that my job was to help her learn to swim more and more effectively, even in choppy water or storms when necessary. I was her swimming instructor. And I told her that, in addition, she sometimes needed a lifeguard, when conditions were too rough for her to swim, someone to rescue her so that she could continue. She needed both a swimming instructor and a lifeguard. I explained that if I were her swimming instructor, I could not be the lifeguard. There are lifeguards in the community, as I told her; emergency rooms, crisis hotlines, other resources, and I needed her to rely on those resources so that I could be devoted to helping her learn to swim. She could call me for coaching when entering a crisis to help her to apply her skills, but that was different than calling a lifeguard. The discussion opened the door to a more extended exchange about how her various needs could be met, and what she could expect of me.

Coming up with a *metaphor* for a situation that is too highly charged, complex, or confusing in order to allow for ordinary collaborative consideration can provide the vehicle to clarify matters and to move things forward. As I discussed in Chapter 9 regarding case conceptualization, I have made it standard practice to include a metaphor, in conceptualizing a case, which captures the central dilemmas as I see them. If effective, this metaphor allows the entire team to have an integrative understanding of the case, which promotes dialogue and creativity in problem solving. For instance, on several occasions I have likened the step-by-step treatment plan to a staircase. With the patient, we start on the bottom step and climb, step-by-step, to the top, where there is a life worth living. We define the top step, our ultimate goal, as clearly as possible, and then we define each step on the way to that life. Each step is crucial to the whole climb, and we must focus attention to each step, one at a time. The metaphor represents the tension between focusing attention on the life worth living at the top as well as focusing attention on each step.

In another case, the patient underwent repeated hospitalizations for her suicidal behaviors, even while various community resources were being used to help her build a life outside the hospital. Typically, she improved during a hospitalization, and then she would be discharged to a plan involving several modalities—psychotherapy, psychopharmacology, supported housing, a DBT skills group, a day program or other daily activity, and a crisis plan. Within days or weeks she began to exhibit crisis behaviors in the context of each modality, her suicidal behaviors intensified, and after two or three visits to the emergency room, she was hospitalized again. She was notorious among providers in the region where she lived, and when we met for consultation, there were about 20 providers present, ranging from her therapist, psychiatrist, and group skills trainer to the crisis team, a case manager, her inpatient providers, and even a captain from the local police force. With such a complex treatment arrangement, it proved useful to find a *metaphor* weaving them all together with the patient. Likening the situation to a large game of pinball, the patient was represented by the ball. When the ball rolled to the "lowest point of gravity" at the bottom of the game, it represented the patient's admittance to the hospital and settling in there for a time. The paddles that were activated in order to keep the patient from falling to the low point (hospital) represented the efforts in the emergency room to send her back into the community rather than hospitalizing her. Even if the paddles succeeded in sending her back up onto the game board (community treatment system), she would inevitably fall back to the emergency room, as if pulled by gravity. After a short time in the hospital, she would be "shot" out of the hospital back into the community, where she would bounce around from one provider location to another, as if bouncing off of each of them. Like the movements of the ball in the pinball game, her movements in the community became more intensely driven and hectic. The metaphor allowed each provider in the room to see his or her own part in how the overall pinball machine functioned. Using the *metaphor*, the group was able to discuss options for "changing the game." We had a productive discussion about ways to tilt the game so that the lowest point of gravity, the "resting place," was not the hospital, but was a desirable location in the community. We came up with several ideas, and the metaphor served as a framework and a reference point for months.

The DBT therapist can find a multitude of metaphors throughout the treatment manual and particularly in the chapter on dialectical strategies. But what is more difficult to describe is how a therapist or a team creates one that fits a clinical situation. For some people metaphors come easily, for others, not. The therapist need not dream up metaphors during the session (although it can be helpful if the therapist has that facility). Finding herself stuck in one of her cases, the therapist can present the details to the consultation team and ask if anyone can think of a metaphor to represent the predicament. If possible, the therapist and team find the dialectic(s) that are embedded in the impasse and try to imagine a synthesis of the opposing forces. Armed with a way of describing the oppositions and possible syntheses, a team brainstorming process can search for a picture or a story—an analogy in which similar forces are embedded—ideally a metaphor to which the patient could relate. The athlete could benefit from sports metaphors, the musician from musical metaphors, and so on.

Let's walk through an example. What if the patient communicates suicidal thinking during sessions. The therapist becomes preoccupied with fear about the patient's possible suicide. As a result, the therapist's attention is narrowed, more focused on preventing suicide than on building a viable life for the patient. From the patient's point of view, the suicidal preoccupation serves as a solution, defining a way out of misery. For the therapist, the patient's suicidal thinking is a problem that actually interferes with her therapeutic capacities. How could we state the dialectic? On the one hand, the therapist needs to be able to feel secure and balanced enough to do good therapy, and on the other hand, the patient needs to be able to communicate his pain, distress, and suicidal preoccupations. If the therapist is not balanced and secure, therapy gets worse. If the patient can't communicate the intensity of suicidal feelings, those feelings grow in strength. In search of a *metaphor*, the therapist might look for a similar scene in which she finds one individual trying to help another with his distress, while becoming unbalanced by that very distress. A scene comes to mind in which one person is drowning in a lake and the other person is trying to rescue him. The drowning person, desperate to stay alive, clutches at the rescuer, potentially pulling her under. Both individuals are at risk. Lifeguards learn techniques for approaching the drowning individual and for saving him without being pulled under water. This leap into a metaphor could point the way for a discussion about safe and effective ways to approach and address the patient's suicidal preoccupations without "being pulled under."

In another *metaphor* for the same clinical situation, the team might liken the predicament to the situation in which a suicidal person (the patient) is standing on the ledge of a building, threatening to jump to her death, while the rescuer (the therapist) is leaning out of a window, trying to forge a connection within which the patient feels listened to and understood. If the rescuer can remain safe and remain engaged with the patient, perhaps a safe resolution can be found. In yet another *metaphor* for the same situation, a soldier (the therapist) in a war zone encounters a bomb (the patient's suicidal urges) that could explode if handled insensitively. How could the soldier approach the bomb and disarm it without getting blown up? As you can see, any of these are possibilities and each harbors strengths and weaknesses. To find the "right" metaphor is a needlessly impossible pursuit; a therapist and team can feel the freedom to play, create, and find a metaphor that matches the circumstances.

USING DIALECTICAL ASSESSMENT

The final dialectical strategy in the treatment manual, though perhaps the one driving all others, is that of *dialectical assessment*. When we feel stuck and the usual work of problem solving and validation fails to create movement, we can deliberately ask ourselves, "What am I missing? What is left out of my understanding of the situation?" Having tried various solutions without success, and having grown more frustrated, we sometimes get stuck in our thinking and believe we have exhausted the possible ways to understand the problem. We get convinced that if only we could make a little adjustment, if only we were a little smarter, if only the patient were a little more willing, we would get the change we need. It is as if we were operating a microscope to view something that remains somewhat blurry, but we only use one level of magnification. If we stop, step back at that moment, and ask, "What am I missing? What is left out of the equation?," we might shift to a different level of magnification, opening our eyes to other options of understanding. We might realize that we have not been considering the impact of the therapy relationship, the influence of family dynamics, the role of cognitive impairment or a learning disability, the pressure of an undiagnosed psychotic process, the erosive presence of a medical condition, or a hidden aspect of the patient's environmental context. Maybe we are failing to take into account that the patient never really made a commitment to the work at hand, but we are acting as if he did. Maybe we are overlooking the fact that the patient lacks the skills to accomplish what we are asking, and yet is too ashamed to tell us. Or perhaps the intensity of the underlying shame or fear is greater than we know. Or, in some cases, as beleaguered therapists ask themselves, "What am I missing in this situation?," we might realize that we are not receiving sufficient support from our consultation teams and that we need to ask for more. The possibilities go on and on. We are always missing something—some perspective, fact, dynamic, treatment-related factor—so if we are stuck at an impasse in treatment, we should automatically ask, "What am I missing?" We might not find any satisfying answer, certainly not immediately, but simply to ask the question, and perhaps to change the level of magnification, alters everything and can provide a turning point.

I was working with an individual in her late 30s with anorexia and borderline personality disorder. It seemed that every week she would have another life crisis—housing, relationships, medication, finances, accidents, etc. Session by session, we worked on each one. Any plans she made to improve her life situation were eclipsed by her latest crisis. She would learn skills in the skills training group, but her poor judgment and repetitive crises interfered with practicing the skills. She dated men with severe problems, one of which was usually substance abuse, which ushered in more crises. It became frustrating. Sometimes I felt that we were finally "turning a corner" and collaborating on a good plan. But in each case, another crisis would appear, and our work would be undone. I asked myself the question, "What am I missing?" I spoke with my consultation team about it, and I posed the question to my patient. I wondered aloud with her, "Do you have any idea why we were not making progress?" Her answer was telling. "I think you care more about my progress than I do. I'm not really sure I want to make progress. It is hard to imagine a life that goes smoothly. I think it would be totally stifling." I was completely surprised. She had put on a good show of engagement around identified goals, and I had completely missed her ambivalence about improving. She was then able to articulate a variety of fears of what life would be like if she were to make progress. Suddenly it made sense that she was not likely to make progress unless we addressed her underlying fears of success.

Another way to ask the question "What am I leaving out of my current understanding?" is to ask which relevant links in the behavioral chain we are missing. We can never have awareness of all relevant emotions, thoughts, actions, and environmental events in the chain leading up to and following a target behavior. We can assume that we are missing links— sometimes, important ones, and sometimes the most important link. It keeps us curious, humble, and leads us to understand that while *dialectical assessment* can be particularly helpful when treatment is stuck, it is also a strategy that we use constantly—since things are *always* left out.

If we keep in mind that a dialectical way of thinking is systemic, holistic, and transactional, we can always expand our "field of vision" to include another set of transactions, another subsystem of the larger system, and we might thereby locate the relevant transactions and systemic factors that we have left out. At the very moment that we think we have run out of options, a widening of our "visual field" reveals hundreds or thousands of interconnections that could give way to an intervention.

Sometimes the patient is stuck because of a connection to an important family member who is stuck. I was supervising a therapist who was treating a 15-year-old boy who was refusing to go to school. He didn't seem depressed; he seemed angry. He would not say why he was not attending school. The therapist began meeting with the patient in the context of his family, which included his parents and a younger sister. The boy was silent during the sessions, staring down at the floor in front of him. After two sessions, during which the parents shared their concern, exasperation, and worries about their son, the therapist asked the parents about their own relationship with each other. The father looked down. The mother looked at him and asked why he was looking away. He became quiet. The son looked at the father (I was watching behind a one-way glass). The mother tried to redirect the conversation back to her worries about her son. The husband's withdrawal was obvious and troubling, but the session ended with no real resolution.

At the beginning of the next session, the mother announced that the father had moved into the attic, was not sleeping with her any more, and was not joining in other family gatherings. He started to speak, with an edge of anger toward his wife, then began to cry, and admitted that he felt lost, depressed, and had little hope about the future. As it turned out, he was clinically depressed and was profoundly unhappy about his marriage. Within the next week, the son spontaneously returned to school without saying anything further about it. The son and daughter were dismissed from sessions and the treatment focused on the father's depression and hopelessness and the marriage itself. As it turned out, for reasons that remained unclear, the boy's refusal to go to school appears to have been in transaction with his father's state of mind. We are wise always to maintain humility, remain open to hidden explanations, and realize that the answer to the question "What am I missing?" may pave the way to problem solving.

MAKING UP YOUR OWN
DIALECTICAL STRATEGIES

Once we appreciate that the essential nature of dialectical strategies is to create movement where there was impasse and to find synthesis among opposing forces, we realize that the nine dialectical strategies identified by Linehan (1993a, pp. 199–220) and discussed in this chapter are just a few of thousands of potential strategies. Competent DBT therapists who embrace the underlying essence of dialectical strategies keep movement going in the face of stasis, continue to widen the field of inquiry in reaction to rigidity and narrowing, keep their eyes on the transactional nature of behavioral phenomena, and always continue to ask what is being left out. Such a mindset leads to "being dialectical" rather than just using dialectical strategies.

To illustrate how a therapist might invent and use new dialectical strategies, I mention two here that have worked for me: *drop the rope* and *be the dog*. *Drop the rope* is, of course, a metaphor itself. When I realize that I have fallen into a struggle with a patient in my problem-solving efforts, and that the struggle has become nonproductive and tiring, I imagine that the patient and I are involved in a tug-of-war, each holding opposite ends of a rope and pulling against each other, with neither side winning. Then I simply imagine dropping my end of the rope. Stated more prosaically, I let go of my attachment to my side of the argument. This concept can be found within other dialectical strategies, such as *allowing natural change*. But sometimes I just find it useful, all by itself, to imagine the tug-of-war and to let go of my end of the rope, to see what will happen next.

I was treating a teenage girl who would barely speak during the first 3 months of therapy with me. She actually would talk in the family sessions I held with her and her parents, where I taught skills to them, but not in individual sessions. She sat sideways to me, had long hair, and I almost never saw her face. She always seemed angry and resentful, treated me as if I were ridiculous and useless, and yet she continued to come to sessions—whereas she had dropped out of school. I tried everything I could think of just to get her engaged in conversation, including some of the dialectical strategies. Nothing worked. It was becoming difficult to go on as her therapist. One day I came into the session in a different frame of mind. I just felt that there was no point continuing to try to engage her in dialogue. I just started talking, and told her about something that had happened to me the previous day:

THERAPIST: Yesterday I took my 2-year-old son with me to get the snow tires put on the car. He wanted to watch them as they hoisted the car up and changed the tires. I was standing in the parking lot behind the building, holding him in my arms, as we watched the mechanic do his work. Suddenly, this boy, who was backing up in a car, hit me from behind. I was slammed forward to the ground.

PATIENT: (*Suddenly she turns her head toward me, her hair flies to the side, and I can see her face for almost the first time.*) What happened to your son?

THERAPIST: (*I'm a bit shocked, and I can tell that the question is heartfelt.*) I was very lucky. The guy knew he hit something or someone, and he stopped backing up. I fell forward and hit my knees hard on the pavement. I held my son up as high as I could, and my elbows hit the pavement too. My son was fine. In fact, he thought it was pretty cool that within minutes there was an ambulance, a police car, and a fire truck from next door. They took me in the fire truck and bandaged up my knees, but I didn't have to go to the hospital.

PATIENT: (*She looks cautious, even suspicious, of me.*) Let me see your knees. (*She wants proof.*)

THERAPIST: OK. (*I roll up my pant legs, and, thank God, the bandages were on my knees.*)

PATIENT: (*She acts as if I have passed a test.*) OK.

This proved to be a turning point in the therapy. I tried to figure out what had broken the logjam in that session, so that I could understand the "formula" that got her more engaged. Maybe she felt more comfortable when I spoke with her more like a friend talks with a friend, different than a therapist talking with a patient. Or maybe it made a difference to her that I provided an example in which I was hurt and vulnerable, and in which my son's well-being was in jeopardy. I was never to know for sure, but I knew I had stumbled onto something that worked, and I tried to replicate it. I started the next few sessions talking about episodes from my own life in which I was vulnerable, in which I did things wrong, or in which people close to me were in jeopardy. She noticeably softened in her reactions to me, she sat facing me, and she began to open up about her own life. Within a few weeks we were working on her problems.

I have labeled this dialectical strategy *being the dog*. Rather than thinking of the patient as a dog and myself as a trainer, using learning principles, I thought of myself as the dog and her as the trainer. As the dog, I was looking for reinforcement. Reinforcement came in the form of the patient's willingness to speak with me. As a good "dog," I kept generating new behaviors until one of them was rewarded; then I tried to do more of the same. This strategy, which relies on the principle of opposites—in that I preserve the tension between myself and the patient, but think of myself as the "dog"—also follows from systemic thinking, in that new behaviors arise when roles are reversed. It has served me well in very stuck situations.

DIALECTICAL STRATEGIES IN THE CONTEXT OF THE CHANGE AND ACCEPTANCE PARADIGMS

Naturally, dialectical strategies represent the synthesis of the change and acceptance paradigms. In each one, the therapist is at the same time pushing for change and accepting what is. This is obvious in *balancing treatment strategies*. In *eliciting wise mind*, the "place" for finding synthesis is the wise mind. In *making lemonade out of lemons*, in a manner of speaking the therapist "accepts" the distressing or dysfunctional moment, while at the same time reframing it in an optimistic, change-oriented light. In using both *devil's advocate* and *extending*, the therapist not only accepts the patient's dysfunctional position, but takes it even further, in the hopes that the new imbalance will precipitate the patient's willingness to adopt a more change-oriented position. In *allowing natural change*, the therapist accepts the current alteration of the treatment frame, rather than trying to push it back into place, and in so doing establishes a new frame, which might lend itself better to a push for change. In *entering the paradox*, typically the patient experiences the therapist as siding with her, accepting her, at the same time as "siding against her," insisting that she change. (For instance, "I care too much about you [acceptance] to allow you to continue to make phone calls to me [change].") In *using metaphors*, the therapist finds a way to represent the dialectical tension, usually between acceptance and change, which allows for dialogue and creative discovery of a synthesis. In *using dialectical assessment*, the therapist who finds that she cannot facilitate movement by using either change or acceptance strategies, asks, "What am I missing? in my current understanding, in order to augment the case conceptualization and to open doors for other interventions.

We can understand the maneuvers of dialectical strategies from the perspective of the principles underlying the change paradigm. After all, the intent is to generate change: movement where there is paralysis, synthesis where there is polarization, or a wider perspective when thinking is narrow and rigid. We want to shake things up, even if temporarily, allowing for a new outcome. Whatever the nature of the particular impasse, we can understand it as a segment of a behavioral chain that has become rigid and predictable. If we look at it from the perspective of classical conditioning, we may be inserting a different cue into the equation (e.g., "Are you sure you want to commit to this treatment?"), which then generates a different behavioral response. Or, still within the model of classical conditioning and exposure procedures, we may be blocking the patient's escape from his emotions by eliminating struggle with the therapist (e.g., "Maybe it is best for you to continue to refuse to complete the diary card, so that we can work on that problem").

Or we can view the rigid segment of the behavior chain from the perspective of operant conditioning. In this case, some dialectical interventions remove reinforcement from a particular problem behavior and provide reinforcement for a different response. For instance, by "turning the tables" in using *devil's advocate* or *extending*, the patient who has been reinforced for opposing the therapist's position is now in the confusing position of having to generate pro-treatment behaviors in order to remain in opposition. Reframing things in a surprising or temporarily confusing manner (e.g., in *entering the paradox*), removes the predictable outcome that may have been reinforcing the predictable sequence, opening the door for a change in pattern.

Most dialectical strategies will highlight or challenge a pattern of dysfunctional thinking (cognitive mediation of behavioral change), modeling a new way to think or at least opening the door to one. *Eliciting wise mind* suggests and models that one can refer to one's wise mind to shift a process of thought. *Using metaphor* reframes a thought process that has grown stuck and problematic, and opens doors to new ways to think. *Allowing natural change* suggests that sometimes one can adapt and adjust one's cognitions rather than insist that reality adjust itself to fit one's assumptions and beliefs.

Finally, from the perspective of the change paradigm, the use of dialectical thinking and "finding the middle path" with dialectical strategies can be presented as a skill for a patient to learn. If the patient can understand dialectical approaches "from within," learning to use the skill, it can create more fertile soil for these interventions.

Awareness of the principles underlying the acceptance paradigm shapes the use of dialectical strategies as well. Effective use of dialectical strategies require that the therapist experience a significant degree of freedom along with an attunement to the patient's thinking, both explicit and implicit. For a therapist to be fully present in the moment and to be unattached to what "should be" sets the stage for more freedom and improvisation. For a therapist to "lower the boundary" between himself and the patient in the moment, to sense what is going on in the patient, helps him to find the right wording and balance for delivering dialectical strategies. This is akin to the skill of a good stand-up comic who can accurately read the explicit and implicit responses of the audience. The therapist is further enhanced by letting go of a sense of purpose and direction in the moment, using the strategies to highlight hidden factors or to unbalance the current situation. Once the dialectical strategy has had its effect, it may then be possible to return to problem-solving strategies driven toward targets and goals. Finally, for a therapist to accept that things are as "they should be," even if they are distressing, helps to liberate him from judgmental thinking that can interfere with the optimal nonjudgmental position from which to deliver dialectical strategies.

CONCLUDING COMMENTS

Dialectical strategies are a perfect fit for individuals with severe and chronic emotional dysregulation. The tendency toward rigid thinking and polarizing processes finds its antidote in strategies that help to shake up the status quo, find the wisdom on both sides of an argument, and work toward synthesis. These strategies include *balancing treatment strategies, making lemonade out of lemons, extending, using devil's advocate*, and *entering the paradox*. The tendency toward simple narratives and narrow perspectives is countered by complex, realistic, systemic thinking that comes from a broader perspective. We incorporate systemic thinking through *balancing treatment strategies, eliciting wise mind*, and *using dialectical assessment*. The tendency to become stuck is addressed by the recognition that reality is always in flux and therapy is always moving. The fact that DBT has so many strategic options from which to choose, and that the dialectical strategies in particular provide additional interventions especially designed for stuck situations, makes this therapy workable.

To use these strategies effectively requires something different of us than the effective use of problem-solving and validation strategies. We must encounter stuckness, experience impasse, be "up against the wall," recognize the opposing positions in the dialectic, and in that context, let our minds relax enough to leap to creative interventions that may or may not work. These strategies emerge, at their best, from a sense of freedom in the face of paralysis. I have found it helpful, when experiencing a difficult and polarized clinical encounter, to try out these strategies in my mind or in role plays. There is no substitute for practice and a willingness to try, fail, try again, fail again, learn, and adjust.

CHAPTER 14

Skills and Skills Training

FROM PSYCHOANALYTIC THERAPIST TO SKILLS TRAINER

When I first learned about DBT in the late 1980s, I was intrigued by the skills. Given my 10 years of psychoanalytic practice, I was skeptical regarding the claim that something so "superficial" could truly result in enduring behavior change. Still, I visited Seattle and while sitting behind a one-way glass, I watched Marsha Linehan teach a skills training session to six women with borderline personality disorder. Several things drew my attention. First, in contrast with the objective, technically neutral psychoanalytic stance, she was so warm, direct, and encouraging. She acted very natural, much as she acted with me. Second, while the patients were obviously anxious (it was the first session of a new group), some of them barely able to speak, Marsha was personable and optimistic. She acted as if she were surrounded by ambitious, comfortable, excited students, and she persisted with that tone throughout the group until group members began to loosen up and actually act like interested students. Third, though her style was casual, she was rigorous in teaching skills and insistent that the patients learn them. Her overview of the modules was well organized, precise, and motivating. She balanced her welcoming style with a structured and meticulous agenda. In sum, she blended the empathic and reflective skills of a psychotherapist with the structuring and demanding skills of a good coach.

In retrospect, I realize that seeing Marsha in action opened a door for me. Although I had chosen a career path through psychoanalysis, I

328

had abandoned any efforts to pursue another passion: to coach basketball. Through DBT I could imagine finding my own synthesis of therapy and coaching.

Back in New York, not everyone was so pleased with my new direction. As I mentioned in the Preface to this book, when I attempted to bring DBT elements into my long-term inpatient psychoanalytic psychotherapy program, members of my senior staff forcefully objected to "diluting" our approach. The obstacle was temporary. I was allowed to develop a different inpatient program using the principles of DBT. Our implementation efforts began with learning the skills ourselves and then teaching them to the patients in groups. As we became more adept and confident in teaching the skills, the patients provided positive reviews, reinforcing us to keep going.

The identifiable steps in our journey as we became skills trainers paralleled the steps of skills training itself. *The first step in skills training is skill acquisition, brought about through instruction and modeling.* After teaching ourselves the skills, we worked on ways to instruct them to the patients. We even wrote up a lecture for each skill to make sure we could articulate how to do each one. And we quickly recognized that in addition to instructing the patients, we had to model the skills. We had to show them how to do the skills, or for the skills that are more internal (e.g., mindfulness skills), we had to "talk through" the practice of them. Of course, this meant we had to know the skills from the inside and use self-disclosure in teaching. We watched segments of popular films in which the skills were used, or not. This was not a "seminar" about DBT skills, it was a coaching session punctuated with watching films and modeling the skills ourselves.

We had to get the patients' attention. We learned quickly that our interest in the skills did not necessarily translate into the patients' interest. If they were to acquire the skills, they would have to pay attention, and we realized we had to work hard to get their attention. The content of the skills, wonderful as it was, would not get their attention. It helped when we tried the skills ourselves, applying them to our personal and professional lives. We could then teach with more conviction and sympathy. Still, we often felt like we were a group of bold generals marching our troops up the hill into battle, except our troops lagged back at the bottom of the hill. I thought back to the first group I had witnessed, in which Marsha brought steady, optimistic energy and a sense of ease into a scene filled with moodiness, irritability, reluctance, and frank noncompliance. She gently but steadily pushed her troops toward the top of the hill—supporting them, cajoling them, connecting with them, winning them over little by little. We tried to imitate Marsha, balancing our teaching with charm, entertainment, and humor, and our sense of urgency with infinite patience.

It usually proved deadly to begin a group by saying something like, "Everyone, turn to page 27," or "Tell me what you think of this skill." Responses were stiff and minimal. We were forced to be creative, connected, and even dramatic at times. We learned to introduce the topic of emotion regulation skills by calling for a down-to-earth and personal discussion about emotions in our lives (ours and the patients). We might begin by asking, "Does anyone here have any emotions?" Once we had a down-to-earth discussion about our emotions, we could transition into the teachings. At other times, we tried introducing the Emotion Regulation Skills module by asking everyone to sing a rousing and familiar song, something like "Take Me Out to the Ball Game." We would get boisterous and silly. Immediately upon ending the song, we would ask each person to notice whether singing the song had changed his or her emotions. Typically emotions changed for the positive. We would quickly move on to teaching how we all have the capacity to change our emotions voluntarily, by choosing our actions and thoughts. Suddenly we had arrived at the central idea of the whole module, and the teaching of specific skills could follow.

Sometimes it was difficult to get the patients' attention when beginning the Interpersonal Effectiveness Skills module, especially given that the first handout is generic and boring. I once arrived, took my chair in the group, and started to teach the module. Within a minute, my coteacher (and our clinical psychologist), Cindy Sanderson, arrived and took a seat opposite me. She greeted the group, opened her skills manual, and announced, "OK, group, it's time to start!" I quickly stopped her and told her that I had already begun. She quickly retorted, "But it's *my* turn to teach!" I responded with an edge in my voice: "Cindy, we met this week and agreed that I would teach this module." Cindy came back at me with more than an edge: "That's just not true, Charlie. You and I explicitly decided that *I* would teach this module. I can't believe you are doing this to me in front of this group!"

I was unrelenting, as was she. Back and forth, our voices rising, the rhetoric became more accusatory. The patients' eyes grew larger; they could hardly believe that they were witnessing a fight in public between two unit leaders. We definitely had their attention. It was staged in advance, but once underway, it was intense. Suddenly we stopped the argument. I stood up next to the blackboard and asked the patients if they could identify problems with how Cindy had tried to convince me to allow her to teach. They listed many. I asked them if they could see problems with the way in which I had refused her. They listed many. We wrote them down. We were well into the essence of the module—how to skillfully ask for what you want, and how to skillfully say "no"—before they realized it.

The second step in skills training is skills strengthening, which comes about through behavioral rehearsal (practice) with specific feedback and coaching. Having learned the content and practiced the skills ourselves, having begun to master the arts of instructing and modeling, and having improved in our capacity to get the patients' attention, we began to attend to whether the patients were actually integrating the skills into their daily repertoires. We must have assumed that if we "sold" the skills well enough, they would buy them and use them. It simply was not true. At times I quizzed patients who had completed our skills training sequence, and I was both astounded and discouraged by the outcomes. What was the point of excellent teaching if the skills didn't get incorporated? My training as a psychoanalytic therapist had not prepared me to insist that patients change their behavior and practice the skills. A turning point for me was when I realized that skills training is more like basketball practice, during which instructions and modeling are followed by insisting that the players practice the new moves, and then coaching them with detailed feedback. Taking on the challenge with the zeal of a convert, I held myself accountable to prescribe practices for every skill, and then coached the patients in their practice. The process began to be fun! As obvious as it seems now, it was a revelation for me that in order to change behavior, one has to *change behavior.* Insight is not an end in itself; it is a step toward behavioral change. Linehan's (1993a) emphasis on "dragging new behavior" out of the client in every session made a big impression on me.

The third step of skills training is skills generalization, the process of applying new skills to all relevant life contexts. It comes about through generalization programming, followed by practice and coaching in the relevant environments. As new skills trainers, we had effectively integrated the first two steps (procedures) of all skills training, acquisition and strengthening, but needed to focus more on the third and final one, generalization. A personal experience, in the context of teaching mental health professionals how to teach DBT skills, helped me to move forward in this crucial step. (One of the great values of teaching others is to finally understand, personally, the lesson one is teaching.) Around that time, I was preparing to teach a 2-day workshop on DBT skills training along with my friend and colleague Alec Miller. We were in Detroit, Michigan. We had an audience of 400, and the event manager was a rather formal, obviously very professional young woman whom I had not met before. As was common for me, I woke up early on the first day, ruminating about the workshop and pondering one of the huge challenges in skills training: We teach all the skills in the curriculum, week after week, whether or not patients need them. I knew from personal experience that no one learns a skill unless he or she sees and feels the need for it.

For instance, during my second year of medical school I had studied "acid–base balance." It was complex stuff, hard to grasp. It seemed rather academic. I could pass the exam but knew I had not mastered the material. During my third year of medical school, I was assigned a patient who had an undiagnosed acid–base balance problem. Late that night he was in acute distress. I talked with him, took his blood pressure and pulse, did a physical exam, drew blood for laboratory evaluation, studied his urine, and did a "blood gas" to determine the oxygenation of his blood supply. As I put together the data, I realized that the man had an acid–base balance problem, possibly based on kidney failure. He was declining, and my insufficient mastery of acid–base balance suddenly seemed like a life-threatening deficiency of my own. With heightened concentration, I sat down for an hour with my medical texts, rapidly and intensively reviewing the material on acid–base balance. Within that hour, I "got it." I learned it. *I learned it because I needed it.*

As it neared 8:30 A.M. that morning, I committed myself to sharing this insight with the workshop participants. We had to help our patients realize why they needed the skills. In the best spirit of modeling this lesson for the participants, I wanted to demonstrate to them that *I* needed DBT's emotion regulation skills while teaching the workshop. How could I show them that I needed the skills while I taught them the skills? Having taught so many workshops, I had grown comfortable with the process. How could I create emotional discomfort in myself while I taught, so that I would need to practice the skills? Suddenly I remembered that as a child I used to dream of finding myself undressed, naked, in the middle of a classroom. It always caused me great distress (and relief when I woke up). I knew that if I were to be undressed in front of the audience while I taught, I would be very self-conscious, embarrassed, and emotionally distracted. I decided to undress down to my waistline while I began the workshop (I was still aware of certain boundaries of decorum, thank God!).

I thought I should tell Alec Miller as my co-teacher, or tell the event manager of the workshop, but I knew that if I told them in advance, I would not be as anxious. So I kept it to myself. As I began the workshop, standing at a podium, I took off my tie. I put it at the table next to Alec. I then took off my sports jacket and placed it with the tie. I paused. Then I unbuttoned my dress shirt and took it off, placing it on the chair next to Alec. He looked at me with shock and concern, put his hand on my arm, and said, "Charlie, are you all right?" I told him I was fine. I was not really fine, in that I was thoroughly embarrassed and self-conscious. I began to teach the morning segment, beginning by explaining that no one ever learned a skill if they didn't need it, telling them that I was going to use my emotion regulation skills that morning while I taught, because I needed them. I had their attention! In the service of modeling the skills for the participants, I had found a way to generalize them, myself, to that context.

For those therapists who are new to DBT, and who ask me how to get started, I generally suggest learning the skills and then teaching them to an individual or a group. In that process, you learn that in order to change behavior, you have to change behavior; that to teach the skills, you have to learn them yourself; that to teach the skills to others, you must get their attention; and that people do not learn to use new skills unless they perceive themselves as needing them. In the learning curve when becoming a skills trainer, you discover, firsthand, the necessity of all three steps of skills training: skills acquisition, skills strengthening, and skills generalization. Finally, you learn a great deal about behavioral treatment in general by starting out by learning and teaching the "replacement behaviors."

THE PATH TO A LIFE WORTH LIVING IS PAVED WITH SKILLS

Over the past 15 years, beginning with research on the use of DBT skills training (without individual therapy) for patients with eating disorders (Safer et al., 2001) and a study on the use of skills training (without individual therapy) for the elderly depressed population (Lynch et al., 2003), it has become increasingly clear that "stand-alone" DBT skills training is efficacious. Our current understanding of the research is that the acquisition and use of DBT skills reduce emotional dysregulation, which mediates reductions in primary target behaviors such as suicide attempts, self-harm behaviors, substance use behaviors, eating disorder behaviors, and so on (Neacsiu et al., 2010). Between this research, the recent publication of the second edition of Linehan's (2015b) skills manual, and the recent publication of the DBT adolescent skills manual (Rathus & Miller, 2015), the value of skills training has moved into the foreground in DBT.

If we formulate the entire treatment in light of the research proving the central importance of skills, we can see that each of the various structures, protocols, and strategy groups are concerned with the acquisition, strengthening, and generalization of skills. The ultimate goal of DBT is to build a life worth living. To build a life worth living takes place in steps, and each step involves behavioral changes. Behavioral change results from the replacement of maladaptive behaviors by skillful behaviors. At its core, the prescription for getting a life worth living in DBT boils down to a lengthy sequence of steps, and each step involves the replacement of maladaptive with adaptive behaviors: *instead of this . . . that.* Instead of being mindless . . . be mindful. Instead of being submissive . . . be assertive. Instead of emotional dysregulation . . . regulate. Instead of avoiding discomfort . . . approach. Instead of being hijacked by the past . . . observe, accept, let go, and move on. Instead of believing and acting on dysfunctional cognitions . . . mindfully generate realistic and wise mind cognitions. Instead of self-damaging behaviors to relieve distress . . . use crisis survival strategies.

Far from being an "add-on" or "one of many choices," a careful look reveals that skills are integrated throughout the treatment package. For instance, each of DBT's five stages of treatment centers around the use of skills to achieve sequential goals. During pretreatment, the goal is to get the patient committed to the treatment plan, which requires an increase in the skills for making a commitment in the face of hopelessness, avoidance, confusion, fear, and other problematic behaviors. During Stage 1, the goal of which is to replace behavioral dyscontrol with behavioral control, the work involves the replacement of maladaptive life-threatening, treatment-interfering, and quality-of-life-interfering behaviors with behavioral skills. As part of this work, we attempt to replace the maladaptive patterns known as *dialectical dilemmas* (emotional vulnerability, self-invalidation, active passivity, etc.) with skillful behavioral patterns (emotion modulation, self-validation, active efforts to seek help as needed). The central organizing strategy during Stage 1 is behavioral chain analysis, which consists of the microscopic elucidation of links in the chain, highlighting the presence of maladaptive behaviors, the use of skills, and deficits in the use of skills. The goal is to locate maladaptive links and skills deficits and then to replace them with skills.

The goal of Stage 2 is to replace anguished emotional experiencing with nonanguished experiencing of emotions. Using ongoing reinforcement of behavioral skills while engaging patients in exposure procedures, we help them to gain and strengthen the skills required in approaching emotionally evocative cues rather than avoiding them, allowing for the experience of an emotion rather than escaping from it. Although several strategies are used to bring this about, all the strategies are aimed at the enhancement of emotion regulation skills.

Stages 3 and 4, although less well defined, also can be understood as enhancing skill sets for the overarching goals: to solve problems in the service of building a life of "ordinary happiness and unhappiness" (Linehan, 1993a) and to experience more sustained joy, meaning, and freedom in daily life.

Linehan, in workshops over the past few years, proposes four ways to address any given problem. Each of them involves the application of a set of skills.

1. To solve the problem requires problem-solving skills, often from the interpersonal effectiveness skills.
2. To change one's emotional response requires emotion regulation skills.
3. To tolerate distress more effectively requires distress tolerance skills.
4. To stay miserable involves the continued use of maladaptive behaviors rather than replacement with skills.

Skills training is one of four change procedures in DBT, the other three being cognitive modification, exposure, and contingency procedures. Cognitive modification comprises the acquisition, strengthening, and generalization of a set of skills that targets problematic cognitions and errors in information processing, attempting to replace them with more realistic and functional processes. Exposure procedures promote skillful responses to evocative cues and painful emotions. Instead of reflexively avoiding cues and escaping from subsequent emotional responses, the patient learns to avoid avoidance, block escape responses, and remain in contact with the cues long enough for new learning to take place. And instead of being overwhelmed by emotional responses or globally dampening responses to cues, the patient is taught to skillfully use certain emotion regulation skills and certain distress tolerance skills to allow an optimal level of exposure to take place without resulting in further trauma. Contingency procedures do not teach new skills per se, but they involve reinforcing skillful behaviors while extinguishing and occasionally punishing nonskillful behaviors. And, in fact, in the second edition of the skills manual, in the context of teaching "middle path skills," Linehan (2015b) teaches patients to understand these learning principles so they can use them skillfully for themselves.

One other essential framework for DBT is the partitioning of all DBT interventions into five functions of a comprehensive treatment. This format can also be understood as centering around the acquisition, strengthening, and generalization of skills. (1) By enhancing capabilities, we increase patients' skillful behaviors. (2) By generalizing skills to patients' natural environments, we add interventions to promote the use of skills in relevant contexts. (3) By improving patients' motivation, we increase their motivation to use the skills. (4) By structuring patients' environments, we find ways to ensure that their use of skills is reinforced there. (5) And by enhancing therapists' motivation and capabilities, we are increasing their set of skills for maintaining motivation and doing therapy correctly—which, in turn, eventuates in increasing the skill sets of patients. There can be little question that DBT, through its stages, goals, targets, functions, modes, and behavioral change procedures, is, at its core, a treatment for replacing maladaptive behaviors with skills.

SKILLS ARE COMPLICATED

Our familiarity with skills can create the illusion that skills training is the "easy" part of DBT. But the ease with which we can identify the skills needed and use the manual to present them to the patients belies the actual complexity of teaching—and learning—even one new skill.

For the patient (for any of us!) to learn even one skill—*acquiring it, strengthening it, and generalizing it*—involves the coordinated application of a number of very specific behaviors in real time, despite constantly changing internal pressures and micro-environments. Just as the understanding of particle theory in physics was made richer and more complicated with the discovery of subparticles, the practice of skills training in DBT is enhanced and complicated by realizing that each skill consists of a synchronized aggregate of *subskills*.

For instance, consider the skill of asking your companion for some time to yourself by saying "Please let me have some time to myself." In fact, to make this request skillfully requires an aggregate of several subskills. First, you must gain awareness of the desire to have time to yourself. However, if you reflexively subordinate your own desires to those of others, it may be impossible to become aware of wanting time for yourself—in which case, the whole skill is impossible to learn. Second, although you may be aware that you want time to yourself, a host of factors could interfere with the subskill of having a willingness to ask for it. Maybe you think you don't deserve to have that time to yourself, or you are convinced that you should not inconvenience your partner. Third, even if you are aware of your desire and willing to ask for what you want, to successfully do so, you need to integrate several other subskills: You need to be tactful, use good timing, and find the optimal posture and voice tone with which to deliver your request. Choosing the words that will most effectively convey what you want and influence your partner to agree with you is another subskill in itself. All of this undertaking rests as well on the skill of "reading" the mindset of your partner, before and while making your request. It is a complex and subtle skill set to respond, in real time, to your partner's responses as you make the request, since you may need to adjust as you go. It may seem rather tedious to enumerate all of the subskills that are involved in making one skillful request, and in most contexts it is pointless to do so. But when teaching a skill to an individual for whom that skill is difficult to use, you may need to break it down into the subskills in order to diagnose and treat the impediments.

The person who is deficient in skills, and whose life does not go so well as a result, almost never attributes her disappointing outcomes to skills deficits; she almost always assumes that there is something more damnable wrong with her or the people around her. How difficult it is to solve a problem when you cannot see its infrastructure! The skills trainer who understands that the "devil is in the details"—that the details are skills deficits (and deficits in subskills), that skills deficits can be replaced with skills, and that to do so requires diligence, accuracy, and compassion—can change the patient's life. And that skills trainer will realize that he cannot diagnose the impediments to a skill without seeing, or hearing about, the patient's practice of the skill. He needs to see it, break it down, make specific coaching suggestions, have the patient do it again, and work toward a more integrated, smooth, and effective practice of the skill at hand.

Supporting the practice of a skill when the patient is generalizing it to her environment requires an equal level of diligence. I once had a patient in a skills training group who was just beginning a job as a barista in a coffee shop. She had been through most of the skills training curriculum, and we were identifying which skills would help with her intense social anxiety when dealing with customers. She planned on using "one-mindful" to do just one thing at a time in order not to become overwhelmed. In addition, she planned to regulate her emotions and tolerate distress by observing her breath and taking occasional breaks. Still, the patient and I expected serious challenges implementing these skills in her "real world." It was a busy job, and she did not want to tell her boss how much difficulty she had with simple encounters. One of the patients in the skills group suggested that they all take turns coming there to see her, ordering coffee, and providing support and reinforcement. In fact, they set up a schedule so that during her first 2 weeks on the job, someone from the group would come there about every 2 to 3 hours. This helped her to use the skills and to establish momentum on the job during the early stages. If only we could come up with that kind of support for skills *generalization* all the time!

SKILLS, LINKS, AND THE BEHAVIORAL CHAIN

I was working with a young woman who entered treatment for suicide attempts, suicidal ideation, binge-eating disorder, and severe interpersonal dysfunction. Her repetitive interpersonal patterns were of two types. When she thought someone was competent or admirable, she experienced self-hatred and shame. When she thought someone was less competent than she was, she grew intensely irritated with that person. The outcome of either pattern left her distant from others and unable to bridge the gap. As a result, she was isolated and lonely.

After her suicidal patterns and binge-eating behaviors diminished early in treatment, we increasingly targeted the interpersonal dysfunction. In analyzing the chains related to all of her treatment targets, from suicidal behaviors to interpersonal dysfunction, it was possible to identify a certain pattern. We discovered that early in each chain, an antecedent event triggered the conviction that something was deeply wrong with her, so much so that she wanted to end her life. The associated shame could be temporarily dampened through binge eating followed by purging. It was in this context that we understood the origins of her irritability with others who were more or less competent than she: When the conviction that something was deeply wrong with her was activated, she deflected her self-hatred onto others. It became clearer that the *"there-is-something-deeply-wrong-with-me"* self-statement was a discrete and predictable link, a kind of "switch point" through which her behavioral chains would pass on the way to undesirable social and emotional outcomes. We began to assess and target this link. We identified numerous prompting events that would activate the *"there-is-something-deeply-wrong-with-me"* belief and the typical consequences of that link. Understandably, the patient wanted to understand early life influences that had led her to feel this way, and we did explore some relevant aspects of her learning history. Shedding light on the historical context was interesting, but it did not lead to behavioral change. I recognized that we needed to become very specific about the chain of behaviors leading up to and following this dysfunctional cognitive response, to "script" a more adaptive response pattern and to help her to actually replace the adaptive response for the dysfunctional one.

Fortunately, on some occasions this dysfunctional pattern arose during sessions with me, in response to something I said or did. In fact, as we paid closer attention, we could see that it came up somewhere in nearly every session. Her conviction of her "badness" was triggered so silently and automatically that she had no idea it was happening until it was too late. By the time we noticed it, she already felt demoralized, had already withdrawn from our interaction, was convinced that she was a "bad person," and could see no way out. We had to find a way to change the course of the chain leading up to the problematic link. For her to clearly see the all-consuming role of this previously unidentified one-sentence conviction was a powerful moment of insight for her.

Of course, this one particular link, the self-statement that *"there is something deeply wrong with me,"* became gradually linked to a more complex response that included emotion and action components. The self-statement exerted a paralyzing impact, operating the way a sliver eventually leads to an inflammatory response that can no longer be ignored. It sometimes came into view as rage toward the other person, which disguised the hatred toward herself. At other times, she became inexplicably inarticulate, cautious, and rigid in her thinking when something had happened between us that activated her self-hatred. Still, the solution had to involve removing the sliver—that is, seeing the hidden but damaging self-statement and replacing it with adaptive alternatives. Over time, even before the self-damning process came into awareness, she and I began to be able to "feel" the presence of this inchoate, self-doubting, self-hating complex as it entered the conversation.

By "catching it" sooner, she gained a greater measure of control. At the point at which she could see it and feel it as it happened, when she could "hold it" rather than proceed down the old patterns, it became possible for us to brainstorm skills for her to use to modify her thinking that *"there is something deeply wrong with me."* Over time she tried several skills. One skill was to observe and describe whatever prompting event had triggered her belief that she was bad, and then to find a nonjudgmental way to reframe her interpretation of the prompting event. For instance, one bout of intense self-criticism was triggered during a therapy session when I suggested something for her to read. She grew inhibited and more rigid. I pointed out the pattern. Immediately she "caught herself in the act" of hating herself. She quickly identified the prompting event: She had automatically interpreted my suggestion of something to read as an indication that I thought she was stupid. She stopped, stepped back, and observed her self-hatred, her shame, the associated bodily sensations, and she described her observations to me. By seeing the process as it passed through her, the negative impact was already tempered. I prompted her to reframe my suggestion in a nonjudgmental, nondamning manner. Once she could see that she had options, she reframed my communication. Rather than saying to herself, "He thinks I'm stupid, so he's assigning me something to read," she said to herself, "He respects me enough to suggest something for me to read."

At other points when her self-hatred was activated, she used the skill of "checking the facts" of the situation, scanning for evidence as to whether or not she was a "bad person" who had done something wrong. Although she was sometimes able to identify ways in which she was disappointed in herself, rarely could she find evidence that she was indeed a bad person. By becoming more familiar with her own behavioral chain, by locating the dysfunctional links or sequences in the chain, and by having a set of skillful options at hand for replacing the dysfunctional links, this patient became more versatile at breaking up the invisible and rigid process before it solidified and did its damage. She grew more able to think of herself objectively and realistically, and to catch herself early on the way to the old self-critical patterns.

This example brings us into the skills-related work that occurs within the mode of individual therapy. The therapist helps the patient bring skills into his life and into the sessions. She breaks down the skills into subskills when it will help the patient understand impediments and point the way to solutions. The therapist finds where and how the patient can "insert" particular skills into the behavioral chain as it unfolds. This often requires careful, compassionate, accurate, and dedicated work. Typically, in order to provide the full value of skills training, the therapist has to "get into the trenches" with the patient, hold the situation steady, shed light on the process, remain engaged, and intervene in replacing links and in studying and changing the interlink dynamics. The work is incremental and sometimes tedious, yet when a patient learns even one skill to replace one dysfunctional link in the chain, it can transform a life.

EVERY SKILL FOR EVERY SITUATION

In workshops, Linehan has explained that the highest test of a DBT skills trainer is to find a way to use any given skill in any situation. In other words, she is proposing that DBT skills are "multipurpose tools." For heuristic purposes, we categorize the skills modules as either "acceptance modules" (Core Mindfulness Skills, Distress Tolerance Skills) or "change modules" (Emotion Regulation Skills, Interpersonal Effectiveness Skills). This categorization is congruent with the overarching dialectic of acceptance and change in DBT, and provides a user-friendly way to present the skills to patients. Yet, the proposition that there are "change skills" and "acceptance skills" is overly simplistic and limiting. In fact, skills are aggregates of specific behaviors (subskills) conducted in synchrony. A given skill may serve a multitude of functions in different contexts, and within a skill there may be subskills with differing "subpurposes."

Skills are highly versatile. A skillful person has a great deal of flexibility. Mindfulness skills, presented as an acceptance module, can be powerful change agents. Validation, packaged within the change-oriented Interpersonal Effectiveness Skills module, provides acceptance in the service of changing someone else's behavior. Validation in another context, in which we validate someone's primary emotion, can result in greater exposure to that emotion with the outcome of improved (and changed) emotion modulation. "Acting opposite" the urge associated with an emotion (one of the change-oriented Emotion Regulation Skills), although it can be used to change emotional responses, may also help the individual act with acceptance toward an unpalatable reality from which he has the urge to flee. Reality is too complex and dialectical in nature, and the skills too versatile and complex themselves, for us to stay with oversimplified categories of acceptance and change skills. Change requires acceptance. Acceptance requires change. Any given skill can help with acceptance, with change, and with dialectical synthesis. DBT's multipurpose skills curriculum is versatile, with each skill having the potential to be used toward change, acceptance, or dialectics.

USING DBT'S PARADIGMS AND PRINCIPLES
IN SKILLS TRAINING

The job of a skills trainer is structured and scripted, spelled out in Linehan's (2015b) *DBT Skills Training Manual*. First, he must know the skills himself. Second, he orients the patients to the goals of skills training and the guidelines for participation. He organizes the session agenda according to three prioritized targets: (1) stopping therapy-destroying behaviors, (2) increasing skills acquisition and strengthening, and (3) decreasing therapy-interfering behaviors. He follows a predetermined syllabus, and in each session he takes the group through a format that moves sequentially through a mindfulness practice, homework review, break, teaching of new skills, homework assignment, and wind-down. He learns the preferred means for dealing with diary cards, reviewing participants' homework, addressing homework noncompliance, and managing problematic behaviors in the group.

In addition, the DBT skills trainer brings the arsenal of DBT strategies to her work in the group. She implements the manualized group skills training protocol with problem-solving strategies, irreverent communication strategies, validation strategies, reciprocal communication strategies, and dialectical strategies. Furthermore, her interventions arise from the same paradigms and principles that inform the work of the individual therapist when implementing targeting, behavioral chain analysis, case conceptualization, commitment, and other strategies. In so doing, the group is based on the same foundations as the rest of DBT, which creates a synergy between the group format and other modes. Given that the skills trainer is working to keep a group of emotionally dysregulated individuals on track to learn all the skills in a timely manner, she faces pushes and pulls, lively moments and dead segments, and behavioral dyscontrol and overcontrol. By grounding herself in the principles of DBT, out of which the strategies flow, she brings more flexibility, fluidity, and confidence to her group work. By informing and backing up the protocols and strategies with principles, the therapist can enhance the precision and rigor of skills training; deliver it with more presence, awareness, and acceptance; and navigate the challenges with greater speed, movement, and flow.

Principles from the Change Paradigm

Just as is done in individual therapy, the group skills trainer organizes the session agenda in keeping with prioritized targets. His highest-priority target, necessarily, is the reduction of group-destroying behaviors. When these are not present, his highest-priority target is the acquisition and strengthening of skills by the patients in the group. This is the preferred target, in that the trainer would prefer, if possible, to spend 100% of the session time on this one. The third prioritized target is the reduction of therapy-interfering behaviors by group members, meaning those behaviors that interfere with the individual's learning even if they do not contribute to destruction of the group for others. We might consider the process of targeting to rise to the status of a principle in that it is constantly providing direction to the group. Accompanying the focus on targeting is a focus on monitoring behavioral progress. This takes place with the assistance of the diary card, whereby the skills trainer can review each patient's progress in utilizing skills each week.

Having established direction and persistence through targeting and monitoring, the skills trainer pushes the group, and each member within it, toward the maximal possible commitment to learning and using the skills. She works to (1) gain group members' attention to the lessons, (2) establish a rapport and culture that encourages participation and hope, and (3) utilize DBT's commitment strategies as needed with each member. Many interventions by group leaders, and the tone with which they are delivered, are driven by the continued focus on targeting, monitoring, and commitment.

Beyond this agenda, in the service of helping each patient notice and overcome obstacles to the acquisition and strengthening of skills, the skills trainer is informed by the behavioral change principles that under-lie the four change procedures in DBT.

1. The skills deficit model proposes that deficits in the skills rep-ertoire of the individual account for problematic processes and outcomes, and that skills training is the solution.
2. The model of cognitive mediation of emotions and actions posits that problematic cognitions lead to problematic behaviors, and it suggests cognitive modification procedures as the remedy.
3. The model of classical, or respondent, conditioning proposes that the pairing of stimuli in the mind of the individual results in intense emotional reactions to relatively neutral cues, and those intense emotions lead to problematic behavioral responses; stim-ulus control strategies and exposure procedures are prescribed as the treatment.
4. The model of operant, or instrumental, conditioning proposes that targeted problematic behaviors are reinforced by conse-quences, and that the effective use of contingency procedures is the solution.

Skills Deficit Theory

Keeping this model in mind alerts the therapist to certain types of phe-nomena and directs him toward certain types of interventions through-out the group. The skills trainer who is routinely scanning for deficits in emotional and interpersonal skills as they occur in the group setting is more likely to notice them as they happen and to address them on the spot. Insofar as DBT is fundamentally a "replacement model," help-ing the patient to do "this instead of that," the skills trainer develops "replacement reflexes," reflexively highlighting skills deficits and imme-diately suggesting or brainstorming replacement behaviors. The therapist might say, "Why don't you look at me while you talk to me about your homework so you can see what my reactions are rather than assuming that I am criticizing you?" or, "Do you think you could express your anger at me about this assignment without shouting or cursing at me?" The therapist not only seizes opportunities in the moment to elicit more skillful behaviors from the patient but also takes every opportunity to reinforce whatever skillful behaviors emerge on their own. In other words, while following the curriculum and teaching the skills, the skills trainer is simultaneously applying principles of skills training when defi-cits become noticeable and when skills are applied. At its best, the result is a skills training laboratory, in which new behaviors are tried, skillful behaviors are immediately reinforced, and morale goes up. At its worst, if done too stiffly and without balance, this kind of relentless focus on replacing deficits with skills can feel oppressive. The application of skills principles must be balanced with responsiveness, timing, and tact.

We apply the skills training principles not only with each individual, but also in establishing an optimal atmosphere for the entire group, trying to create a culture based on practice. Not only does the therapist recommend *in vivo* practice between sessions and follow-up with review of practice assignments; she sponsors a routine of "do-overs" within the skills group. "Now that you've received some feedback on your role play, try it again." Or, "Now that you all have had a chance to see what it's like to continue to 'observe' while we walk around the room, and to hear each other 'describe' the experience, let's do it again for 2 minutes and see what you notice this time." The practice of do-overs in the group setting creates the sense that there are also do-overs in life, that life can be more forgiving and modifiable than previously thought, that opportunities for change are everywhere, and that "mistakes" can be opportunities for change and improvement rather than embarrassment and self-hatred.

The three steps of skills training discussed earlier in this chapter—acquisition, strengthening, and generalization—need not be used in stepwise fashion. They are highly interdependent, do not need to be done in a strict sequence, and together shape the entire skills training enterprise. For instance, attention to the third step of skills generalization from the beginning of the sequence provides a rationale for acquiring and strengthening a skill. In other words, linking the teaching and strengthening of the skill (acquisition and strengthening) to its ultimate destination (generalization) from the beginning strengthens the whole process. This is akin to the math teacher who links the equation under discussion to real-life problems as a way of heightening the sense of relevance, thereby enhancing motivation. In sum, the atmosphere of the group that is conducted with skills training principles in mind is pervasively influenced by replacing deficits with skills, by practicing new behaviors, and by linking the new skills to the relevant contexts of the patients' lives.

Cognitive Mediation Theory

Keeping the cognitive mediation model in mind alerts the skills trainer to the presence of problematic cognitions as they occur in group members. Much as the skills trainer develops replacement reflexes to notice skills deficits and suggest more skillful replacements, he also has "cognitive reflexes" for noticing problematic cognitions as they occur, highlighting them immediately in one way or another, and sometimes suggesting replacement cognitions on the spot. He might respond to the patient who says "I just can't do it" by saying, "That kind of thought certainly won't help you change; how about trying 'I think I can do it, but I know it will be really difficult'?" At other times, his intervention might be as brief as a brushstroke, momentarily highlighting that a patient's pessimistic conviction is a thought rather than a fact, and then moving on. The trainer's emphasis that "thought errors" such as judging, blaming, catastrophizing, overestimating, and overgeneralizing are natural accompaniments of difficult moods and anxiety, and are natural outcomes of invalidating environments, creates a validating context for the recognition of problematic cognitions while pointing out that they are "nothing more than thoughts." Treating problematic thoughts as behaviors that can be recognized and changed, much as deficient actions can be recognized and changed, adds further to the laboratory atmosphere mentioned above.

Classical Conditioning Theory

In classical (or respondent) conditioning, a given cue, which might be relatively neutral in an objective sense, automatically triggers an intense emotion because the cue is paired in the patient's mind with prior stimuli that set off painful experiences indeed. For instance, having an objectively "tame" conversation with a man might trigger intense fear because it is paired in the mind of the patient with prior experiences with men in which supposedly tame conversations preceded abusive behaviors. The individual may reflexively seek to avoid any proximity to the evocative cue and to escape any experience of the painful emotion. Avoidance and escape prevent further encounters with the cue and the emotion, which in turn prevents corrective learning opportunities. Exposure procedures block the avoidance and escape responses and help the patient establish and maintain contact with the cue and the emotion long enough for new learning to take place. This new learning then leads to a more reasonable and objective response to the cue.

Viewing the skills group through this lens alerts the skills trainer to similar phenomena as they occur in the group. First, she realizes that in working with individuals who experience chronic and pervasive emotion dysregulation, cues are *everywhere*. The group context presents neutral stimuli that can set off anxiety, panic, startle, disgust, rage, sadness, love, and other intense responses. The presence of several other patients, or one particular patient with particular characteristics, can set off panicky feelings, associated with memories of having been trapped, teased, bullied, or otherwise mistreated by others. The delivery of constructive critical feedback, even if couched in gentle terms, can set off memories and feelings of being accused, shamed, and dismissed earlier in life. The expectation to review practice assignments in the group context can set off memories and feelings in patients of being exposed, shamed, and physically abused earlier in life. The list goes on and on. The skills trainer remains alert to these possibilities, realizing that due to prior learning, a "stick" to one person can be a "snake" to another person. She takes each person's responses seriously, is ready to validate a range of different reactions to the same experience, and is ready to suggest that each individual, within the group setting, find ways to manage the normative group cues and to cope with the emotional responses without having to interfere with learning by engaging in avoidance and escape behaviors.

The individual who routinely avoids such cues and thereby escapes from cued emotional responses, when in fact the cues are not inherently dangerous to her life or well-being, is inadvertently perpetuating those patterned responses. The implications for the skills trainer are several. For one thing, she needs to establish an objectively safe and supportive group environment, so that overwhelming emotional responses take place in a context that is not, in fact, aversive. Accordingly, the skills trainer maintains a baseline demeanor of ease, friendliness, and responsiveness. Furthermore, while validating the strong emotional responses of the patients and their urge to avoid and escape, the skills trainer acts consistently in favor of nonavoidance and nonescape, of "hanging in there" and skillfully coping with cues. She is reluctant to modify the actual cues unless they are indeed problematic, as doing so only reinforces avoidance and escape and communicates the message that the patient is too fragile for the normative life of a well-conducted skills group. The skills trainer creates a group atmosphere that supports everyone working together to notice and confront classically conditioned cues and reactions by consistently (1) scanning for cued emotional responses and for avoidance and escape behaviors; (2) recognizing and validating cued responses and urges; (3) keeping the cues in place if they are normative and not dangerous; and (4) encouraging each patient to skillfully lean into the cues and emotions rather than to run away and hide. An atmosphere of courage and resilience for the entire group will translate into courage and resilience for each member.

It may be obvious, but may also bear mentioning, that the use of principles of exposure procedures, flowing as they do from classical conditioning theory, are part and parcel of skills training. Asking a patient to give up a habitual maladaptive behavior and replace it with a new, more skillful response automatically exposes the patient to emotions and thoughts that may be uncomfortable and distressing. At that point, the skills trainer wants to help the patient *stay with* the new behavior, encounter the feared responses, avoid avoiding, avoid escaping, and bring about new learning by staying in contact with the cues. The skills trainer conveys an attitude of "You can do this," "Hang in there," and "I can support you in coping with these cues" through comments and actions. This is another reason why group practices and exercises, such as role-play exercises, can be so useful. They provide the perfect opportunity to help the patient *lean in to* a feared situation, to act opposite the action tendency. Equally important, the skills trainer assures each patient when being asked to do something new and frightening, that he can opt out, defer, or do it at his own pace. Patients need to be in control of their own exposures.

Operant Conditioning Theory

Keeping the operant conditioning theory in mind heightens the therapist's awareness of the ongoing presence and power of reinforcement, extinction, and punishment. Not a minute goes by in a skills group without the influence of contingencies upon current behavior. As such, the skills trainer tries to establish a culture in which skillful behaviors are routinely reinforced and maladaptive behaviors are not. Reinforcement should be available for effort applied, risks taken, participation, and practice; for supportive intragroup collaboration, validation, and supportive responses with respect to one another. It helps if the skills trainers are optimistic (without being unrealistic), operate with a sense of ease and interest, and work toward a group atmosphere that includes humor, warmth, and fun. These qualities of a group culture, consistently cultivated by the trainers, create a learning environment that reinforces attendance, effort, participation, collaboration, and the learning of new skills.

Realizing that different individuals are reinforced by different responses, it can be challenging in a group setting for a leader to know how to reinforce different members. In fact, what reinforces one individual might even be aversive to another. For instance, the therapist might use praise for one group member because it serves as reinforcement for her, whereas another individual in the same group, for whom praise is aversive, might shrink back from participation because "praise is in the air." Although there is no simple answer to this issue, the skilled group leader who maintains an appreciation of the principles of contingency management will gradually get to know each patient well enough to reinforce each one accordingly.

Principles from the Acceptance Paradigm

I have previously identified and discussed five principles associated with DBT's acceptance paradigm: (1) present-moment awareness, (2) nonattachment, (3) interbeing, (4) impermanence, and (5) "perfect as it is." Pervasively weaving these principles into the conduct of a skills training group contributes to a context in which present-moment awareness and acceptance are promoted, and in which validation strategies and reciprocal communication strategies are used frequently.

Present-Moment Awareness

The mindfulness practice that begins each skills training session, in addition to modeling the practical use of a mindfulness skill, brings everyone's attention into the present moment. This effort to let go of the past and the future in favor of inhabiting the present moment sets the tone of acceptance and awareness as the group begins. It serves as a threshold through which all individuals in the room enter the session, and the skills trainer works to extend the present-moment, acceptance-oriented baseline into the remainder of the group session. Whether the group is pleasant or unpleasant is not the point. Akin to those mindfulness practices focusing on present-moment awareness—for example, "This moment is the only moment," or "Just this one . . . [during the in-breath] breath [during the out-breath]"—the leader works to bring the group entirely into the current group session. He does what he can to get everyone's attention and to convey that this group is meaningful, relevant, even precious. Although the agenda of the group is always full and there is the tendency to rush, present-moment awareness helps to create a sense of spaciousness that is reinforced by pauses, reflections, and brief experiential practices.

Nonattachment

These groups can be difficult. Even if the group is well structured and well managed, and even if the skills are well taught, there are always challenges when we assemble six to eight individuals with emotional dysregulation, black-and-white thinking patterns, problematic interpersonal functioning, and a tendency toward judgments about self and others. The atmosphere can be fraught with anxiety and tension, boredom and restlessness, pessimism and cynicism—a far cry from the optimal optimistic, collaborative atmosphere. The skills trainer has an opportunity to model ease and flow as a counterpoint to tension and anxiety, patience and compassion as a counterpoint to restlessness and judgment, and acceptance of the current moment as it is as a counterpoint to the urges to avoid and escape. Given that groupwide emotional dysregulation may create an impetus to push away the reality of the moment and cling to "how things *should* be," it is the perfect opportunity for the therapist to model non-attachment. She can "let go" of her attachment to the "ideal group" and truly embrace the group *as it is*, with all of its flaws. She can (metaphorically, and in some cases, actually) smile at the discomfort, smile at the judgments, and embrace the moment with all of its tensions and all of its promise. In addition to teaching the skills of the day, the trainer has a chance to demonstrate skillful, tolerant reactions to dysregulation, thereby providing a corrective experience. Practicing nonattachment in the current moment with the group-as-patient can provide the equivalent of the therapist who, while treating a phobia, models approaching the phobia with calm in contrast to the patient's avoidance, escape, and terror.

Predictably, the moment when the skills trainer initiates patients' reviews of their practice assignments sets off heightened anxiety and self-consciousness. Patients may anticipate being put on the spot, exposed for noncompliance, or criticized for being less than perfect. It's an opportunity for the therapist to model nonattachment to "homework practice as it should be," while accepting and working with the patients' actual performance.

Interbeing

The skills trainer who can remain aware of the profound moment-to-moment interrelatedness and mutual influence among all individuals in the room, and who can see how the group operates as one organism, without boundaries and without separate selves, can contribute toward the sense that "we are all in it together." Through this lens, the skills trainer is made up entirely of group members, and group members are made up entirely of the skills trainer and each other. Everyone is treated as equal to everyone else. Everyone is treated as an individual who is on the path of building a life worth living, acquiring and strengthening skills; all paths are intertwined and mutually influential. Everyone matters. If someone is absent, everyone is partly absent. If someone participates willingly, then to some degree, everyone participates willingly. By envisioning the group in this manner, as a team, working toward the same ends, with members influencing each other minute by minute, pushing everyone toward his or her life-worth-living goals, the therapist helps the group members to experience themselves as meaningfully interconnected. Feeling themselves to be integral parts of a positive whole—not just separate selves but part of something bigger—offers patients an antidote to isolation and stagnation.

Impermanence

The principle of impermanence emerges naturally in concert with the other principles discussed to this point. We recognize that the present moment, the present group session, is the only moment, the only group session. Nonattached, we attempt to let go of judging that "it should have been otherwise." All participants in the group arrive at the point where they feel mutually influential with each other, where they feel themselves as part of a larger whole. Just as each of these principles serves as an antidote to experiences of pain, tension, aloneness, avoidance, escape, and judgment, the awareness of the impermanence of the group, of each group session, and the passing of each moment of each group can be an antidote to the hopeless sense that everything (bad) stays the same, that nothing ever changes. The therapist keeps the group moving forward, commenting on the progress made in the curriculum. He highlights changes that patients make and the differences among points of view expressed in the meeting. While listening to patients, he underlines their contributions, their discoveries, and their unique ways of describing their observations. He creates a sense of movement, discovery, and change. He connects a certain patient comment to a prior one made by that patient or a different patient. Now and then he comments on the uniqueness of the particular group, implicitly or explicitly communicating the sense that this group is special, that everyone in the group is working to change his or her life, and that time is passing. In spite of the feeling of some individuals that "nothing is happening," or that the same things happen again and again, the group leader reinforces the idea that actually things are constantly changing, that nothing is the same. It's very important for the group skills trainer, when feeling as if the group is stuck and nothing is happening, to remember that it is actually constantly changing, that more is happening than meets the eye, that opportunities are present, and that if things feel difficult, "this too shall pass."

Perfect as It Is

The group is "perfect as it is," filled with individuals, each of whom "is perfect as he or she is." Everyone in the group is doing the best he or she can do, given everything up to the moment. How could it be otherwise, when we take history—everything up to this moment—into account? We work repeatedly to acknowledge, accept, and validate the current functioning of the group and each person in it. Antidotal to the tendency to judge and control each other and ourselves, the individual and group that can embody this realization can settle in to the current moment, let go of judgments, need not grasp or cling to "what should be." They can allow the interdependency of everyone in the group and can focus on the work at hand: the acquisition and strengthening of skills.

To the degree to which the group skills trainer can embody and promote these five principles in leading the group, she has a chance to move everyone in the direction of awareness and acceptance, reducing judgment of self and others, simply doing the work of the group, and bringing about a culture in which it's "all for one and one for all."

Principles from the Dialectical Paradigm

As noted previously, four principles are associated with the dialectical paradigm, as follow:

1. Oppositions are inherent in reality; truth evolves through synthesis.
2. Phenomena are interrelated in a holistic, systemic manner.
3. Everything is transactional, including identity.
4. Change is constant; flux is the rule.

The skills trainer who can embody these principles will promote tolerance for difference and conflict; the search for synthesis rather than determining who is right; the sense of speed, movement, and flow; and the feeling of each member as being part of the larger whole rather than alone and separate.

Reality Is Filled with Oppositions; Truth Evolves through Synthesis

As is the case in all group processes, the skills group will experience the emergence of one conflict after another. Oppositions are the rule, not the exception. A tense disagreement arises between a patient and a skills trainer, or between two patients. A conflict between a patient and her psychotherapist or her psychiatrist is brought into the group, and different patients align themselves with different sides of the disagreement. Some patients want to "go deep" in explaining their circumstances, whereas others want to stay on the surface. Or, as in the case of one of my groups, all the patients want to do more heart-to-heart sharing, whereas I'm trying to keep us on track with a focus on the skills. There is the ever-present conflict between the amount of material to teach and the amount of time available. A patient may want to remain silent and withdrawn to protect himself, but greater participation results in more learning. Two group members want to deepen a private relationship, but this could come into conflict with a group guideline about private relationships. It goes on and on. One thing is for sure: Conflict is to be expected. The skills trainer who understands this is not thrown off balance as conflicts arise. She has the opportunity, again and again, to model a dialectical approach to opposition: to specify the two sides of the conflict, to search for the validity on each side, and to move the discussion toward finding a synthesis that preserves the validity on both sides. The process of valuing opposing forces and finding synthesis is reinforced again and again, creating a sense of confidence in the group that everyone's point of view will be valued and that differences are normal and need not be destructive. It is another aspect of the corrective experience of being in the group.

Phenomena Are Related to One Another in a Holistic, Systemic Manner

This principle overlaps with the acceptance-oriented principle of inter-being. Everyone in the group is part of a larger whole and is defined, to some degree, by the whole. The whole of the group is defined by the contributions of the individuals. A change in one results in a change in everyone. Much as the family therapist may approach the "identified patient" by addressing other family members, the group skills trainer can address one member of the group by addressing others or by addressing the group as a whole. Linehan (1993a, 30) has explained the dialectical balance between patient and therapist through the metaphor of a teeter-totter balanced over a tightrope above the Grand Canyon, in which the movements of one party intimately influence the experiences and movements of the other. One needs a group version of this metaphor to capture the exquisite and immediate interrelationship among the individuals and each other, the individuals and the whole. We might consider the group to be traveling together on an inflated rubber raft moving down a river with whitewater. The group, with the leader at the helm, must navigate ever-changing conditions that could lead to the loss of one member or the capsizing of the entire raft. Keeping this metaphor in mind, the skills group leader is likely to think systemically in coming up with ways to respond to tensions and obstacles within the group process, and to keep all members in the raft and keep the raft afloat.

In one of the first groups I co-led, in the context of a day treatment program, we had a patient who was in the manic phase of a bipolar disorder. He showed enormous excitement about the group and was enthusiastic about each skill and each group member. His pressured, excessive speech and euphoria became a disruptive influence. It was easy to sense that he was alienating everyone. On the one hand, he was an enthusiastic group member who truly wanted to learn the skills. On the other hand, his pathology led him to be disruptive. On the one hand, he wanted to participate fully. On the other hand, other members of the group wanted him to be quiet. I had the impression that everyone else would be happier if we asked him to leave the group, but clearly he wanted to be there. As the group leader I searched for a synthesis. I had to do something to change the status quo, but I did not want to expel him from the group. I discussed it with my co-leader and my consultation team. We came up with a plan that represented a synthesis. He was allowed to be in the group, at the table with everyone else, until he became too overwhelming verbally. He would be given one request to suppress his urge to speak. If he couldn't comply, he would be asked to sit on a chair against the wall, away from the table. In that chair, the rule was that he could not speak, but he could hear everything that went on. That way he could continue to learn. When he felt that he could be at the table without overwhelming others with his speech, he could return. He was pleased with the plan because he had been ejected from many groups in the past, and our approach honored his desire to learn. He came back and forth to the table several times in coming weeks, and it seemed to work for all. We kept him in the raft with the others.

Everything Is Transactional, Including Identity

This principle is interrelated with the prior one emphasizing the holistic, systemic way of understanding group interaction. The identity of a given individual is not static and isolated; it is part of a transaction. I am a teacher insofar as I am in transaction with a student. Without the student(s), I am not a teacher. The identity of each group member is not static and isolated; especially once the group has formed, the identity of each individual in the group is based on a set of transactions. In relationship to some groups I feel like an excellent teacher. I soar with confidence, teaching seems easy, and everything I do seems to work. In other groups I feel clumsy and ineffective. My confidence plummets, I lose confidence in my teaching choices, and the whole experience feels like pushing a boulder up a hill. It is remarkable how much different I can feel about myself based on the transactions. It helps me when I realize how much my sense of myself is dependent on transactions. I can observe my internal ups and downs, try to notice them without judgment, try to notice how they are influenced by transactions in the group, and stay focused on the teaching agenda. Wondering how I came to feel so ineffective, I might notice that one patient in the group treats me as if I am dumb, and that this one person has a disproportionate impact on me. I come to feel that this one patient's response to me is defining my identity with respect to the whole group. If I can objectively see that this is happening, I can address it within myself. Or, I might realize that the group as a whole seems withdrawn, with low motivation, and then realize that their withdrawal has led me to feel ineffective. I find myself working increasingly hard to get everyone involved, but it doesn't work. I feel like a failure. Once I can see objectively that there is a problem to be solved, but without attributing the problem to my ineffectiveness alone, I have a better chance to address the groupwide slump with greater ease and confidence, averting a downward shift in my identity.

Realizing how much my own sense of self as teacher can fluctuate depending on transactions with one group member or with the entire group, I assume that this is the case for every group member. If a patient feels recognized, validated, and valued within the group, she is more likely to operate effectively. If the skills trainer can keep this understanding in mind, he can watch for the kinds of transactions that might explain the behavior of each member. The patient who acquires the identity of the "problem patient," the "outlier," or the "prima donna" is likely to suffer from the resulting transactions. The therapist who notices the nature and impact of transactions on the identity and behavior of each member can find ways to intervene to balance or shift the transactions.

In one of my skills groups in which there were six patients, only one of them was in individual therapy with me. All others had other therapists. When the group started, my therapy patient played a constructive role with others and took an active stance in learning the skills. Two months later, she seemed more withdrawn in the group, more irritable, and less active in her homework practice. She had said nothing in individual therapy that would help me to understand the change. I noticed that during the break, she was often busy on her cell phone when other patients were talking with one another. I wondered whether transactions that she had with others in the group could explain the change in her behavior. In individual therapy I pursued the question. At first she didn't know how to explain the change in her behavior. She said she felt less involved in the group and not very well liked. She just assumed she wasn't very likeable. As we reviewed the 2 months, we could see that her sense of self in the group had changed, as had the transaction with other members. After a positive start in the group, other members apparently had begun to distance themselves from her. She sensed that they resented her for being an eager student, a "show-off," in particular because she was my only patient among them. I recalled that she had made comments in the group about discussions she'd had with me in individual therapy, which excluded the rest of them and may have led them to resent her. She could cite comments from them that supported this hypothesis. It was helpful to her to realize that her declining sense of self may have resulted from this transaction rather than from something inherently bad about her. She worked on changing the transaction, becoming part of the group, giving positive feedback toward other members, and distancing herself from me during group sessions. The transaction changed, and her feelings about herself became more positive.

Change Is Constant

This principle of dialectics has its counterpart in the acceptance-oriented principle of impermanence. Within the group everything is moving, everything is changing, everything is in motion, nothing stays the same for a minute, in spite of the sense sometimes that things are static and stuck. Oppositions are rising and falling, syntheses are occurring, everyone is influencing everyone else, and everyone's sense of self is evolving in response to group interaction. The skills trainer who thinks that the group is stuck and stagnant may feel that it is up to her to create movement. As she challenges the group to become more active, she might think of herself as the force of movement, while thinking of the rest of the group as united behind stasis. If instead she remains aware that change in fact is occurring, that forces are at work "under the surface," she can "let go" of pushing so hard, while observing and intervening with less pressure and more imagination. Rather than assuming that the forces of change are located in her, in opposition to the forces of stuckness located in the patients, she assumes that change is indeed underway and that it is her role to assess the situation and facilitate that change toward effective skills acquisition and strengthening.

When I was teaching interpersonal skills to a constricted and withdrawn group, I found myself working hard to teach in a livelier and more entertaining manner. Still, I felt as if I were trying to drag a battalion of reluctant soldiers into battle. I felt frustrated and ineffective. I was covering the material but not successfully engaging the group. Just as I mentioned above, I came to feel that it was up to me to get the group moving, as if I had to inject them with energy. I reminded myself that in spite of all appearances, the group was filled with energy and was constantly changing. I pictured it as a river in the wintertime with a surface of ice that seemed solid and stuck but with a strong current of water flowing underneath. I had to figure out how to break the ice and allow the energy to move the group members into greater involvement so they could learn more actively. Once I framed the problem in that metaphor, an intervention occurred to me. I realized that I might be participating in the stagnation by pushing them to get involved. Instead, I began the next group, with no further introduction, by engaging each of them in role-playing exercises in which I played the role of a detached and stubborn father, while they played the roles of children asking their father to get involved with them. They liked the exercise. It was fun, it became quite lively, and we were able to identify more and less skillful ways to ask someone to change. By placing myself in the role of the immovable object, and placing them in the role of the force for change, the ice was broken and the change was visible and productive.

CONCLUDING COMMENTS

Tension and opposition are inherent in group settings. Although the structured agenda of a skills training group, focused on the task of learning and practicing skills, helps to establish the order of a well-managed classroom, the tensions and oppositions are still present all the time. Linear problem-solving strategies, including a wide range of options, will help keep the group on track. Acceptance-oriented strategies based on mindfulness and validation help patients reduce suffering and tolerate distress. Still, tensions bubble up within and around each group session. The skills trainer who is conversant with the principles of opposition moving toward synthesis, with systemic thinking, with the way in which transactions can influence identity, and with the principle of flux (constant movement and change) has a multitude of tools to allow for conflict, validate both sides of a conflict, find syntheses, widen his perspective on current conflicts, and maintain speed, movement, and flow in the group. Group members learn a great deal by being part of a process in which polarization is handled dialectically.

CHAPTER 15

Prevention and Treatment of Therapist Burnout

Treating individuals with chronic, severe emotional dysregulation, poor judgment, and impulsivity would challenge the capacities of any therapist to stay present, connected, and involved. As any DBT therapist would attest, we are repeatedly exposed to evocative patient-related cues in and out of sessions. Patients' relentless hopelessness can elicit our own hopelessness, sadness, and helplessness. Their passive approach to problem solving can be demoralizing and frustrating. Threats of suicide can set off our fear, anxiety, and sometimes our anger. When patients direct their anger at us, we can experience fear, anxiety, resentment, and frustration. Patients whose ongoing dysfunction is known within the surrounding social–professional community can cause us shame and embarrassment. We might fear that our reputation is under threat, that our failure to help such patients has become "public," and sometimes we may even face potential legal or professional consequences. Emotionally disconnected, high-risk patients can elicit our anxiety and uncertainty, and cause us to make frantic efforts to connect. Such experiences may lead us to detach in the face of our seeming failures to engage the patient.

How we cope with painful, valid emotional responses influences both the quality of the treatment and our own balance and resilience. Our coping style is shaped by our personal histories as individuals and therapists, our values, and our treatment philosophies. Beyond these personal factors, our behavior and attitudes will be shaped by the responses of others with whom we interact around the care of our patient.

I have been consulted by many seasoned therapists who admitted they felt off-balance from working with patients diagnosed with borderline personality disorder. One midcareer female therapist, highly regarded within her community as an empathic and wise therapist, was treating a man from a large working-class family in which conflict, physical threats and fights were the norm. The treatment focused on his "anger management problem." He had been arrested several times for violence toward his brothers, triggered when he felt that they didn't treat their mother with sufficient respect. Although psychotherapy was a new experience for him, he seemed willing to assess his angry episodes and to try out solutions. Still, he brought an "edge" into therapy that was vaguely threatening at times, and his anger flared when the therapist challenged his interpretations of his brothers' behaviors. She was intimidated by his irritable style and implied threats, and steered away from challenging him any further.

Even though his behavior showed little change in the first 6 months of treatment, he repeatedly praised and thanked the therapist for her compassion and understanding. His gratitude helped her to persist, perhaps helped her to tolerate her fears and anxiety. She was not presenting this case in supervision of any kind, nor was she interacting with a consultation team. When she realized that this patient had made no visible progress in 6 months of treatment, she consulted me. When presenting the case to me, she seemed calm and rational, but as she aired her experiences and reactions to this patient, her strong feelings surprised both of us. She quickly realized that she had been suppressing her emotions. She recognized, for the first time, that she had been dreading the sessions with this patient. She felt frightened of him and ashamed of her ineffectiveness. She felt helpless and hopeless. She anticipated the day on which he was scheduled with anxiety that affected other sessions as well. As she talked with me, she looked down and acted as if she had committed a crime or a sin.

Although the treatment of this patient was difficult, and would have been so for most therapists, her level of burnout was not simply due to this case. And her experiences of anxiety, fear, powerlessness, and shame were not, in themselves, the cause of burnout. These were natural, valid, primary emotional responses to cues within the therapy relationship, which all of us face in the treatment of some patients. The germination of burnout began the moment she suppressed her first negative emotional responses. Her approach became unbalanced. In the service of suppression, she avoided some of the cues by refraining from any confrontation, by minimizing the importance of her emotional responses, and by overrelying on soothing, validating interventions. By avoiding statements that would inflame him, and empathically exploring the precursors to his angry episodes, she hoped that she would garner his trust, which would then allow for more change-oriented work. Instead, his irritability persisted, and he took little responsibility for his angry episodes. In fact, she grew more passive and timid, became the target of more of his anger, and came to feel trapped in the relationship with him. She was unable to act on her own behalf.

The suppression of her growing emotional responses had led to their proliferation, as is typically the case. As she came to realize how emotionally dysregulated she actually was, and how much distress she had been quietly suppressing, she was gradually able to make sense of her predicament, to resurrect her confidence, and to directly address his intimidating style and his failure to take responsibility. I responded to her with uninterrupted respect and without judgment, which allowed her to open up. From one perspective, the essence of the treatment of burnout is that the therapist has the opportunity to tell the "burnout story," to experience and express the associated (previously suppressed) emotions in a nonjudgmental context where the anticipated negative consequences are not actualized. It is easy to imagine that had this therapist not sought help, her emotional responses to this patient may have further immobilized her capabilities, the treatment would have come to a bad ending, and the therapist's confidence would have been scarred. Therapist burnout exacts a high cost for everyone involved. Fortunately, in this case, it was caught early enough.

This vignette allows us to document steps on the way to therapist burnout in all of its variations. As a therapist, supervisor, and DBT consultation team leader, I have experienced and seen this story unfold countless times. The common sequence of events proceeds approximately as indicated. The therapist:

1. May already be experiencing emotional vulnerability due to professional or personal circumstances unrelated to the patient.
2. Finds that she is exposed repeatedly to evocative patient-related cues related to that particular patient.
3. Experiences a range of painful negative emotions.
4. Thinks she should be able to handle them by herself.
5. Attempts to suppress the growing emotions.
6. Makes adjustments and compensations in therapy to cope with growing internal pressure but without facing his emotional responses.
7. Doesn't recognize the proliferation and increasing intensity of the suppressed emotions.

8. Engages in behaviors (errors of omission and commission) to escape the painful emotions that are arising, which causes a problematic imbalance in the therapeutic relationship.
9. Feels increasingly shaken by her lack of confidence in her own capacity to treat this patient.
10. May go on to find her avoidance tactics begin to impact her overall functioning with other patients, which leads to a loss of confidence in her therapeutic work in general, and can even spill over into her personal life. At this point the therapist is suffering from a full-blown case of therapist burnout.

Not uncommonly in cases that proceed to burnout, the therapist's areas of difficulty or vulnerability seem, in retrospect, like a perfect match with the patient's areas of difficulty or vulnerability, creating a "perfect storm." In the case of another therapist who consulted me, the problem began when a 25-year-old female patient with PTSD complained that she felt unsafe everywhere in her life, but claimed to feel safe with him. She complimented him for his steadiness and compassion, which was a source of pride for the therapist. Nevertheless, he began to feel rather drained and somewhat resentful of the patient's frequent requests for support outside of sessions. He was frustrated by her passive approach to solving problems in her life, which did not change much when he challenged her. Despite her claims that therapy helped her, her behavior did not change. He tried to keep his discouragement, resentment, and frustration in check. He was encouraged that she, at least, seemed to feel safe with him. He did not share his negative reactions with her, as he thought it would interrupt her feelings of safety. He did not share any detail of his difficulties with his DBT consultation team because, in his opinion, this was not a challenging case compared to many others being treated by team members.

In the third month of therapy, the patient began one session by asking if she could sit closer to the therapist. In fact, she wanted to sit right next to him, facing in the same direction that he was facing. She explained that it would make her feel closer to him, more "with him," and therefore stronger to tackle her life problems. He felt uncomfortable with the new seating arrangement but agreed to it, based on her obvious appreciation and increased level of comfort. In the next session, she attributed some gains she had made to his willingness to let her sit next to him. She asked him politely if he would please go a step further and allow her to hold his hand during sessions. She assured him that it was nothing sexual, that she knew it went beyond the "usual boundaries of a therapy," but argued that it would lead her to feel safer, more trusting, and "held." She communicated to him that she felt on the verge of a positive breakthrough in her life, and this added support would help her take the next step. The therapist felt acutely uncomfortable about the direction of things. That may have been the first moment in which he realized he had accommodated too much, had suppressed too much, and now was "in trouble."

He recounted this part of the story with a sense of humiliation, but it paled in comparison to what happened next. He felt incapable of saying no to her request in spite of his discomfort, and he agreed to let her hold his hand during the session. In retrospect, he felt as if he had been "under her control." He explained to me that his actions were not associated with any overt sexual feelings toward the patient, but were fueled more powerfully by a growing sense of impotence in relation to her. She had reinforced him again and again for his willingness to violate his own personal limits, had punished any of his more confrontational interventions, and he had lost control of the treatment.

Having progressed to this point where he was suppressing strong reactions and doing what was necessary in order to avoid the patient's anger at him, he became aware of an additional emotion: fear. He was afraid to challenge her, and feared for his reputation if his boundary violations were to become known to others. Feeling like a failure and as if he had become a victim, having difficulty sleeping, and beginning to doubt whether he should continue in this career, he set up a consultation with me. He and his patient had one more session before our meeting. In that session, talking as if she were a young child making a benign request of her daddy, the patient asked the therapist if he would allow her to sit on his lap in order to feel "even safer." For the first time, he rejected one of her requests. The patient silently stood up, went to the windowsill, grabbed hold of a two-by-four that was holding up the window, and tried to attack him with it. Fortunately, he was able to block the attack and escort her to the waiting area. After she berated and threatened him, he called the local crisis team and the patient was hospitalized.

Upon hearing a story like this, many assume that this therapist must differ from the rest of us, must be psychologically impaired. We separate ourselves from him. Yet this was a highly skilled therapist with good experience and an early but solid grasp of DBT. He had never had anything like this happen in treatment before, and he was thoroughly humiliated. Given the "right" patient and circumstances, any one of us can suffer from burnout in therapy and can make decisions that seem unimaginable in the moment. The more we can understand the "formula" for burnout, the more likely we will be able to find and use antidotes.

BURNOUT RESULTS FROM EMOTIONAL DYSREGULATION OF THE THERAPIST

As illustrated by these examples, the pathway to burnout begins when the therapist suppresses important, valid emotional responses to the patient. In the first example, the therapist suppressed her fear of the patient's anger; in the second, the therapist suppressed his awareness of his resentment of her demands and his frustration with her passivity. The suppression, in each case, led to imbalance as the therapists tried, heroically, to foster trust and engagement but without acknowledging or addressing their own negative emotions. Meanwhile, they each became more emotionally distressed, and tried to handle it without seeking help from others. The proliferating negative emotions led to broader difficulties, affecting the therapists well beyond the sessions. Each therapist grew more sensitive and reactive, emotionally fatigued, and ashamed. Self-confidence plummeted.

These steps in the progression toward therapist burnout show a striking resemblance to the steps outlined in DBT's biosocial theory for explaining the causation and maintenance of borderline behavioral patterns. Although biosocial theory posits a chronic and pervasive emotional regulation dysfunction affecting multiple life domains, we may be able to use the same theory in looking at the emotional dysregulation of the therapist with respect to the particular case. We might borrow the theory to explain how the therapist develops some of the borderline behavioral patterns within the relationship to the patient. The wide variety of problematic therapist behaviors associated with burnout, which we could call *burnout behaviors*, either follows directly from the therapist's patient-related emotional dysregulation or from efforts to cope with it. Framing our understanding of burnout in terms of DBT's biosocial theory provides us with a DBT-compatible conceptualization that opens up the possibility of using DBT's principles and strategies to prevent and treat it. As I argue, this approach provides the consultation team with a framework and "treatment plan" to help the therapist with burnout.

BIOSOCIAL THEORY AND THERAPIST BURNOUT

Biosocial theory posits a transaction between two factors and the results of that transaction. The first is a "person factor" and the second is an "environment factor." The person factor is the therapist's emotional vulnerability, in particular, his emotional vulnerability as activated in the treatment of the patient. The environment factor includes the invalidating or nonvalidating features of the environment related to his treatment of this particular patient. Over time, the transaction results in the therapist's emotional dysregulation, which affects his emotions, actions, thoughts, and physiology. His tendencies to avoid, suppress, and escape from the emotional responses, rather than face, express and process them, only exacerbate the problem.

The Therapist's Emotional Vulnerability

Following DBT's biosocial theory, we can identify three features of the person factor, the therapist's patient-related emotional vulnerability: (1) high emotional sensitivity to patient-related cues, (2) high emotional reactivity once the emotions are elicited, and (3) slow return to emotional baseline.

The heightened emotional vulnerability may or may not have been a prominent factor in the therapist's development or her personal life in general, but it is hypothesized to be present with respect to the treatment of the patient in the context of whom her burnout occurs. She has become highly sensitive and reactive to cues associated with the patient. Stressors in her personal or professional life, unrelated to the patient, may contribute to her vulnerability. In addition, she may have found that features of this particular patient uniquely engage her intense emotions, whether positive or negative or both. We have all come across certain patients (and other people in our lives) who "strike a chord in us," "get under our skin," "push our buttons," or just happen to provide a perfect match for some sensitivities based on history or biology. Once the therapist's sensitivity is activated with respect to the patient, the cues set off high-amplitude reactions. After a number of these, the therapist's emotions in response to this patient are slow to return to baseline, increasing the likelihood that the next patient-related cue will elicit a strong response. After awhile, the therapist's overall response to this patient is shaped by her need to manage her vulnerability, which can be enervating and stressful.

When I refer to *patient-related cues*, I include not only interactions in or out of sessions with the patient, but contact with family members, other professionals, fellow therapists, agencies, and requests for documentation about this patient. In our DBT day treatment program, a young postdoctoral fellow in psychology was treating one highly suicidal patient in DBT. He took part in one-on-one supervision and the DBT consultation team. As it was his only DBT case, and because he cared deeply about making a good impression on his supervisor and the team, he was highly sensitive about whether his work was viewed favorably. He oriented his patient to the telephone coaching policy, with which she was encouraged to call him for skills coaching in a crisis. He began to receive more and more phone calls from her during days, nights, and weekends. Beyond her calls, he began to take phone calls from the patient's mother, who was worried that her daughter would die. He did not feel that his coaching was helping her use skills, but he knew it was an expected practice in DBT. He did inform the consultation team about the phone calls, but fearing that he might be taking more calls than he should, he failed to convey the extreme frequency of the calls, their ineffective nature, or the additional calls by the mother. He made it sound as if everything was going OK, even though privately he was growing more and more distressed.

Fairly soon he was dreading the prospect of another phone call from her. In the terms of biosocial theory, his emotional vulnerability with respect to this patient had become pronounced: He was highly sensitive to any cue related to her, his emotional reactions to her (kept private by him) were intense, and even with "time off" from the program he could not reduce his distress. As we subsequently learned, his anxiety about the patient was accompanied by his doubts about his own abilities. He felt ashamed to be keeping information from the team, and came to feel like a "phony." Although he had team members willing to support him, he felt trapped and alone in his treatment of this patient. He dreaded even going home to his apartment at the end of the day because he anticipated that a voice mail message would be waiting for him from this patient or her mother.

During a consultation team meeting, other therapists noted that he was more withdrawn during meetings. One was worried about this therapist's "morale." Team members expressed concerned and asked him how things were going. Unable to maintain his business-as-usual facade, he shared, reluctantly and tearfully, that he was taking more than a dozen phone calls per day from this patient and her mother, that he felt very ineffective and isolated, and that he feared that if she killed herself it would ruin his career. He was thoroughly embarrassed, but with the team's encouragement and validation, he was able to express all the reactions he had been suppressing. With some additional help in individual supervision, he was able to reframe the treatment within his personal limits and with a well-defined crisis protocol. The patient was distraught about the changes, but with some validation, soothing, and problem solving by the therapist, was able to remain in treatment and ultimately to benefit from it.

The Therapist's Invalidating Environment

We have considered the features of the person factor of the theory. The other factor pertains to the environment around the therapist, in particular, the *microenvironment* surrounding the therapist's treatment of this particular patient. This microenvironment is likely to include other members of the consultation team, any individual supervisor on that case, administrative personnel related to the patient, other professionals outside the DBT team who work with the patient, family members of the patient, and the patient herself. The therapist may have transactions with any and all of these parties regarding the patient, his treatment of the patient, and his emotional responses to the patient. Of special relevance to the theory and the progression to burnout are those transactions in which members of the environment are invalidating him (usually inadvertently) or not validating him, especially for his vulnerabilities. The therapist suffering from emotional dysregulation regarding his treatment of a patient is usually keenly aware of the responses of the environment to the treatment, the patient, and his reactions to the treatment and the patient. Being vulnerable puts him on a state of *alert*. He is likely to notice if his communications about the patient are treated, whether subtly or not so subtly, with disregard or criticism. Whereas the nature of invalidation of the individual with borderline personality disorder may involve rather severe neglect and abuse, the nature of invalidation of a therapist by those around him is likely to be more subtle, even if quite pervasive.

Certain characteristics of the typical culture of clinical settings can add to the experience of invalidation and vulnerability. First, therapy takes place in private, rarely seen by anyone else. Second, although DBT is an evidence-based treatment, and the therapist and team may be gathering and documenting outcomes, the therapist is understandably uncertain about whether her work is adherent to the model and efficacious with the patient. Third, the therapist works in a social environment in which self-sufficiency is valued; the therapist may think that she should not need much help. Finally, these are very difficult patients and problems to treat, and the risks can be high. In sum, in most clinical settings the context itself, before even starting with a given patient, may be filled with factors that heighten therapists' vulnerability. Linehan (1993a) defined DBT in such a way that every therapist must be part of a consultation team. Teams encourage all members to share the vulnerable aspects of their work, and all team members make six agreements, including a "Fallibility Agreement," affirming that everyone on the team is fallible. By trying to increase connection and sharing, and decrease defensiveness, the team works to establish conditions in which therapists are more likely to accurately express difficulties they are having in their work.

As mentioned, invalidation in a team context might not be obvious. In one way or another, the therapist may experience himself to be invalidated by fellow team members. For instance, if he has a strong emotional response to a patient and expresses it to fellow professionals, his response might be considered to be "excessive" or "inappropriate." This critical view will rarely be stated outright, but the therapist might sense this subtle criticism nonetheless. Disapproval, criticism, and judgment can be communicated more in what is not said than in what is said, or more in the subtly judgmental tone of questions and suggestions. Because the therapist may tend to act self-sufficiently and competently even when not feeling that way, and the team members may act respectful and nonjudgmental even when not feeling that way, the therapist who is expressing strong, negative, emotional, patient-related responses to the team might sense that team members' respectful and validating comments lack authenticity and depth. He could feel "invalidated through faint empathy," akin to the feeling of being "damned by faint praise." The nonverbal feedback from the team could amplify his sense of being isolated and incompetent. Given his strong emotional responses, he may feel stuck amid three options, none of which provides a solution: (1) to express the feelings in team and risk invalidation, (2) to express them to the patient and risk invalidating the patient, or (3) to suppress them with the risk of increasing emotional dysregulation. The consultation team is in the key position to help the therapist find a better option: to provide genuine validation when the therapist expresses his feelings, and to help the therapist assess and problem-solve the controlling variables underlying his reactions.

In the latter two examples above, one in which the therapist proceeded step-by-step toward seriously inappropriate behaviors that included physical contact, driven by his fear of the patient; and the other in which the young therapist tolerated an unbearable number of telephone coaching calls without informing his team, the consultation teams were, in fact, genuinely respectful and supportive. They did not appear to be harsh, critical, neglectful, or actively invalidating. Still, there was something in the transaction among the therapists, the consultation team "culture," and the broader professional environment that reduced the two troubled therapists' emotional openness, increased their suppression of intense emotional responses, and blocked their willingness to request help from the team. It is wise for consultation teams to assume that therapists may withhold emotional vulnerabilities and present themselves as confident and capable even when burnout is occurring. In this respect, teams should take a proactive stance in seeking evidence of burnout and addressing it.

Accompanying this "syndrome" of pervasive invalidation or nonvalidation in our field, and further elaborated in some clinical environments, there is an unstated oversimplification of the often very difficult task of regulating our emotions in response to our clients. Most people act as if therapists "should" be able to tolerate and productively manage patients' anger, threats, suicide attempts, violent behaviors, and passive way of addressing life problems, without much need for validation or support themselves. The subtly but pervasively invalidating clinical environment inadvertently reinforces therapists for acting as if they feel competent, and for suppressing negative emotional responses unless and until they escalate to the point where they cannot be suppressed any more. When a therapist "breaks down" or "blows up," thereby finally receiving recognition and support, the team is reinforcing escalated therapist presentations with an intermittent reinforcement schedule. The resulting pattern tends to reinforce escalated therapist behaviors in the team setting while suppressing a more routine expression of negative emotions.

Consequences to the Therapist

This transaction between the therapist's patient-related vulnerabilities and the subtly but pervasively invalidating professional, clinical, and team environment has several consequences. First, having adapted to the invisibly invalidating environment in which she finds herself, the therapist is then prone to invalidate her own responses. She becomes self-critical and cautious, doubting her abilities. She becomes unsure about her clinical judgment and intuitions. Second, she is likely to oscillate between suppressing her emotional responses to her patient much of the time, whereas on some occasions being overcome with extreme responses. Finally, she may follow the environment's lead in oversimplifying the therapist's task of emotional regulation regarding her patients.

The ongoing transaction between the therapist's emotional vulnerabilities and the invalidating environment causes distortions and excesses in the therapist's approach to the patient. He may begin to avoid patient-related cues to which he has become sensitive. By evading certain topics in therapy, avoiding certain kinds of interventions that will elicit the patient's emotional responses, "accidentally" forgetting appointments or failing to return phone calls, neglecting the need to follow up with patient-related collaborations or documentation, and by skirting discussions about his patient in team meetings, he drifts from the treatment model. Even with all of this avoidance, team members might not realize that the therapist is becoming dysregulated in his treatment of a particular patient.

In particular, the therapist on the road to burnout may find it increasingly difficult to validate the patient's own emotional responses. Validation comes from a position of awareness and compassion, both of which might be compromised, and requires an active effort to empathize with the patient's experiences when, in fact, the therapist may be averse to hearing about them. Because of not wanting to "get into it" with the patient by probing or confronting him, the therapist might show little attention or reaction to the patient's significant but less than extreme emotional behaviors. The therapist might even begin to criticize the patient's lack of self-control or extreme emotional responses—a reaction that mirrors the patient's previous invalidating environments. The patient recognizes all of these dynamics implicitly or explicitly, and occasionally will generate more extreme behaviors that will get the therapist's attention, resulting in the intermittent reinforcement of the patient's escalated behaviors.

In addition to avoiding patient-related cues, the therapist may engage in other behaviors to escape his painful emotional responses. He may find himself detaching from the patient, forgetting what has been said even a minute ago. He may engage in a more superficial rendition of therapy, retreating into safe topics or platitudes. A psychiatrist or other prescriber might shift the discussion into the realm of psychopharmacology and medical problems rather than sticking with emotionally evocative material. The therapist might overreact to some incidents in sessions while underreacting to others. He might be looking at the clock when there are still 20 minutes left, thinking about what will be happening after the session. Outside of sessions, when the process toward burnout is far along, the therapist may try to avoid thinking about the patient, but actually experience intrusive thoughts about the patient that extend into his personal life and may result in insomnia.

The Impact of Therapist Burnout on the Patient and the Treatment

In sum, the emotionally dysregulated therapist acts in many ways that provoke further emotional dysregulation in the patient, whose reaction patterns then further provoke the syndrome in the therapist. *A transactional burnout spiral ensues.* Unchecked, the therapist might proceed in the direction of near or total detachment, may harm the client, may want to end therapy, and even might want to change her career path. Therapy is often dead long before anybody knows, which harms both parties.

IT IS UNIQUELY THE ROLE OF THE DBT CONSULTATION TEAM TO PREVENT AND TREAT THERAPIST BURNOUT OF EACH MEMBER OF THE TEAM! I have yet to convey that therapist burnout is normal. Just as firefighters must prepare for the likelihood that they will, at some point, suffer some burn or smoke inhalation injury, DBT therapists must prepare for the likelihood that in working with emotionally dysregulated individuals, they will, at some point, become emotionally dysregulated. It is necessary to assume this as an expectable possibility at any time for any therapist on the team. One of the primary functions of a DBT team is to anticipate and actively manage therapist burnout, ideally preventing it whenever possible, detecting it when it happens, and treating it when it has occurred.

APPLYING DBT PRINCIPLES TO THE PREVENTION AND TREATMENT OF THERAPIST BURNOUT

Fidelity to the model of DBT requires regular meetings of all therapists on the consultation team, conducted according to certain guidelines and agreements. It is not an optional supervision, as is the case in many treatment models; it is part and parcel of the program. The function of the team is to attend to therapists' motivation and enhancement of their capacity to conduct DBT therapy with adherence to the manual. Given that the therapist's emotional dysregulation can disrupt therapy and damage her self-confidence and well-being, a high priority for the team is to anticipate, detect, prevent, and treat emotional dysregulation in each team member. This is a substantial part of what it means to say that the DBT consultation team provides "therapy for the therapist," drawing from the DBT treatment model and its principles. I consider three steps in team-based burnout prevention and treatment: (1) detection of the process of burnout; (2) prevention of burnout through consistent application of DBT's principles; and (3) treatment of burnout once it has taken root, also by use of DBT's principles and associated strategies.

Detecting Burnout

The consultation team members should not wait for the overt presentation of burnout, but instead should proactively screen themselves and each other for evidence of burnout. Active screening is important because of the typical atmosphere of clinical settings, in which therapists get the consistent message to manage patient-related emotional distress privately.

Metaphorically, team members should search each other for indicators of burnout in the loving way that monkeys groom one other, searching for bugs in the fur and picking them out. What are the indicators of the presence of burnout? Some are direct indicators, announcing the presence of burnout, and others are indirect, suggesting that burnout may be under way. None of these provides convincing evidence that burnout is present, but they are indicators of the need for further inquiry and observation.

DIRECT INDICATORS

1. *"I'm burned out."* The therapist reports the problem to the team in no uncertain terms.

2. *Premature urge to terminate.* The therapist, wanting to escape from the cues and emotions, presents a recommendation that he stop with the patient when there is little evidence to support that suggestion.

3. *Blatantly judgmental statements about the client.* These statements indicate that the therapist is reacting to her own difficult emotional responses to the patient by packaging them in criticism of the patient.

4. *Marked imbalance in the therapy.* Team members notice that the therapist is adopting what appears to be a markedly unbalanced response. He may be (a) extremely focused on behavioral change while attending little to validation, (b) extremely empathic and validating while ignoring the push for change, (c) approaching the patient with rigid demands and limits with minimal flexibility, or (d) offering extreme flexibility and nurturance in the context of almost no demands or limits.

5. *Therapist burnout is suggested by the patient.* Sometimes the patient is the first to "blow the whistle" on burnout, directly asking the therapist why she has changed so significantly and whether she "cares" any more. Sometimes the patient brings this to the attention of the skills trainer or some other team member rather than directly to the therapist.

INDIRECT INDICATORS

1. *Therapist seems emotionally vulnerable.* Team members notice that the therapist is more sensitive, reactive, moody, irritable, sad, or otherwise emotional than usual. This might come up in the context of one case, or may have gone beyond the one case and is more general.

2. *Therapist seems subtly judgmental/disrespectful/imbalanced toward a particular patient.* Team members note the change in the therapist, which is significant but not as extreme as the direct indicator noted above. Team members gently inquire about their perceptions.

3. *Therapist evidences imbalance with respect to the team.* When discussing the patient in question, the therapist may evince extreme or maladaptive responses in the team meetings: He is more withdrawn, more argumentative, more erratic, or in some cases, surprisingly protective toward the patient. Team members gently note the shift and inquire about causes and conditions. Therapist burnout is one possible explanation.

4. *Therapist deviates from DBT's assumptions, agreements, or biosocial theory.* DBT's assumptions, agreements, and biosocial theory define guidelines and a practical philosophy that help the therapist to walk the "middle path" between acceptance and change, resulting in care that is compassionate and effective. The therapist who usually operates within these guidelines is noticed to have drifted from them in one direction or another, and is therefore moving out of compliance with the treatment manual. (Note that this point means that all DBT therapists should be familiar with the assumptions, agreements, and theory!) Team members gently inquire about the changes, wondering whether they are early manifestations of burnout.

5. *Therapist allows repeated violations of his personal limits.* It is up to team members to support each other in defining and observing his personal limits. When team members recognize that a therapist's personal limits seem to have become broader or narrower than usual, or notice that his limits are extreme enough to result in dysfunctional consequences for the patient or him, they inquire as to whether the therapist might like consultation on the case or on the limits, in particular.

Preventing Burnout

DBT's three paradigms and the use of the principles flowing from each provide all the needed tools for the team to help prevent emotional dysregulation in each therapist. The team establishes an atmosphere of acceptance in keeping with the five principles of the acceptance paradigm. Within that context, when a therapist asks for the team's help, she is received in an alert, nonjudgmental, and validating manner that encourages an open, accurate rendition of the story leading up to her dysregulation. Given that part of the problem is due to suppression, avoidance, and escape responses, the team's response already offers relief and compassion, which promotes self-acceptance on the way to improved emotion modulation.

Within the validating context, the team is guided by principles of the change paradigm to target the problematic behaviors, secure a commitment from the therapist to join in problem solving, work with the therapist to assess for the controlling variables, arrive at a case conceptualization of the burnout behaviors and syndrome, select solutions among the possibilities present within the four behavioral models in DBT, and implement solutions with follow-up in subsequent team meetings. The therapist with burnout benefits from the team's active use of the acceptance principles, and the use of the principles of change and a rational problem-solving sequence can also engender hope where faith that there is "a way out" may have been lost. I discuss the role of the change principles in more detail when we turn to the *treatment* of established therapist burnout in teams.

Through the principles of the dialectical paradigm, the team injects a different set of "ingredients" into the process that can help with burnout prevention and treatment. These principles provide a framework for recognizing and successfully resolving opposition in treatment, for broadening the perspective on the systemic factors contributing to the therapist–patient impasse, and for acknowledging that change is always happening regardless of the appearance of paralysis and stagnation. Dialectics provides ways to deal with the kinds of rigid positions and conflicts, narrow perspectives, and stasis that accompany burnout syndromes. Dialectical principles are discussed below insofar as they help with burnout prevention, and then further in the next section insofar as they help with treatment of established therapist burnout.

The Acceptance Paradigm in the Prevention of Burnout

It cannot be overstated that the therapist whose team members are open, present, awake, alert, gentle, and compassionate will be more likely to open up, to share vulnerabilities, to express emotions generated in treatment, and to ask for help. It is challenging to establish an atmosphere of openness, but it should remain the ideal for every team. It begins by applying the principle of *being in the present moment*. The team starts its meeting with a mindfulness practice designed to help therapists let go of preoccupations and settle into the present moment. Team members practice DBT's core mindfulness skills: observing, describing, participating, remaining nonjudgmental, remaining one-mindful, and interacting effectively. Some teams designate an "observer" within the team, who monitors mindful participation in the team meetings and sounds a mindfulness bell to alert everyone to moments of judgment and nonmindful behaviors. Inviting all team members to repeatedly return to the *present moment* creates an expectation that if anyone raises delicate matters and vulnerable emotions, he or she will be received with "all eyes and ears."

Members are likely to be alert and attuned to each other, and will naturally practice the first three levels of validation (wide awake listening, accurate reflection, and articulating the unarticulated). Because manifestations of burnout might not be recognized or volunteered by the affected therapist, the wide awake, alert team members grounded in the present moment are more likely to notice subtle changes in each other, screening for burnout and taking care of burnout manifestations in each other.

Given that DBT is an evidence-based treatment packed with a wide range of different elements, it is the job of each therapist to practice the entire treatment with fidelity. Accordingly, it is a task of the team to help each member practice correctly. However, in some teams, the push for adherence can result in an atmosphere that stifles openness, the sharing of vulnerabilities, and the presentation of work that violates elements in the manual. If the therapist becomes excessively preoccupied with adherence to the point where he sheepishly omits some of his emotions, thoughts, and actions with respect to the patient, he fails to acknowledge the reality of his responses, fuels his own shame, and loses the opportunity to get help. An unbalanced, excessively compliance-focused team atmosphere can worsen burnout rather than resolve it.

Those teams that are overly change-focused are actually not adhering to the manual. Since a balance between change and acceptance represents good DBT practice, the consultation team should reflect this balance as well. It is not a small challenge. Teams need to focus on adherence, performance, and improvement of each therapist and simultaneously maintain an atmosphere of presence, warmth, genuineness, openness, and compassion. The team meeting should shift back and forth from acceptance to change, change to acceptance, over and over again. The acceptance principle of *nonattachment* can be most helpful for everyone in pivoting between change and acceptance. When team members begin to listen to a fellow therapist as she presents a difficult case situation, which may require sharing her vulnerability, therapists often need to temporarily "let go" of the attachment to "what should be" and just listen for "what actually is." Letting go of the urge to correct, criticize, or improve their colleague, team members listen for the accurate description of what is happening, listen for what the therapist wants from the team rather than what she "should be" asking, and find the validity in the therapist's responses. Therapists will respond to this kind of respect and openness with greater willingness to share honestly even if they are not proud of their responses. After the initial part of the consultation, involving accurate listening and assessment, team members can help the therapist improve her therapeutic handling of the situation if she so desires.

To the degree that team members can apply the principle of *interbeing*, by recognizing the deep interdependence of everyone on the team, they are more likely to act as part of one team organism rather than as totally separate beings. As a result, the power of the team and the resources available to each member increase. Each therapist is on the team and in the team; the team is in each therapist. Each patient of each therapist is the patient of all. In making themselves vulnerable by presenting potentially painful material to each other, each therapist is a patient sometimes and a therapist to his fellow therapists at others. Role definitions shift; everyone plays all parts. Participating in the spirit of *interbeing* allows each therapist to share meaningfully, to "lean in" to the team, and to depend on the team as a trusted partner. Emotional dysregulation in one therapist becomes a point of concern for all; becomes, in a sense, everyone's emotional dysregulation. The intimate quality of support stays with each therapist, so that even when he or she is doing therapy, it is, to some degree, as if the team were doing the therapy. In fact, Linehan has recommended that if one therapist on a team is called into a court hearing as a result of a patient's suicide, the entire team should attend, making it clear that all are one in the team. Obviously, the chances of recognizing indicators of burnout and helping a therapist to process the emotional response is much more likely to happen in this team context than in a collection of separate, unrelated individuals, each one wary of the others.

Recognizing the principle of *impermanence*—stating that everything, including things that we treasure and things that we fear, is transient—promotes a desire to live within, appreciate, and treasure the present moment. Every moment of every team meeting is fleeting, precious, unique, and will pass on immediately. If team members are practicing according to this principle, they are more likely to "show up," to share vulnerable material, and to take good care of each other. In short, each moment matters. Even if the present moment is unpleasant, and is not yielding a desirable solution, team members know that it is temporary, that things are changing, that "this too shall pass." Therapists might be able to inhabit the precious moment, recognize it, and let go of the need to control it. It becomes easier to allow, and even trust, the emergence of possibility. *Impermanence*, in concert with *present-moment awareness* and *nonattachment*, helps each therapist to simply *be* in the moment, to let go of controlling it, recognize its transient nature, and engage in practicing the treatment. For the therapist who is "on the fence" with respect to sharing vulnerable feelings and difficulties in therapy, the resulting atmosphere will be more conducive to his or her "jumping in." Burnout prevention becomes the natural consequence.

"The world is perfect as it is." Everything has a cause. Each therapist is doing the best he or she can do, given everything that came before. The team looks for the validity in the therapist's behavior in therapy and team meetings. The behaviors might be valid in the context of history or biology, that is, the therapist's previous experience. They might be valid with respect to the current context in that her behavioral response might be the same as that of many in the circumstances. Her behaviors might be valid with respect to her ends-in-view. Whereas there is a place for understanding a therapist's behaviors by assessing the controlling variables that are causing a progression toward burnout, there is no place for judging the therapist. The therapist who is considering whether to present events from her treatment of a patient, including her fallibility and vulnerability, is much more likely to do so if the team truly acts as if *"the world is perfect as it is."*

In sum, the consultation team that creates an accepting context for all by combining the principles of present-moment awareness, nonattachment, interbeing, impermanence, and "perfect as is" has created a context that includes everyone; that values difference over conformity; that listens and assesses rather than assumes; that supports the kind of interdependency that strengthens each participant; and that allows for discussion of sensitive, painful, and poignant matters. Every therapist, and every patient of every therapist, is the recipient of this bounty. The morale and resiliency of each therapist goes up, and the risk of burnout goes down.

The Dialectical Paradigm in the Prevention of Burnout

Implementing principles of the dialectical paradigm also serves to strengthen the consultation team. Using these principles will add a flavor of flexibility, creativity, and inclusiveness of all perspectives; movement, speed, and flow; and a willingness to allow for the full expression of opposing positions in a dialectical process that moves toward synthesis.

DBT team members often disagree, which can be productive or destructive. One therapist argues that another therapist is too strict or too flexible with his patient. One therapist believes that the team spends too much time on chit-chat and mindfulness practices, and too little time on consultation. Or, one team member suggests that the team leader is being too rigid about DBT fidelity, and the team leader counters that this is just the goal! Just when one disagreement is solved, another one arises. And the ones that do not get solved can become chronic festering wounds within the team, growing over time until things become very uncomfortable and the environment feels unsafe.

In fact, when team members have different responses, ideas, and styles, this diversity, if tolerated and valued, will expand team resources and possibilities. Optimally, each therapist will feel free to be him- or her self in team, even as each therapist is participating within team guidelines and the principles covered in this book. But if team members are uncomfortable with conflict among them, this is not the case. As noted, one principle of the dialectical paradigm holds that reality is composed of *opposites*; that a proposition, or thesis, will elicit the opposing proposition, or antithesis. For instance, the ambitious team leader, wanting everyone to practice DBT as perfectly as possible, will elicit an opposing opinion from someone in the team, that it is important to apply DBT with flexibility. Once a conflict exists, the dialectical approach is not to choose which is correct. Dialectical thinking is not "either . . . or" thinking but a synthesis that emerges from two valid perspectives. In team meetings, implementing dialectical processes provides a way to increase the comfort with conflict and to see the enormous value in it. It's the perfect process to apply to situations in which differences have led to impasses, which is part of the burnout formula. If the team can handle conflicts dialectically, members will know that differences are not only safe, but also desirable. When a dialectical process is in place, therapists express more perspectives, come up with more solutions, and take more risks with each other.

When the team accepts conflict, it helps to prevent burnout in several ways. First, if all members feel included and find that their contributions are valued and not rejected, there is an enhanced sense of safety and collaboration in the team. Second, if someone on the team would otherwise fear that her experiences or viewpoints are either incorrect or unusual, an accepting atmosphere encourages her to communicate, trusting that in a dialectical process, the validity of her position will be respected. If a therapist is suffering from emotional dysregulation, but is too ashamed to share his emotions or behaviors with the team, he may be more likely to do so if he anticipates an inclusive and respectful response. If it can operate dialectically, responding to opposing positions by seeking synthesis, the team is ultimately more flexible and safer.

I have consulted with a number of teams that were, by their own admission, "too nice for their own good." Therapists did not intentionally submerge conflicts and differences, but would do so almost automatically. And it can be pleasant to be on a team in which everyone always seems to agree with one another. Still, it is unimaginable in an endeavor as complex as DBT, with challenging patients and therapists prone to emotional dysregulation, to think that everyone truly shares the same perspective all the time. I believe it is worth it for a team to work on the capacity to disagree, to contain opposing positions in a manner that makes it safer and more productive to do so. In consultations and training, teams can work deliberately on expanding their dialectical capacities by staging disagreements, using formats such as formal debating or role playing, wherein team members deliberately take opposing positions and then work on how to validate opposites and search for synthesis. A little bit of practice goes a long way in strengthening the capacity to manage disagreements productively and thereby increasing safety and flexibility in the team.

Systemic thinking helps to generate new angles on a stubborn problem: new perspectives on formulation and new avenues of approach. The realization that any given entity (a patient, a therapist, another team member, a family member, etc.) is always part of a larger whole, and that a change in any one part results in a change in all other parts, opens up a universe of options that might have been overlooked. For instance, sometimes when a therapist has gotten stuck in treatment, he can feel like a failure. He's closed to other options. His thinking narrows, and he feels alone and discouraged. But in DBT, perspectives can be expanded by "handing over" the patient to the team. This can be done via role playing in a number of ways: (1) The therapist could play the patient, and a different team member plays the therapist; (2) the therapist could play herself as therapist, while someone else plays the patient; or (3) the therapist could watch as one team member plays the therapist while a different one plays the patient. New perspectives arise, new solutions emerge, and the team begins to "own" the treatment. The entrapped individual therapist emerges with new ideas and an expanded vision. Even more concretely, the therapist could invite a team member to join him for a session with the patient, to consult with the two of them together. He might even ask a different therapist to meet with the patient for a couple weeks as part of consultation.

In my treatment of a 17-year-old boy, it seemed as if we spoke different emotional languages. I liked him and tried to help him with his depression, suicidal intentions, and substance use behaviors, but somehow we always ended up getting stuck. If I made a suggestion to him, however gently, he acted as if I was criticizing him and trying to "remodel" him, as he put it. With the help of the team, I tried different interventions, including several different problem-solving strategies, validation strategies, and some dialectical strategies such as the use of metaphor and making lemonade out of lemons. No matter what, we would end up at the same standoff: it seeming as if I were criticizing him or trying to control him. I was getting frustrated, somewhat hopeless, and was at risk for a more advanced condition of therapist burnout.

One of my team members wondered whether I was somehow unknowingly "playing the role" of someone in the boy's family, possibly the father, with whom the boy barely spoke. She suggested that I meet with the boy and his father, just to see what would happen in that constellation. I followed her suggestion. In the meeting, I found myself at odds with the father again and again, no matter what we discussed, as if we were siblings in a perpetual quarrel. The boy commented on my conflict with his father and made some insightful comments and skillful suggestions. The boy's comments reflected a deep understanding of the process of quarreling and of the damaging impact of criticism. That session led to a refreshing shift in our one-on-one relationship. Systemic thinking and systemically informed interventions direct attention to the larger whole and its various parts, which can open up unexplored territories and keep the process moving.

When a therapist is stuck, or a team is stuck, it can seem as if time goes on forever, with frustration and hopelessness ever increasing. In fact, from the perspective of the third dialectical principle, *flux*, the experience of being at a standstill is an illusion. The therapist, and team, that can call this principle of reality to mind at the moment of a perceived impasse can escape from the illusionary entrapment. If we stand still, things will change. If we move, things will change. We can count on it; we just can't always see it when it is happening. When a team is consulting on a stubborn problem that one therapist is having in individual therapy or that team members are having among themselves, burnout-promoting predicaments, problems can seem unsolvable and time can feel unbearably long. It is at those moments that one team member can remind the others that, in spite of appearances, actually everything is moving and changing every moment and that options will emerge with time. This perspective can ease the sense of entrapment, facilitate greater patience, and help everyone freshly consider how to create movement, speed, and flow. Sometimes it can be the case that frantic efforts to bring about change can actually interfere with change, whereas truly "letting go" of trying to change things allow movement to occur and new perspectives to emerge.

Finding validity in opposing positions, searching for synthesis of what is valid from each, expanding our field of observation with systemic thinking, and allowing ourselves to remember that flux is constant, at every level of every system, promotes resolution of conflict, opens up interventions addressing the larger system, and allows for greater patience and movement. The dialectical principles facilitate a more flexible frame within which to detect and prevent therapist burnout and its manifestations in consultation team. Finally, I now address principle-based approaches to the resolution of therapist burnout once it is well established.

Treatment of Therapist Burnout by the Consultation Team

We now move on to the step-by-step application of change principles when working in team with a therapist who is suffering from a moderate to severe level of burnout.

The Change Paradigm in the Treatment of Burnout

The explicit work on burnout begins with the process of *targeting*. Not surprisingly, the highest-priority target for the team will be consultation with a therapist whose patient is exhibiting high-risk life-threatening behaviors. The second highest target priority for the team is consulting with a therapist who is experiencing or demonstrating evidence of burnout. In some cases, a therapist will place herself on the agenda, asking for help with burnout or emotional dysregulation. On other occasions, the therapist himself might not recognize or might not volunteer that he is on a path toward burnout, but team members may notice indicators and inquire about them. The active search for signs of burnout in team members, if handled with respect and validation, may help to catch it early and prevent it from proceeding to the transactional therapist–patient burnout spiral discussed above.

In one team, a highly capable DBT therapist, who was in charge of a DBT day treatment program and who usually asked the team for help, grew more and more silent over several weeks. When directly asked if she had anything for the agenda, she would just say, "Everyone is doing fine." It was so unlike her and so unlikely to be true, given the stressful nature of her program, so that her team members became puzzled and worried. As we established the meeting agenda, we inquired if she needed help, to which she responded with resentment and a firm refusal to be on the agenda. One team member persisted, and she grew overtly angry and told her to "Back off!" It was difficult to either inquire further or to let it go. The team sat in silence. When the team member who was personally a good friend of hers asked "How can we help?," she burst into tears and her concerns came pouring out. For one thing, she had a very high-risk patient in her program and she was frustrated with the patient's therapist. She went on to express discouragement about her program as a whole and about her competence as a leader. She finished by stating that she "always knew" that she was in the wrong field and was thinking about leaving mental health altogether. Nothing in what she said was totally new to team members, but the level of intensity and hopelessness was way beyond what anyone had known. It was as if an abscess was lanced and intense pressure came pouring out. After another silence, she thanked the team for being patient, and it became possible to begin to assess the controlling variables of her pressure and despair. For our purposes here, it is important to note that the process of targeting is not always simple in cases of burnout, because suppression of responses and shame about one's effectiveness are often part of the story.

Furthermore, it is important to realize that sometimes what appears to be a process of burnout around the treatment of one patient or a group may have sources far away from the clinical environment. In one example, team members noticed that a therapist seemed very distressed and unusually judgmental when talking about her work with one patient. She was reluctant to talk about it. When a team member pushed her a little bit, she nearly shouted out the news, which was new to everyone on the team, that she had been diagnosed with cancer. Her burnout was not the result of therapy, but it was affecting her treatment of everyone, most notably her most difficult patient. Team members, stunned and worried, asked if they could be of help. They volunteered to help with any cases, any groups, and to support her more personally if that were possible. She expressed appreciation, but informed team members that she had good supports, and had other places to manage her feelings. She asked if she could just continue to participate on the team to the degree possible because she found it "normalizing." This example may help to clarify that when we talk about the consultation team as "therapy for the therapist" in DBT, this does not mean that it is a form of "personal therapy." It is "therapy for the therapist" insofar as we are helping each other within the context of conducting treatment of patients.

Once teams have ascertained that a therapist is asking for help with problems associated with burnout, the therapist will ideally provide a detailed description of the situation, including events, thoughts, actions, and emotions. At this point, one of the most common mistakes that team members make is to begin making suggestions. They may have had a similar challenge in cases of their own and are eager to share their solutions. They may know the patient, either through prior contact as a therapist or within a skills training group, and they have an immediate impression of the problem and what needs to be done. It is quite possible that the suggestions are right on target, and the intention is honorable, but quick and easy ideas can engage a defensive response from the therapist. What needs to come next is a thoughtful assessment. Most of the time, after the therapist describes the problem in some detail, it is best if someone on the team says something to the therapist such as, "Now that you have explained the problem, tell us what you think we can do to help you."

Sometimes a therapist does not want suggestions, she just wants to be heard and understood, and that is enough. At other times, a therapist wants ideas about how to conceptualize the situation. At times, a therapist actually wants suggestions about how to solve the problem with the patient. And occasionally a therapist asks specifically for help on how to regulate his own emotions, which may have become overwhelming. The team members' job is to find out what kind of help the therapist seeks, not to provide everything that occurs to them.

Targeting and monitoring go hand in hand; once a therapist's progression toward burnout is addressed in a team meeting, it should be revisited on the agenda in future meetings to get updates and to allow for continued problem solving.

Commitment is essential as part of problem solving on a consultation team just as it is in the conduct of individual therapy. This point refers both to the level of commitment of the team to each therapist and the level of commitment of the therapist to target her problematic behaviors and distressing treatment-related emotions. Participating on a DBT consultation team requires "signing on" to the six consultation team agreements and arranging to be on time and consistent with attendance. In the meetings themselves, therapists are expected to be fully present and attentive to one another, not distracted by other work, cell phone communications, or sideline discussions. In the past few years, when explaining her latest insights about consultation teams during seminars, Linehan has argued the importance of everyone who participates on a consultation team being "vulnerable," by which she means that everyone is practicing DBT in one mode or another. No one is sitting "outside" the vulnerable circle of therapists who are sharing their work. To have one, two, or more "observers" who are not practicing DBT can inhibit the willingness of some therapists to share their fallibilities. For instance, having administrators on the team to keep them abreast of team developments or having non-DBT therapists attend to learn about DBT can interfere with the optimal atmosphere. In short, the DBT team is more like a "fighting unit" dealing with combat than a seminar or administrative meeting. Time is precious, attendance is precious, and being "all in" is crucial. In the presence of this kind of manifest commitment, therapists will be more likely to commit as well. It is not unusual for problematic interpersonal dynamics within the team to interfere with therapists' full-fledged commitment to the team. If that is the case, it would constitute pervasive team-interfering behavior, and it should be put on the agenda for targeting in order to assess it, solve it, and restore a full sense of commitment and participation. In my experience, problematic dynamics can occur in typical (non-DBT) interdisciplinary team meetings in mental health, where the discussions are usually less personal and members are not likely to share vulnerability, and good work can still occur. But these processes seriously interfere with the work of consultation in DBT teams.

The subsequent steps depend on what the therapist wants and needs. If he wants help with assessment, conceptualization, and problem solving of his difficulties with burnout, the template provided by *behavioral chain analysis* becomes useful. Team members try to get clear about the burnout behaviors of the therapist, such as avoidance of patient-related cues, withdrawal from the patient in sessions, judgmental attitudes and statements toward the patient, unaddressed violations of his own personal limits, crippling levels of anxiety or shame associated with the patient, and so on. In the scheme of behavioral chain analysis, as we picture the "burnout story" proceeding from left to right on the chain, the burnout behaviors occupy the same spot on the chain as the primary target behaviors of the patient in individual therapy. For instance, in the earlier example of the therapist who acceded to his patient's requests for increasing physical closeness during sessions, the team would analyze the therapist's dysfunctional decision to allow the patient to hold his hand. That would be the burnout behavior under assessment, and the goal would be to identify controlling variables of "hand-holding behavior." Just to make this point very clear: Although the core issue with burnout is the emotional dysregulation of the therapist, we engage the therapist in a behavioral chain analysis of at least one of the problematic therapist behaviors that follow from dysregulation. This is more focused, more aligned with behavioral treatment, more congruent with the kind of behavioral chain analysis we do with patients in DBT, and overall more productive than doing a chain analysis on larger constructs such as *burnout* or *emotional dysregulation.*

The team listens for vulnerability factors. Were there factors in the therapist or the environment, with respect to this patient or unrelated to this patient, that rendered the therapist vulnerable to the challenges of treating this patient? If so, the remedy might include addressing those factors. These might include recent stressors in the life of the therapist, stressful circumstances at the treatment setting, the therapist's excessive case load, or a recent suicide or other adverse outcome in cases, and so on. With respect to the particular patient, the therapist may be vulnerable in relation to certain aspects of the patient's presentation, such as a tendency toward threats and violence, or frequent suicide threats or attempts. The therapist could experience vulnerability because the patient presents with problems that are similar to problems the therapist has had, or the patient may have connections in the community that overlap with those of the therapist, heightening a sense of visibility and self-consciousness. Any or all of these factors, which predate even 1 minute spent together in therapy, could be significant biasing factors in burnout.

The team is on the lookout for prompting events, for those nodal moments in the therapy relationship that set off the trajectory toward the therapist's increasing dysregulation. For instance, when I noticed that I was on a trajectory toward burnout with respect to the treatment of a particular patient of mine, I quickly could identify a nodal moment in that trajectory, a prompting event, as the morning when she broke a lamp in my waiting room prior to a session with me, claiming that she was frustrated with life. It caught me by surprise. While I did immediately insist that she have the lamp fixed and pay for it herself, I realized later that emotionally I suppressed my response and underreacted to my own anger. I held her feet to the fire about repairing the lamp, but at a more intimate level between her and me I was more withdrawn and lenient. From that point on, a spiral took place between us in which she violated various agreements and limits and I continued to provide insufficiently firm contingencies. Soon she was behaviorally out of control and I was burdened with strong negative emotions. It proved useful to me to locate the "beginning of the chain" and then to see how that chain proceeded, link by link, to the burnout behaviors such as the strong desire to stop working with her.

As the team works with the therapist to spell out the links in the chain that eventuated in burnout behaviors, certain links stand out as important, and patterns emerge. As patterns emerge and are noted by the therapist and team, hypotheses may be generated and tested. In the example above, a pattern emerged in which I was underreacting to the patient's willful behaviors. The team and I knew that that was not a pattern with all of my patients, raising the question about my reaction to this patient, in particular. Was I frightened of her, and therefore too lenient? Was I careful with her because of an assumption that she was fragile and couldn't tolerate confrontation? Was I afraid that if I were to challenge her in a manner that was appropriate to her behaviors, she would quit therapy? These are the kinds of hypotheses and questions that will come up in assessing the path to burnout, and the answers determine the search for solutions. As came to light in the assessment of my evolving burnout in this case, I was being unusually careful in handling this patient. She was a college student who was showing increasing behavioral dyscontrol in her life, her brother had recently committed suicide, and the esteemed colleague who referred her to me was a close friend of the patient's family. I came to realize that my unbalanced handling of the patient's dyscontrol in my office was a product of these various factors, and was a link in the chain to my own emotional dysregulation and burnout. I was able to restore the balance in the treatment with a wider awareness of the contributing factors.

By reviewing the chain with the therapist and finding relevant links and patterns, the team works with the therapist toward a *conceptualization* of the particular burnout phenomenon. Again, it requires discipline and objectivity for therapists on the team to refrain from jumping in with their favorite proposed solutions before doing the assessment.

The case conceptualization integrates principles from the four behavioral models that are part of DBT. Associated with each model are possible solutions. It may be that the therapist's intense emotional responses have been triggered by patient or patient-associated cues, as in *classical conditioning*. Aligned with the model of *operant conditioning*, a therapist might be reinforced by the patient for therapy that soothes and validates, while being punished when she pushes for behavioral change in the patient, and as a result the therapist has become unbalanced. The therapist may have been reinforced for violating her own personal limits, which has resulted in an intolerable situation for her. The therapist in the burnout mode has often arrived at dysfunctional assumptions or beliefs about the patient, about therapy, and/or about herself, as expected in the model of *cognitive mediation*. Finally, *skills deficits* in the therapist might be highlighted—deficits either in the skill set for conducting DBT therapy (treatment strategies) or the skill set taught to the patients in DBT. Lacking a full and active set of strategies and skills appropriate to the situation, strategies and skills that could help the therapist maintain therapeutic control and balance, the therapist may fall back on automatic reaction patterns that deviate from DBT. Each of the four behavioral models brings with it a theory of change, including a repertoire of solutions, which might be helpful to the therapist. Next, I consider the use of each model in the treatment of therapist burnout.

Classical Conditioning Principles in the Treatment of Burnout

As can be seen in the examples I have given, the therapist with burnout is likely to be highly sensitive to certain recurring patient-related cues. These cues automatically trigger the emotional reactions in the therapist that are painful and difficult to manage. The team might help the therapist become more aware of the nature and impact of the cues, and the involuntary nature of his responses to them. With this kind of understanding and support, the therapist might engage in stimulus control strategies, deliberately avoiding some cues and modifying others. For instance, he might shift the timing of a patient's session to a time of day when the therapist is most resilient, or work directly with the patient to modify certain therapy-interfering behaviors that are crossing his personal limits.

Sometimes, once the cue-driven behavioral pattern is more apparent, the team may work with the therapist through exposure procedures, deliberately presenting similar cues to the therapist in team meetings or through assignments in therapy with the patient. For instance, I once had a patient who would respond to every one of my interventions as if I were interrupting her, throwing her off track, and ruining her treatment. I decided to do less talking and more listening, with the assumption that as our relationship grew and her trust in me increased, my input would become more acceptable and important to her. Over the next few weeks this pattern continued. Still, once in a while I would intervene, and in every instance she would ignore, dismiss, or counter my input. Her reactions to my interventions became an evocative cue for me. I anticipated her responses with anxiety, and when they happened, I felt immediately annoyed and resentful. I knew that things were getting worse when I began to resent the sound of her voice. Sessions became onerous, and I would long for her to cancel.

During the assessment of this pattern, team members hypothesized that I was particularly triggered by her dismissive treatment of my interventions. This hypothesis rang true to me, since I knew that I typically had strong reactions in my personal life if I was ignored. I agreed to a suggestion that in a role play within the team, one of them would play a patient who was dismissing my interventions. We did this several times, which actually became rather fun, while I began to desensitize myself to the impact of dismissive responsiveness and played with different ways to respond. In therapy with the patient, I nearly looked forward to her dismissive treatment of me, and I became more balanced and straightforward in response. This process played a significant role in reversing my trajectory toward burnout.

In almost every burnout experience, certain cues related to the patient have acquired the power to trigger strong negative emotions in the therapist. It may be the patient's angry outbursts, irritable responses, expressions of hopelessness, or passivity in the face of challenges. What might have once triggered curiosity in the therapist eventually becomes a trigger point for intense, unmanageable emotional responses. In most significant team-based treatment of the syndrome of therapist burnout, the model of classical conditioning and the procedures of stimulus control and exposure with response prevention can play a useful role. The trick is to find a way to match the patient-related cue with some stimulus in the team meeting, to elicit the full emotional response in the team meeting, and to explore various options for the therapist to experience the response and to act opposite the urge that goes with that response.

Operant Conditioning Principles in the Treatment of Burnout

In therapist burnout, it sometimes becomes apparent that the contingent consequences of the therapist's behaviors have shaped her toward maladaptive responses, including emotional suppression—the formula for burnout. If the team can help the therapist to see these processes more clearly, and can reinforce adaptive therapeutic responses, balance can be restored and burnout reduced.

For instance, the therapist may recognize more accurately that he has been inadvertently shaped in the direction of violating his personal limits "for the good of the patient," suppressing his inevitable emotional responses. The team can consult with the therapist about modifying the limits to match his own comfort zone. In so doing, the therapist receives reinforcement from the team for behaviors that are subject to punishment from the patient. In addition, the team can help the therapist determine effective ways to present his modified limits to the patient. The therapist must settle on limits that work for him; clarify them to the patient; soothe and validate the patient; reinforce the patient consistently for staying within those limits; and use shaping, extinction, and punishment procedures with the patient to bring about a workable solution. This can be difficult. The therapist might be ashamed to have extended his limits to the degree that he has, and requires a nonjudgmental team approach to become clear about the problem before solving it. He is likely to fear the patient's reactions to the narrowing of his limits. He may still believe that the patient benefits from wider limits. It may be hard for him to objectively weigh the long-term benefits to him of defining the limits that he needs, versus the short- and long-term benefits to the patient for keeping the wider limits. The team's efforts can be crucial at this juncture in helping the therapist to weigh the pros and cons, while remaining consistent in reinforcing the therapist for effectively observing his limits. As noted, the long-term negative consequences of burnout can be severe, and once it is well established, it is difficult to turn around.

The team's use of contingency procedures goes well beyond using them in the context of reinforcing personal limits. In every consultation with every therapist, the team is reinforcing some therapist behaviors and extinguishing and punishing others. Team members should be thoughtful about reinforcing therapist behaviors that are aligned with the treatment model and effective in therapy. Since the therapist is subject to a set of contingencies from the patient, or from others associated with the patient, the team needs consistency in reinforcing good therapy behaviors when others might be reinforcing ineffective therapy. I was once treating an adolescent who would not speak with me. After a couple months

I began to think I should consider stopping with this patient since she seemed totally uninterested in me. I found it to be exhausting to endure the sessions and what I perceived to be her silent and cynical disdain toward me. As I presented my "urge" to stop with her to my team, one of the therapists insisted that I had no way of knowing for sure how the patient felt about me and whether she was benefiting, even in her silence. He suggested that I imagine that the patient was attached to me, choosing to come when she didn't have to be there, and he and others on the team reinforced my persistence, patience, and imagination of attachment. As it turned out, a short time after that I found a way to get her engaged in conversation, and some of the team's approaches were confirmed.

Cognitive Mediation Principles in the Treatment of Burnout

This example also demonstrates the application in the team of another behavioral model and its principles: *cognitive mediation*. In arriving at the belief that this patient was not attached to me and only had feelings of disdain, even though she did not explicitly share her thoughts with me, I eventually found myself feeling discouraged and hopeless. When team members noted that I was pessimistically interpreting her behavior and reminded me that I did not have access to the actual facts, I realized that they were correct. My emotions and urges in relation to her were being driven by a set of beliefs about her, not facts. I was then able to recognize my pessimistic thoughts in the upcoming sessions and to entertain other interpretations of her behaviors. It eased the pressure on me to "get her to engage," which ultimately allowed a process of attachment and engagement to slowly unfold. In every case of therapist burnout that I can remember, the therapist's dysfunctional assumptions and beliefs about the patient, the therapy, and/or him- or herself, even if they were not the initial drivers toward burnout, became important maintaining variables. In the assessment and treatment of burnout, team members need to be alert to the cognitions of the therapist, willing to highlight them as thoughts rather than as facts, and to suggest alternative interpretations.

During a team meeting, one of the therapists on my team was discussing a patient with suicidal ideation. I had the impression that the therapist was overestimating the likelihood of a lethal suicide attempt, in that the patient had never attempted suicide. I realized that I had heard this kind of interpretation from this therapist regarding other patients, and it always caused her a good deal of fear, and sometimes resentment of the patient for talking about suicide. I asked her if she could explain her thinking about the patient's high suicide risk. In the course of the discussion in the team, the therapist acknowledged that this was an area of anxiety and confusion for her. As she put it, "I prefer to err on the side of assuming that a serious suicide attempt is coming, rather than be caught by surprise." As we learned, there had been a suicide in her family when she was young, and she was still operating with assumptions that would spare her another catastrophic event, another devastating surprise. The team was then alert to this therapist's "cognitive vulnerability" with respect to suicidal patients, which helped in consulting with her and preventing burnout with her suicidal patients.

Skills Deficit Theory Principles in Treating Therapist Burnout

Finally, the consultation team can implement principles of the fourth behavioral model, *skills deficit theory*, by engaging the therapist in skills training procedures. Team members are on the lookout for strengths and weaknesses in each other's application of DBT, which is an explicit function of the consultation team. In the joint enterprise of acquiring all strategies in the arsenal of DBT; strengthening the practice of those strategies through study, practice, and reinforcement of each other; and generalizing them to the treatment of the patient or the conduct of a skills group, team members strengthen each other's DBT practice. To have at one's fingertips a wide range of strategies, each linked to principles of the treatment, inevitably serves well in the treatment of burnout. Each therapist can use the same sets of strategies whether working with the patient or participating in team meetings. Team members' use of the same language and sharing the goal of mastering the same strategies and skills potentiates a more effective team process. Team members use validation strategies with one another, all the change strategies, and dialectical strategies. For instance, as discussed above, the team uses contingency procedures such as reinforcement of therapist behaviors to help the therapist use contingency procedures, such as observing personal limits, more effectively with the patient. To return to the biosocial theory of burnout, in which the therapist is coping with emotional dysregulation in the context of invalidation or nonvalidation, the treatment of the therapist requires a validating environment, within which the team uses DBT strategies to increase the therapist's effectiveness at coping with emotional dysregulation while treating the patient.

Principles from the Dialectical Paradigm

In this section, I focus on ways in which dialectical principles can help the team help its members break up the protracted "logjams" that characterize most well-established cases of burnout.

On a consultation team in a DBT-based day treatment program, one of the therapists was also an excellent nurse. She prided herself on maintaining her medical knowledge and skills while also being a first-rate DBT therapist. One of her patients had multiple medical problems, including diabetes, seizures, and severe hypertension. This patient often had to miss one of the groups due to medical complaints, and on those occasions she would sometimes seek out her therapist, who would try to help her with the medical problem. It seemed to other team members, some of whom had this patient in their groups, that the medical incidents were increasing and that the patient was leaving groups more often. In a consultation team meeting, one of the group leaders suggested to the therapist that by being so knowledgeable and available regarding the medical problems, she was probably reinforcing more dysfunctional behaviors than she was solving. The therapist was hurt and irate, feeling accused of being inappropriate and thoughtless. She raised her voice: "You think I don't think about that? You think it is easy to treat this person? I tell you what, why don't you take her on as a patient and treat her just perfectly! I am sick of all of you!"

It was a sudden outburst, unanticipated by all team members, as their colleague was almost always steady and composed. It seemed that a problem of therapist burnout was suddenly thrust into the room, and her emotional dysregulation became everyone's emotional dysregulation. Team members sat in silence, trying to collect themselves and to figure out what to do. The therapist who raised the question issued an apology to her colleague, and said that she did not mean to accuse her of anything, but was just wondering. The therapist treating the patient seemed a little embarrassed by her own outburst, but was difficult to console.

Finally someone in the team said, "I wonder if there is a dialectic here," knowing that intense conflicts often resulted from the failure to validate both sides. Another therapist followed her lead: "When you ask that, it makes me wonder if we can say what the opposing sides are. On the one hand, the [nurse] therapist is doing everything she can, trying to figure out how to help a patient who is medically ill and emotionally distressed; and, on the other hand, there is a possibility that she is so good at it that she is inadvertently reinforcing the behaviors. I don't know." The key to this therapist's effectiveness in making this statement was in her truly nonjudgmental attitude; she was really just trying to frame the conflict as resulting from two opposing but equally valid positions. Once the dialectic was identified in the form of *two opposing but valid statements*, the discussion could proceed. The therapist seemed to accept the validation. She explained that she was "worried sick" about reinforcing the medical behaviors, which she had considered, and felt trapped by the very real medical problems that she knew how to treat. She was especially upset when the patient left a group meeting to see her, alleging that her medical symptoms made group participation impossible. She felt she was already suffering from burnout in this case, but was embarrassed because she saw the other team members as more competent than she, and she wanted to figure it out herself. The team, once the dialectic was named and discussed, worked together on a *synthesis* involving a protocol that acknowledged that the patient sometimes needed medical support, but that she would not seek out help from her therapist during groups, based on the inadvertent possibility of reinforcing lower program participation. If she were to leave groups for medical reasons, she needed to seek medical attention but not from the therapist, and report back to group leaders about the outcome. Furthermore, the therapist then asked for the team's help in arriving at her own policy, which would eliminate her from the process of medical treatment altogether, since that was not her role.

Burnout almost always involves an unresolved dialectic, in therapy or in a team, sometimes in both contexts. The patient wants something, the therapist wants the opposite, and the solution either involves the patient's or the therapist's capitulating, leading to the suppression of negative emotions. Then the dialectic enters the team context: The therapist has one point of view, other team members have an opposing point of view; one capitulates to the other superficially, but the conflict is unresolved. The dialectical formula in both contexts is amazingly helpful, even if not easy: (1) Nonjudgmentally identify opposing positions; (2) find and state the validity in both positions; (3) explicitly and collaboratively search for a genuine synthesis honoring both sides; and (4) implement the synthesis and evaluate the outcome.

In this process, a number of DBT's dialectical strategies can play instrumental roles. Balancing treatment strategies can help in honoring both sides of a conflict by applying both acceptance and change. Making lemonade out of lemons, extending, playing devil's advocate, eliciting wise mind, and entering the paradox are all creative vehicles that include the honoring of two opposing sides and creating movement. They have been covered extensively in Chapter 13. It is important to remember that they can be utilized in a stuck consultation team process just as they can in therapy.

Approaching a stalemate, the therapist or team relies on the strategy of *dialectical assessment.* All wonder and seek out what has been left out of the equation. In one case, a therapist on the team described his very frustrating work with a patient who diagnosed herself as having fibromyalgia. In every session, the patient would complain about her pain and disability, and describe one incident after another in which health care personnel dismissed her complaints as being "in your head." She complained about the fact that everyone in her life just expected her to go on as normal. She was constantly angry, and after months the therapist was on the verge of concluding that nothing could bring about change. As the therapist put it, "It is as if she is in a burning building, leaning out a second floor window, and every week I put a ladder up to the window to help her get out, and every week she just pushes the ladder away and continues to complain that she will soon die of heat and neglect." The therapist was just about ready to give up, but could not see a way out.

The team leader asked if the therapist could engage in a role play in which she played her complaining patient while someone else on the team played the therapist. The rest of us watched. We were looking for things that might be left out of our understanding. The role play was illuminating. It proved very frustrating for the individual role-playing the therapist, who found that no intervention worked. This was the best form of validation for the therapist, who also got a chance to "sit in the patient's chair" and see how difficult it was to be so difficult. It increased her empathy for her patient, and her curiosity about the causes of the patient's stance. The therapist felt more joined with the team. They were able to brainstorm together. Thinking dialectically, one therapist suggested a dialectical strategy of extending: "Why don't you validate her experience that the world is cold and hard, that no one understands how frustrating it is, and suggest to her that her complaining might not be forceful enough. You could invite her to make more strenuous and descriptive complaints, including complaints about you as the therapist." She was suggesting that the therapist, rather than withdrawing from the patient's complaints, invite more of them.

The therapist thought that it would simply reinforce the patient's passive, suffering stance. But she was willing to try it, first in a role play and then with her patient. It proved to be interesting. The patient did not know what to say. In one way, she felt more deeply validated by the therapist than any time before, but she also said, "I complain all the time already and it doesn't help. Don't you think I should try to do something about it myself?" It came to the patient as a new idea. Although this one point of dialectical intervention, in which the therapist "played with opposites" in a different way, did not transform the case, it did open a door to a new line of dialogue that made it less exhausting for the therapist. These kinds of interventions in the team, as in therapy, do not necessarily solve the problem, but they create disequilibrium and movement in a situation that has been painfully static for a long time.

Interventions based on *systemic thinking* can also play a transformative role when burnout is the problem. In one team, a therapist confessed that he had made an egregious error with his patient. He was ashamed and halting in his account of what had happened in the previous session. As a young therapist he feared the disapproval of his team and mentors. His patient had a factitious disorder. She presented herself as having various medical conditions, even life-threatening ones, when in fact there was never any evidence of pathology. She drew sympathy from others, but then they would get angry at her when they decided that she had "made up" the condition "just to get attention." The therapist knew that others responded to his patient with scorn, which led him to feel sympathetic toward her, until he realized that she was doing the same thing with him. She told him unequivocally and believably that she had pancreatic cancer and only had a few weeks or months to live. She asked for his help in how to make the best of her final days. He was profoundly moved and agreed to help her focus on the end. He received a phone call prior to the next session with her, in which he learned from her physician that her story was completely fabricated. Only minutes later he was to meet with the patient.

He was shocked, amazed at the compelling and believable nature of her story, and embarrassed by his "gullibility." He wished he had some time to ground himself before the session, but she was already in the waiting room. As a way to buy some time, he told her that something had come up and he needed to start the session later. Back in his office, he sat in his chair with the intention to practice mindfulness and to achieve greater balance and clarity. He fell asleep. He woke up when he heard pounding at his door. It was the end of the designated session time and his patient was angrily pounding to get his attention. He had another patient coming and did not have time to see this one. He went to the door, explained that what had come up had taken more time than expected, and rescheduled with her. He was mortified by his behavior.

In the team meeting, when the therapist told this story and waited for the expected disapproval, no one knew what to say. Someone asked him what he needed from the team. He said he needed to be shot. He was more than half serious. Team members listened with compassion. They validated that falling asleep under the circumstances was understandable. Whatever kind and validating statements were made were rejected. He was convinced that everyone was just avoiding saying what he or she really thought, which was that he was a "loser." The team leader suggested that they get the whole story and do a behavioral chain analysis of the target behavior of falling asleep. The therapist did not want to participate, and then he apologized for being so difficult. Everyone in the room grew silent, realizing they were stuck.

Then a team member proceeded to tell the story of a time that he had fallen asleep in a session when a patient was talking about a time that she was raped. The therapist struggling with her remorse was surprised to hear that someone so competent had done that. Another team member suggested that everyone in the room tell about their worst moments in therapy ever. The effect on everyone, including the humiliated therapist, was palpable. Dramatic errors were acknowledged, the mood lifted. There was implicit acknowledgment that mistakes, even serious ones, were part of the work. It's why one of the six consultation team agreements is the Fallibility Agreement.

For a consultation team to "be dialectical" adds enormous potential to prevent and treat burnout if it is used to augment, and not replace, standard approaches from the acceptance and change paradigms. To *be dialectical* means to elucidate opposing positions when there is a stalemate and then move toward synthesis. It means to expand the perspective of the therapist and the team to take account of systemic thinking. And it means to recognize that movement never stops and that it is helpful to keep things moving in therapy and in the team. It catalyzes creative and improvisational thinking and action that include taking some risks in the face of uncertainty. To realize that the team is a system, and that changes in any one member can bring about changes in all, opens the door to a myriad of dialectically based interventions.

CONCLUDING COMMENTS

The consultation team is a mode of DBT. As such, it is another treatment context in which to use the paradigms and principles that underlie the practice of DBT. Far more than being a meeting in which to talk about the treatment, it is a meeting in which to *practice* the treatment. And of the targets of the consultation team meeting—the identification, prevention, and treatment of therapist burnout as an expected event—is a high priority. By conceptualizing burnout in terms of DBT's biosocial theory, just as we conceptualize our patients' emotional dysregulation, we open up the pathway to use the rest of the treatment to help each other. By practicing principles of acceptance, change, and dialectics in the prevention and treatment of burnout, we not only work on the solution of burnout, we reinforce our capacities for the treatment as a whole.

Afterword

T he process of writing this book over the past 3 years has changed me, demanding from me a disciplined effort to consider how a principle-based focus in DBT expands my options, increases my flexibility, and allows for creativity—all without compromising a focus on adherence. While I have found my own way to describe the ideas herein, using a multitude of case examples, there is nothing in this book that was not already present or anticipated by the brilliant work of Marsha Linehan. If you have found something of value in these pages, I owe it to her, my patients, my consultation teams, and my colleagues.

This afterword is intended to re-present the paradigms and principles in an accessible, concise, memorable form, making it easier for readers to remember them and take them into therapy sessions, as I do. When I focus my attention on the principles, I find that the strategies emerge in my practice without having to look for them. The increased sense of freedom and fluidity has helped me to navigate difficult moments in therapy.

THREE PARADIGMS, FIFTEEN PRINCIPLES

The juxtaposition of and synthesis among the change, acceptance, and dialectical paradigms, or more pointedly the cognitive-behavioral, mindfulness, and dialectical paradigms, provide a powerful foundation for getting our patients out of the hell of chronic, severe emotional dysregulation. It is my suspicion that the three paradigms also provide an excellent basis for solving stubborn problems in life in general: how to cope with chronic illness or care for a partner in decline, how to parent teenagers or manage family life, how to come to grips with adversity at work, and even how to perform at the highest level. Extrapolations of the principles of DBT beyond the clinical situation will have to wait for another book. For now, I focus on each of the three paradigms, presenting the five principles of each.

Change (CBT)

1. *Direction* (targeting)
2. *Force* (commitment, attachment, contingencies)
3. *Persistence* (monitoring, contingencies, consultation team)
4. *Intelligence* (behavioral assessment, case conceptualization, treatment planning)
5. *Technique* (protocols, strategies, skills)

The first five principles are the core components of the change paradigm. They are the keys to solving stubborn problems in therapy. In this section, each of these principles is broadly stated for the sake of brevity. The first is *direction*, manifest in DBT as *targeting*. Working toward a target recruits other problem-solving principles and activities. The patient's targets constitute the treatment plan; the therapist's targets involve moving the patient toward achieving his or her targets. The best targets are compelling, clear, specific, realistic, and collaboratively defined. The absence of a direction is seen in *drift*. By *targeting*, I refer to the establishment, prioritization, and utilization of the primary treatment targets, the recognition and pursuit of secondary treatment targets, and the recruitment of the patient's engagement in therapeutic procedures (e.g., behavioral chain analysis or diary cards).

The second change principle, is *force*, manifest in DBT as strengthening *attachment*, getting a *commitment* to a given target, and *reinforcement* of attachment and commitment. Without sufficient force, we cannot solve the target issue. Many problems in therapy result from insufficient force, and the therapist who can enhance his own and the patient's attachment and commitment has a better chance of achieving the targeted outcomes.

The third change principle is *persistence*, which involves sustaining sufficient force toward identified targets over time. Whereas treatment may begin with a burst of targeting and commitment, persistence requires momentum and endurance. The DBT therapist insists on the practice of *monitoring* progress on treatment targets, by which I refer to the patient's nightly self-monitoring on the diary card, and the therapist's weekly review of the diary card. Monitoring targets and the level of commitment throughout treatment leads to persistence. The DBT consultation team helps the therapist stay on track with the targets, generate enough force in herself and the patient, and persist in the treatment. In part, these efforts are achieved by identifying, preventing, and treating burnout.

Direction, force, and persistence are necessary but not sufficient ingredients to solve stubborn problems. The fourth principle is *intelligence*. By using repeated *behavioral assessments* guided by an evolving *case conceptualization* based on DBT's theory and assumptions, arriving at and adjusting a *treatment plan*, we push toward the targets with force, persistence, and intelligence.

The fifth change principle involves using the proper *technique* to accomplish the goals. For the therapist, technique requires *protocols and strategies*. DBT therapists need expertise in cognitive-behavioral strategies, DBT-specific protocols and strategies, and DBT's set of *skills*. Otherwise, all of the direction, force, persistence, and intelligence in the world will not come together in effecting therapeutic change

Acceptance (Mindfulness)

1. *Presence*
2. *Impermanence*
3. *Nonattachment*
4. *Interbeing*
5. *Perfect as is*

The first acceptance principle is *presence*, by which we refer to the effort to bring attention, again and again, to the present moment, without judgment. Awareness of presence, and the repeated practice of returning to the present moment, communicates to the patient, in so many ways, "My dear patient, I am present, I am here for you right now."

The second acceptance principle, *impermanence*, refers to the therapist's acute awareness that this present and unique moment is the only moment, never to be repeated. It deepens the therapist's participation in the moment, which hopefully activates a similarly heightened engagement by the patient. Through the repeated awareness of the impermanence of everything in this moment, the therapist communicates to the patient, in so many ways, "Join me in this precious moment, this one and only moment."

The third acceptance principle of *nonattachment* refers to the therapist's practice of letting go of attachments to various beliefs and perceptions. Attachment to beliefs of what "should" be happening but isn't, of what we "should be able to do as therapists" but aren't, and what our patients "should be doing" but aren't, leads inevitably to suffering and dysregulation. Letting go of these kinds of attachments, while staying focused on "simply" practicing DBT as prescribed, the therapist cultivates and preserves freshness, freedom, and balance while staying focused on the targets.

As the fourth acceptance principle, *interbeing* refers to several core insights: that from a certain perspective there is no such thing as boundaries, there is no such thing as self, that any entity is made up entirely of other entities (also known as "emptiness" in Buddhist thinking), and that the degree of interdependency among all phenomena is deep and constant. The awareness and practice of interbeing facilitate the dissolution of boundaries between patient and therapist, promote the sense that "we are in it together," and increase the therapist's genuineness and reciprocity. Awareness of non-self helps us realize that our behaviors are influenced by context and contingencies as much as are patients' behaviors. We are able to see reality more objectively and to consider the mutual influences impacting all involved: therapists, patients, and contexts.

The fifth and final acceptance principle, *perfect as is*, refers to the understanding that everything emerges from causes and conditions, and that everything is therefore exactly as it should be. Flowing from the awareness of this reality is a whole set of validation strategies. This principle promotes radical acceptance of reality, reduces the suffering that results from denying reality, and helps the therapist to maintain balance and freshness.

Dialectics

1. *Opposition*
2. *Synthesis*
3. *Systemic thinking*
4. *Transactional processes*
5. *Flux*

The first dialectical principle is that of *opposition*. We recognize that reality consists naturally of opposing forces: that is, that X elicits –X. Tension, conflict, chaos, and confusion usually are manifestations of the presence of opposition between two or more positions. By recognizing the ubiquitous presence of opposition within ourselves, among ourselves on the team, between patients and therapists, within patients, and between patients and their environments, we maintain our balance in the face of opposition.

The second dialectical principle of *synthesis* begins with a search for the valid kernel of truth on each side of an opposition. Rather than decide between the two positions, we look for the validity in both and try to preserve them. We emphasize a process of looking for synthesis rather than getting to the conclusion, even though we may need to draw a conclusion as well. Once we find validity in both positions, we allow synthesis to take place such that both kernels of truth are preserved in a new construction. The search for synthesis is a pervasive, constant target in DBT as we pursue the primary and secondary targets.

With the third dialectical principle of *systemic thinking*, we assess and treat the phenomenon or conflict of the moment by widening our point of view to encompass the systemic variables that impact on the moment. This principle broadens our perspective in assessing the controlling variables and treating the current target or conflict. Every element is one part of a multipart system, probably of several systems, and changes in the other parts will change that element. Every element also has parts within it, and is therefore a "whole," containing parts, as well as a part of other wholes. Every change in every part will change every whole and every associated part.

The fourth dialectical principle is something of a subset of the third one, and involves the awareness and use of *transactional processes*. Every element or phenomenon is in transaction with another one (or more). One's identity does not "stand alone" but rather is determined transactionally. Identity changes when the transaction changes. Recognizing transactional processes as the rule, not the exception, helps us to assess factors that are maintaining a given behavior or identity, thereby pointing us toward ways to change behaviors or identities by changing transactions.

The fifth dialectical principle involves the understanding of *flux*, which overlaps with the acceptance principle of *impermanence*. Everything, at every level, down to every cell, molecule, and subparticle is always moving. When we think that "nothing is happening," that things are stuck, and the same thing is repeated again and again, it is an illusion disguising the fact that movement continues. If we address a phenomenon by doing nothing, change continues. If we address it by doing something, change continues. The DBT therapist, aware that movement is constant, engages the patient in treatment, even in "stuck situations," with speed, movement, and flow.

FINALLY . . .

In this book I have attempted to clarify the understanding and practice of principles in conducting DBT. We have considered the advantages of a principle-based approach and how it augments and strengthens the adherent practice of the model. I hope that by focusing on the principles and providing a range of clinical examples, the reader will be able to strengthen the practice of DBT with increased flexibility.

References

Bateman, A. W., & Fonagy, P. (2004). Mentalization-based treatment for BPD. *Journal of Personality Disorders, 18*(1), 36–51.

Brown, J. (2016). *The emotion regulation skills system for cognitively challenged clients: A DBT-informed approach.* New York: Guilford Press.

Buber, M. (1923). *Ich und Du [I and thou].* Leipzig, Germany: Insel Verlag.

Dimeff, L. A., & Koerner, K. (2007). *Dialectical behavior therapy in clinical practice: Applications across disorders and settings.* New York: Guilford Press.

Feigenbaum, J. D., Fonagy, P., Pilling, S., Jones, A., Wildgoose, A., & Bebbington, P. E. (2011). A real-world study of the effectiveness of DBT in the UK National Health Service. *British Journal of Clinical Psychology, 51*(2), 121–141.

Gottman, J. M., & Katz, L. F. (1989). Effects of marital discord on young children's peer interaction and health. *Developmental Psychology, 25,* 373–381.

Gutteling, B. M., Montagne, B., Nijs, M., & van den Bosch, L. M. C. W. (2012). Dialectical behavior therapy: Is outpatient group psychotherapy an effective alternative to individual therapy?: Preliminary conclusions. *Comprehensive Psychiatry, 53*(8), 1161–1168.

Haley, J. (1973). *Uncommon therapy: The psychiatric techniques of Milton Erickson, M.D.* New York: Norton.

Harned, M. S., Jackson, S. C., Comtois, K. A., & Linehan, M. M. (2010). Dialectical behavior therapy as a precursor to PTSD treatment for suicidal and/or self-injuring women with borderline personality disorder. *Journal of Traumatic Stress, 23,* 421–429.

Harned, M. S., Korslund, K. E., & Linehan, M. M. (2014). A pilot randomized controlled trial of DBT with and without the DBT prolonged exposure protocol for suicidal and self-injuring women with borderline personality disorder and PTSD. *Behaviour Research and Therapy, 55,* 7–17.

Hill, D. M., Craighead, L. W., & Safer, D. L. (2011). Appetite-focused dialectical behavior therapy for the treatment of binge eating with purging: A preliminary trial. *International Journal of Eating Disorders, 44*(3), 249–261.

Kernberg, O. F. (1984) *Severe personality disorders.* New Haven, CT: Yale University Press.

Koerner, K., Dimeff, L., & Swenson, C. (2007). Adopt or adapt: Fidelity matters. In L. A. Dimeff & K. Koerner (Eds.), *Dialectical behavior therapy in clinical practice: Applications across disorders and settings* (pp. 19–36). New York: Guilford Press.

Koons, C., Robins, C. J., Tweed, J. L., Lynch, T. R., Gonzales, A. M., Morse, J. Q., et al. (2001). Efficacy of dialectical behavior therapy in women veterans with borderline personality disorder. *Behavior Therapy, 32,* 371–390.

Linehan, M. M. (1987). Dialectical behavior therapy for borderline personality disorder: Theory and method. *Bulletin of the Menninger Clinic, 51*(3), 261–276.

Linehan, M. M. (1993a). *Cognitive-behavioral treatment of borderline personality disorder.* New York: Guilford Press.

Linehan, M. M. (1993b). *Skills training manual for treating borderline personality disorder.* New York: Guilford Press.

Linehan, M. M. (1997). Validation and psychotherapy. In A. Bohart & L. Greenberg (Eds.), *Empathy reconsidered: New directions in psychotherapy* (353–392). Washington, DC: American Psychological Association.

Linehan, M. M. (2015a). *DBT skills training handouts and worksheets* (2nd ed.). New York: Guilford Press.

Linehan, M. M. (2015b). *DBT skills training manual* (2nd ed.). New York: Guilford Press.

Linehan, M. M., Armstrong, H. E., Suares, A., Allmon, D., & Heard, H. L. (1991). Cognitive-behavioral treatment of chronically parasuicidal borderline patients. *Archives of General Psychiatry, 48,* 1060–1064.

Linehan, M. M., Comtois, K. A., Murray, A. M., Brown, M .Z., Gallop, R. J., Heard, H. L., et al. (2006). Two-year randomized controlled trial and follow-up of dialectical behavior therapy vs. therapy by experts for suicidal behaviors and borderline personality disorder. *Archives of General Psychiatry, 63*(7), 757–766.

Linehan, M. M., Dimeff, L. A., Reynolds, S. K., Comtois, K. A., Welch, S. S., Heagerty, P., et al. (2002). Dialectical behavior therapy versus comprehensive validation plus 12-step for the treatment of opioid dependent women meeting criteria for borderline personality disorder. *Drug and Alcohol Dependence, 67*(1), 13–26.

Linehan, M. M., Heard, H. L., & Armstrong, H. E. (1993). Naturalistic follow-up of a behavioral treatment for chronically parasuicidal borderline patients. *Archives of General Psychiatry, 50,* 971–974.

Linehan, M. M., McDavid, J., Brown, M. Z., Sayrs, J. H. R., & Gallop, R. J. (2008). Olanzapine plus dialectical behavior therapy for irritable women meeting criteria for borderline personality disorder: A double blind, placebo-controlled pilot study. *Journal of Clinical Psychiatry, 69*(6), 999–1005.

Linehan, M. M., Schmidt, H., Dimeff, L. A., Craft, J. C., Kanter, J., & Comtois, K. A. (1999). Dialectical behavior therapy for patients with borderline personality disorder and drug dependence. *American Journal of Addiction, 8*(4), 279–292.

Lynch, T. R., Morse, J. Q., Mendelson, T., & Robins, C. J. (2003). Dialectical behavior therapy for depressed older adults. *American Journal of Geriatric Psychiatry, 11*(1), 33–45.

McCann, R. A., Ball, E. M., & Ivanoff, A. (2000). DBT with an inpatient forensic population: The CMHIP forensic model. *Cognitive and Behavioral Practice, 7,* 447–456.

Mehlum, L., Tormoen, A. J., Ramberg, M., Haga, E., Diep, L. M., Laberg, S., et al. (2014). Dialectical behavior therapy for adolescents with repeated suicidal and self-harming behavior: A randomized trial. *Journal of the American Academy of Child and Adolescent Psychiatry, 53*(10), 1082–1091.

Miller, W. R., & Rollnick, S. (2012). *Motivational interviewing: Helping people change* (3rd ed.). New York: Guilford Press.

Neacsui, A. D., Rizvi, S. L., & Linehan, M. M. (2010). DBT skills use as a mediator and outcome of treatment for borderline personality disorder. *Behaviour Research and Therapy, 48*(9), 832–839.

Ougrin, D. (2011). Efficacy of exposure versus cognitive therapy in anxiety disorders: Systematic review and meta-analysis. *BMC Psychiatry, 11*, 1–6.

Prochaska, J. O., DiClemente, C. C., & Norcross, J. C. (1992). In search of how people change: Applications to addictive behaviors. *American Psychologist, 47*(9), 1102–1114.

Rathus, J. H., & Miller, A. H. (2002). Dialectical behavior therapy for suicidal adolescents. *Suicide and Life-Threatening Behavior, 32*(2), 146–157.

Rathus, J. H., & Miller, A. L. (2015). *DBT skills manual for adolescents.* New York: Guilford Press.

Rogers, C. (1951). *Client-centered therapy: Its current practice, implications, and theory.* New York: Houghton Mifflin.

Safer, D. L., Robinson, A. H., & Jo, B. (2010). Outcome from a randomized controlled trial of group therapy for binge eating disorder: Comparing dialectical behavior therapy adapted for binge eating to an active comparison group therapy. *Behavior Therapy, 41*(3), 106–120

Safer, D. L., Telch, C. F., & Agras, & W. S. (2001). Dialectical behavior therapy for bulimia nervosa. *American Journal of Psychiatry, 158*, 632–634.

Schneidman, E. (1996). *The suicidal mind.* New York: Oxford University Press.

Swenson, C. (1989). Kernberg and Linehan: Two approaches to the borderline patient. *Journal of Personality Disorders, 3*(1), 26–35.

Telch, C. F., Agras, W. S., & Linehan, M. M. (2001). Dialectical behavior therapy for binge eating disorder. *Journal of Consulting and Clinical Psychology, 69*(6), 1061–1065.

Thich Nhat Hanh. (1975). *The miracle of mindfulness.* Boston: Beacon Press.

Turner, R. M. (2007). Naturalistic evaluation of dialectical behavior therapy-oriented treatment for borderline personality disorder. *Cognitive and Behavioral Practice, 7*, 413–419.

van den Bosch, L. M. C., Koeter, M., Stijnen, T., Verheul, R., & van den Brink, W. (2005). Sustained efficacy of dialectical behavior therapy for borderline personality disorder. *Behaviour Research and Therapy, 43*, 1231–1241.

van den Bosch, L. M. C., Verheul, R., Schippers, G. M., & van den Brink, W. (2002). Dialectical behavior therapy of borderline patients with and without substance abuse problems: Implementation and long-term effects. *Addictive Behaviors, 27*(6), 911–923.

Verheul, R., van den Bosch, L. M. C., & Koeter, M. W. J. (2003). Dialectical behavior therapy for women with borderline personality disorder. *British Journal of Psychiatry, 182*, 135–140.

Index